# A Clinician's Guide to
# **Balance and Dizziness**
## Evaluation and Treatment

# A Clinician's Guide to
# **Balance and Dizziness**
## Evaluation and Treatment

*Charles M. Plishka, PT, DPT*
Owner
Posture & Balance Concepts, LLC
Prairieville, Louisiana
Member, American Physical Therapy Association
International Liaison, Vestibular Special Interest Group, APTA
Mentoring Sub-Committee, Neurology Section, APTA
Alexandria, Virginia

Member, Bárány Society
Uppsala, Sweden

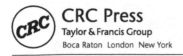

**CRC Press**
Taylor & Francis Group
Boca Raton London New York

CRC Press is an imprint of the
Taylor & Francis Group, an **Informa** business

First published 2015 by SLACK Incorporated

Published 2024 by CRC Press
2385 NW Executive Center Drive, Suite 320, Boca Raton FL 33431

and by CRC Press
4 Park Square, Milton Park, Abingdon, Oxon, OX14 4RN

CRC Press is an imprint of Taylor & Francis Group, LLC

*Dr. Charles M. Plishka* is owner of Posture & Balance Concepts, LLC. He is a consultant for Jintronix and performs contract physical therapy work for Our Lady of the Lake Regional Medical Center.

Library of Congress Cataloging-in-Publication Data

Plishka, Charles M., - , author.
  A clinician's guide to balance and dizziness : evaluation and treatment / Charles M. Plishka.
    p. ; cm.
Includes bibliographical references and index.
ISBN 978-1-61711-060-3 (alk. paper)
I. Title.
  [DNLM: 1. Dizziness--diagnosis. 2. Dizziness--therapy. 3. Postural Balance--physiology. 4. Vestibular Diseases. WL 340]
RB150.V4
616.8'41--dc23
                              2015004388

ISBN: 9781617110603 (pbk)
ISBN: 9781003524434 (ebk)

DOI: 10.1201/9781003524434

Additional resources can be found at
https://www.routledge.com/9781617110603

# DEDICATION

This book is dedicated to the leaders in the field of vestibular and balance research for their efforts to expand our knowledge on these subjects and to you, the reader, for wanting to expand your clinical knowledge into the fascinating world of balance and vestibular evaluation, treatment, and intervention!

# CONTENTS

# CONTENTS

# ACKNOWLEDGMENTS

My goal in writing this book was to present all of the information clinicians need to have in order to perform a comprehensive examination of the patient reporting dizziness or disequilibrium and to do so in an easy-to-understand format. I give special thanks and recognition to those who responded to an endless barrage of emails and calls to answer my many questions, especially Sue Whitney, PhD, PT, and Michael Schubert, PhD, PT. Thank you Debraca Gross, MSPT; Richard O'Quinn, PT; and David Ryerson, MA, for your time and contributions. Thank you Madeline Gyure, PT, for introducing me to vestibular rehabilitation and showing me how it can change people's lives.

# ACKNOWLEDGMENTS

# ABOUT THE AUTHOR

*Charles M. Plishka, PT, DPT* earned his Doctor of Physical Therapy degree from Creighton University in Omaha, NE. He is the owner of Posture & Balance Concepts, LLC, which offers consulting services, program development, and continuing education courses. He teaches courses on vestibular therapy, evaluation and treatment of balance and dizziness, Parkinson's disease, and multiple sclerosis.

Dr. Plishka is a member of the American Physical Therapy Association and is involved with the Vestibular Special Interest Group and the Mentoring Subcommittee of the Neurology Section of that organization. He is also a member of the Bárány Society, which is the International Society for Neuro-Otology.

He is excited to present *A Clinician's Guide to Balance and Dizziness: Evaluation and Treatment* as an easy-to-use reference and instruction for clinicians who evaluate and treat those patients suffering from dizziness and/or disequilibrium.

# HOW TO USE THIS BOOK

This book will walk the clinician through the thought processes and actual mechanics of performing a thorough examination and creating a plan of care for patients who complain of balance issues and/or dizziness. The chapters of the book focus on how their topics apply to the patient populations experiencing issues of balance and dizziness and do not necessarily address other applications or research information.

For quick reference, at the beginning of each chapter is a box that contains the learning goals for that chapter. There are many video examples. This video icon is displayed when a video is available for the topic being discussed: ▶

The following is a complete list of the videos available at www.routledge.com/9781617110603

## Tests

### Oculomotor

1. Cover Test
2. Fixation and Ocular Range of Motion
3. Optokinetic Testing
4. Saccades Testing
5. Smooth Pursuit Test
6. Vergence Test

### Vestibular Function

1. Head Thrust Test
2. Headshake Test
3. VOR-Cancellation (VOR-C) Test

### BPPV

1. Modified Dix-Hallpike Test
2. Side-Lying Test
3. Roll Test for Lateral Canal BPPV

### Findings

1. Direction-Changing Nystagmus With Rebound
2. Gaze Nystagmus
3. Positive BPPV (Patient 1)
4. Positive BPPV (Patient 2)
5. Post Headshake Nystagmus

## BPPV Interventions

### All Canals

1. Brandt-Daroff Exercise

### Posterior Canals

1. Modified Epley Maneuver (for Left BPPV)
2. Modified Epley Maneuver (for Right BPPV)
3. Semont-Liberatory Maneuver
4. Gans Repositioning Maneuver

### Lateral Canals

1. Log Roll
2. Barbecue Roll
3. Lempert Maneuver
4. Gufoni Maneuver
5. Vanucchi-Asprella Maneuver
6. Conversion Methods: Headshake, Quick Head Turn

### Anterior Canals

1. Reverse Semont Maneuver
2. Kim's Deep Head Hang

### Balance Interventions

1. Trunk Sways
2. Weight Shifting

There is a "Quick Reference" section at the back of the book as well, which has bare-bones information. If you are a novice or intermediate practitioner with regard to balance and dizziness evaluation and interventions, reading the entire book will give you the basic required knowledge to evaluate and treat these patient populations. You will know when to include other disciplines or specialists in your team to obtain the best outcome for the patient. Do not rely solely on the quick reference materials. After you have had some experience, the quick references become handy tools for accessing the needed information quickly. For the clinician with experience, this text may serve as a reference book. There are pictures and videos of tests and interventions. This book takes an evidence-based approach, with research findings listed throughout the text.

# INTRODUCTION

Balance evaluation and training are becoming increasingly hot topics. This book addresses the basics of evaluation and intervention choices for the patient complaining of decreased functional mobility, disequilibrium, and/or dizziness. It introduces the reader to the balance system and gives the reader sufficient anatomical, physiological, and clinical information to perform a thorough bedside evaluation of the patient/client who has issues with balance, functional mobility, or complaints of dizziness. It also presents intervention options that are available to address the systems you will examine. When available, evidence-based information is presented to justify evaluation and interventions. Many research studies are referenced, but there is no critical review of each article. Once you have become more familiar with the evaluations and interventions, you may use the book as a reference.

Why are balance and vestibular research and therapy programs becoming so popular? To answer this question, all we need to do is look at the growing segment of our population that is aged 65 or older! As our population of older citizens rapidly grows larger, the need to have clinicians skilled in the assessment of balance, dizziness, and functional mobility increases. In 2011, the percentage of the population that is 65 years of age or older was 13.3%.[1] Looking at CDC statistics, we can see an increase in deaths from unintentional falls as well as increased emergency room visits due to fall injuries in just a five-year period:

|  | DIED FROM ACCIDENTAL FALLS | TREATED IN EMERGENCY ROOMS FOR NONFATAL FALL INJURIES |
| --- | --- | --- |
| 2005 | 15,800 | 1.8 million |
| 2010 | 20,400 | 2.1 million |

As more of the Baby Boomer generation turns 65 and older, these statistics will only get worse as there will be more people at risk. As medical professionals, how well do we recognize signs and symptoms of those at risk of falling? Do we recognize the significance of patient complaints that indicate risk? With increasing frequency, we are called upon to evaluate a patient who has balance problems, gait difficulties, dizziness, trouble performing activities of daily living, or who has recently fallen. Even if they have not yet fallen, if they are presenting with decreased functional movements, a thorough multisystem evaluation to identify and address physical and functional deficits and impairments is warranted. If we can identify the specific deficiencies and issues that are contributing to the patient's disequilibrium and/or complaints of dizziness, we have a better opportunity to introduce interventions that will more effectively address, correct, or reduce these deficits, and thereby reduce the risk of falls and injuries.

Many times we find that if we try to strengthen our patients with therapy, this does not always solve the problem of disequilibrium. This is because there are many contributing systems to balance, and the musculoskeletal system is just *one* of those systems. To get a good understanding of why our patient is off balance, we need to look at each system involved in keeping us upright. If we look at only one system, we are limiting our view and understanding of the balance system as a whole. As with all complaints we investigate, the more information we have, the more insight we will have as to the possible etiologies.

To have postural stability, we automatically integrate the information gathered from the input systems of balance (ie, systems that give us information about our own position and movement as well as information regarding our environment) in order to use the information to choose appropriate motor programs to carry out the desired plan for movement or stability. We use automatic reflexes to help us remain balanced, make quick and needed adjustments while we are moving to respond to environmental demands, and also see clearly while we are doing these things. We must also have the presence of cognition, attention, and reaction time[2-4] and the strength and range of joint motion to carry out our intended actions.

Over the last decade there has been an explosion of research helping us to better understand reasons for complaints of dizziness, imbalance, and falls. While there is much yet to learn, we have some evidence-based guides to help us more effectively evaluate and intervene in those of a patient's functional deficits that result from pathology.

Once we understand the systems involved in maintaining balance, we can better grasp all that may be affecting a patient's ability to perform daily activities and ambulate without falling.

While we have been applying balance and vestibular training to the medical patient, we are just beginning to apply some of these concepts to the healthy and athletic populations. We are now well equipped to identify athletes who are at risk of injury *prior* to the season's beginning and are able to give these athletes training to prepare them for their individual sports while reducing their risk of injury. The use of vestibular training in a healthy athlete is less studied, but early indications are promising that it may help to improve athletic skills. "Sports vision" training has also been used to improve athletic performance. It seems to make sense that the more systems we can improve, the better the potential for a higher level of athleticism.

How do you evaluate and treat patients of any age who have dizziness? How do you evaluate and treat a patient who has instability with gait and balance? While medications reduce symptoms for the typical patient complaining of dizziness, they do not generally improve balance except in very specific circumstances. So sedating patients may make them feel better, but they may remain at risk or even at increased risk of falling. When offered exercises to address disequilibrium, often balance patients are given exercises that do not actually help. The keys to avoiding these traps are to:

- Examine the patient's history, complaints, medications, comorbidities, and past tests and interventions
- Perform a thorough evaluation that includes *all* systems that contribute to balance and movement plans and their execution.
- Address each condition that may be contributing to the balance/movement deficit.

- Use evidence-based treatments and interventions.
- Avoid general *routine* exercises during your intervention that do not address the specific conditions that impact function and are identified during the evaluation.
- Use valid and reliable tests and measures for evaluations and follow-up assessments to determine the patient's baseline and the effectiveness of interventions, revising the plan of care as needed immediately and for discharge planning.
- Refer patients for further testing as needed to better discover the causes of the balance or dizziness problem (ie, know your scope of practice).

Clinicians who know which systems to evaluate, what signs to watch for, and what complaints in the patient history give clues that help focus the examination are much better prepared to provide care. They can easily create a customized plan of care that addresses the patient's needs. They do not hesitate to order or ask for tests that will help rule out various pathologies. They are more likely to have better outcomes and increased patient satisfaction.

Recently a physical therapist who had just completed a continuing education course on the evaluation and treatment of balance and dizziness shared this story. She was treating a patient who had previously fallen and sustained a hip fracture. The patient was treated after the hip fracture using "traditional" therapy approaches and discharged to home. The patient then fell again and sustained another fracture. Fortunately the therapist had just completed the continuing education course and assessed the patient using newly learned techniques that examined each of the systems we use for functional movement and balance. She was able to identify a vestibular deficit, which explained the frequent falls and complaints of disequilibrium while turning, which is the motion the patient was performing when he fell. By addressing the actual causes of system deficits that contributed to the patient's condition of disequilibrium, the therapist greatly reduced the chances of future falls. The vestibular deficit had gone unnoticed by all of the previous clinicians who had treated the patient. Had the therapist not known how to examine each system, the patient would likely have returned home and continued to fall and sustain further injuries. Because she knew how to examine systems that impact balance and complaints of dizziness, the therapist was able to discover what was causing the disequilibrium.

Techniques to screen for balance deficits or system deficits that cause disequilibrium cut across disciplines. Physicians, nurses, therapists, audiologists, ophthalmologists, and trainers all have opportunities to screen and in some cases treat such deficits. As clinicians, we do not need to each be experts in neurology, otology, therapy, pharmacology, and so on. We *do* need to have enough information to identify important signs and symptoms and to know when a patient needs the help of an expert in any of these fields. Once the initial examination unveils the deficits, these professionals may work as a team to make the best possible outcomes available.

The following statistics highlight the need for clinicians of each discipline to be balance- and dizzy-savvy.

## Statistics

As reviewed in more detail later, when the balance system does not work correctly, patients may experience not only disequilibrium but also dizziness. Dizziness is the most common symptom in elderly patients and is a risk factor for falls.[5]

According to the CDC:

- One out of three adults age 65 and older falls each year,[6] but less than half talk to their health care provider about it.
- Falls are the leading cause of injury deaths among older adults.[7]
- Falls are the most common cause of nonfatal injuries and hospital admissions for trauma.[7]
- Most fractures among older adults are caused by falls.[8]
- The chances of falling and being seriously injured in a fall increase with age.[9]
- Some 90% of hip fractures in older adults are caused by falling,[10] most often by falling sideways onto the hip.[11]

Keep in mind that as the population grows older, we will see an increasing need for services to address balance deficits, falls, and complaints of dizziness.

## Sports Injuries

- About 25,000 ankle sprains occur in the United States every day.[12]
- Ankle sprains are common in all sports that involve cutting and pivoting.[12]
- A major determinant of sport-related concussions is a prior history of concussions.[13]
- Overall, the activities associated with the greatest number of traumatic brain injury–related emergency room visits included bicycling, football, playground activities, basketball, and soccer.[14]
- Children up to 4 years of age and older adolescents aged 15 to 19 years—as well as adults aged 65 and older—are most likely to sustain a traumatic brain injury.[15]

While knowing the risks of falling and injury associated with advancing age, an understanding of the causes or risk factors associated with falls is crucial. We know, for example, how the decline or damage of various body systems may impact a person. We examine these closely throughout this book. A 2013 study by Stenhagen et al using longitudinal data on 1763 subjects examined risk factors for falls in the elderly.[16] After three and six years, three main components predicting falls were identified in an elderly population: reduced mobility, heart dysfunction, and functional impairment (including nocturia). The use of neuroleptic drugs was also identified as a risk factor, but with a low prevalence. Knowing these risk factors may help you identify some of your patients at risk more readily. Taking a good history that includes medication use and knowing ways to assess mobility and function, then, will need to become part of your assessment of the elderly person.

# Disclaimer

Research is rapidly expanding our knowledge of the balance-impaired or dizzy patient. Even among the experts, there are many differing ideas about the best way to treat or intervene. The information provided in this book is a good baseline of current knowledge regarding examination and intervention. It is by no means meant to be interpreted as the "only way" to arrive at a good patient outcome. It does offer basic skill instruction as well as presenting research to guide practice. As pointed out by Bhattacharyya et al, clinicians should always decide and act in ways that they believe are in the best interests and needs of their patients regardless of guideline recommendations, which are never intended to supersede professional judgment.[17]

As you assimilate this information, you will most likely want to search for more in-depth continuing education courses and reading materials. Good luck on your journey, and remember to have fun!

# References

1. US Census Bureau. State & county quickfacts. http://quickfacts.census.gov/qfd/states/00000.html
2. Muir S, Berg K, Cheworth B, Klar N, Speechley M. Balance impairment as a risk factor for falls in community-dwelling older adults who are high functioning: A prospective study. *Phys Ther.* 2010;90:338-347.
3. Horak FB. Postural orientation and equilibrium: what do we need to know about neural control of balance to prevent falls. *Age Ageing.* 2006;35(Suppl 2)ii7-iii1.
4. Lord S. *Falls in Older People: Risk Factors and Strategies for Prevention.* Cambridge, UK: Cambridge University Press; 2007.
5. Hansson E, Mans M. Vestibular asymmetry predicts falls among elderly patients with multi-sensory dizziness. *BMC Geriatrics.* 2013;37, 77. doi:10.1186/1471-2318-13-77
6. Hausdorff JM, Rios DA, Edelber HK. Gait variability and fall risk in community-living oder adults: a 1-year prospective study. *Arch Phys Med Rehabil.* 2001;82(8):1050-1056.
7. Hornbrook MC, Stevens VJ, Wingfield DJ, Hollis JF, Greenlick MR, Ory MG. Preventing falls among community-dwelling older persons: results from a randomized trail. *The Gerontologist.* 1994;34(1):16-23.
8. Jager TE, Weiss HB, Coben JH, Pepe PE. Traumatic brain injuries evaluated in US emergency departments 1992-1994. *Acad Emerg Med.* 2000;7(2): 134-140.
9. Centers for Disease Control and Prevention. Injury prevention & control: data & statistics (WISQARS). *CDC.gov.* 2012. http://www.cdc.gov/injury/wisqars/
10. Cummings SR, Kelsey JL, Nevitt MC, O'Dowd KJ. Epidemiology of osteoporosis fractures. *Epidemiol Rev.* 1985;7: 178-208.
11. Hayes WC, Meyers ER, Morris JN, Gerhart TN, Yett HS, Lipsitz LA. Impact near the hip dominates fracture risk in elderly nursing home residents who fall. *Calcif Tissue Int.* 1993;52:192-198.
12. American Academy of Orthopaedic Surgeons. Sprained ankle. *AAOS.org.* 2012. http://orthoinfo.aaos.org/topic.cfm?topic=A00150
13. Sports Concussion Institute. Concussion facts. *Concussiontreatment.com.* 2008. http://www.concussiontreatment.com/concussionfacts.html
14. Gilchrist J, Thomas KE, Xu L, McGuire LC, Coronado VG. Nonfatal sports and recreation related traumatic brain injuries among children and adolescents treated in emergency departments in the United States 2001-2009. *MMWR.* 2011;60(39):1337-1342.
15. Faul M, Xu L, Wald MM, Coronado VG. *Traumatic brain injury in the United States: emergency department visits, hospitalizations, and deaths.* 2010. http://www.cdc.gov/traumaticbraininjury/pdf/blue_book.pdf
16. Stenhagen M, Ekström H, Nordell E, Elmstahl S. Fall in the general elderly population: a 3- and 6- year prospective study of risk factors using data from the longitudinal population study "Good ageing in Skane." *BMC Geriatrics.* 2013;13:81. doi:10.1186/1471-2318-13-81
17. Bhattacharyya N, Baugh RF, Orvidas L, et al. American Academy of Otolaryngology-Head and Neck Surgery Foundation clinician practice guideline: benign paroxysmal vertigo. *Otoryngol Head Neck Surg,* 2008;139(5 Suppl 4):S47-S81.

# 1

# Balance Systems

## CHAPTER GOALS

1. Describe how people balance.
2. Name 3 of the systems used to gather the information needed to assess balance.
3. Identify the anatomical structures of each system.
4. Explain how the gathered information is used to assess balance.
5. Name the part of the brain that deciphers the gathered information.
6. Describe how musculoskeletal limitations affect balance.
7. List changes to body systems that come with the aging process and may affect balance.

A review of the anatomy and physiology required for balance will allow you to better understand the evaluation techniques and intervention options needed to judge balance. While there may be some who enjoy the study of anatomy, for most of us it is a necessary evil. However, by understanding the anatomy and how things work you will have a much easier time maneuvering your way through the many possible causes of a patient's complaint.

Plishka CM.
*A Clinician's Guide to Balance and Dizziness:*
*Evaluation and Treatment* (pp 1-46).
© 2015 Taylor & Francis Group.

Many things impact balance, including the following:
- Cognition
- The function of all of the systems that help to maintain balance
  - Vision, vestibular, somatosensory, cerebellar, and musculoskeletal function
- Infection and inflammation
- Posture
- Strength
- Joint range of motion
- Medications
- Use or disuse of body systems
- Practice and skill of movement

The old adage "If you don't use it, you'll lose it" is true in the case of acquired skills. If you do not stand or walk frequently enough, you will lose some level of skill to perform these activities. There are many steps to complete for performing intended and skilled movements. For planned movement these include the following:
- Having a goal or desire or an externally driven need that provides the incentive to move
- Knowing the body's present position and movements
- Being aware of obstacles that would prevent or challenge the body's movements
- Making a plan to move or remain stable/still
- Having the strength and range of motion to carry out the plan
- Knowing how much muscle force will be required and how far the limbs must move to perform the task
- Assessing and adjusting movements based on feedback or environmental changes
- Having some degree of practice

## OVERVIEW OF THE BALANCE SYSTEM

Before initiating any intentional plan of movement, one must first start by collecting information, so this is where the review begins.

Figure 1-1 is a basic schematic of how the systems of balance interact.

As you can see, there is a lot of information sharing. There is information coming into the brain from the vestibular, visual, and somatosensory systems. Often called the *input systems*, they *give you information* about your own location and position as well as your surroundings. The cerebellum compares and coordinates information flow; in some cases, it alters signals coming from the input systems. It uses the information it receives from the input systems to help make a plan (with help from other parts of the brain) and to carry out the plan.

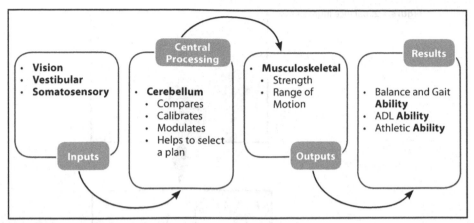

**Figure 1-1.** Diagram of the balance system.

An easier way to imagine how this process works is to compare it with baking a pie (Figure 1-2). In order to do this, you must start with the ingredients, such as apples, eggs, sugar, flour, butter, etc. You must blend these ingredients in just the right amounts to produce what you need—in this case the filling and dough for the crust. Next you need a pie pan in which to place the ingredients before they are baked. If all goes well, once your pie is done you will have a great-looking dessert! To find out how good it is, you will have to perform a taste test.

If there is a problem at *any step* of the process, the pie may either look bad (being burned or misshapen) or taste bad. For example, if you make a pie using rotten apples or rancid butter, it will obviously taste bad. If the blender is not working well, you may find lumps of flour or butter in the pie, and again it will taste bad. If the pan is too thin, the pie may burn. If there are only 1 or 2 small problems, the pie may still be edible. However, if you have multiple problems or even one large problem (perhaps having forgotten to add sugar), your failure as a baker will be obvious.

The balance system is similar to the process of baking a pie. The systems that gather information provide the ingredients of balance—visual, vestibular, and somatosensory information. Like the mixer, the brain (especially the cerebellum) combines the information into a useful plan by using just certain amounts of each system's information, depending upon the given activity needs. Your musculoskeletal system shapes balance, just as the pie pan shapes the pie. Finally, to see how well you balance and perform activities that require balance, you need a "taste test." You do this by using standardized tests of balance and/or the risk of falling. If there is a problem at *any step* in the balance process, it may present itself in the form of disequilibrium, trouble performing the activities of daily living (ADLs), gait deviations, falls, and in some cases complaints of dizziness. The more problems that exist, the worse the individual's balance/function or complaints will be. Just like the pie example, if one small problem exists, the patient may still be able to function. However, the more problems there are or if one very large problem exists, then the impact on functional movement will be obvious.

**Figure 1-2.** Balance ingredients.

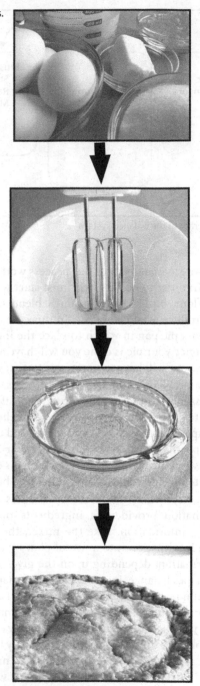

Specific examples of how deficits affect people are as follows:

- *Visual/oculomotor deficits*: These deficits may affect balance, gait, ADLs, and, in the case of the athlete—sports performance. Patients with visual deficits may complain of blurred vision, difficulty reading, or headaches. They may trip on objects in their path, miss stair steps, or find it difficult to keep their balance. For athletes, visual impairments may mean decreased accuracy of depth perception, which causes them to react too soon or too late during sports performance. During throwing or swinging activities, such an athlete may over- or undershoot the target.

- *Vestibular deficits*: Acute and chronic vestibular deficits have both similarities and differences regarding signs and symptoms. During acute episodes of vestibular loss, complaints of vertigo, nausea, and balance disturbances are common. These disturbances may cause vomiting and falls. Chronic vestibular issues do not always present with vertigo (sensations of movement or spinning), but common complaints include dizziness or disequilibrium during quick turns, while in dark environments that rule out use of the visual system, or the presence of nausea provoked by visually stimulating environments such as grocery store aisles, ceiling fans, moving cars, action movies or video games, crowds of people, etc. When questioned, many patients who have chronic vestibular loss admit to avoiding these settings. It is also not uncommon for them to avoid head turns while they walk, since otherwise they tend to deviate or stumble.

- *Somatosensory deficits*: Those lacking somatosensory information often are balance challenged and stumble/fall more frequently than others. Disequilibrium may be more common in the dark or on compliant (soft) surfaces.

- *Central processing deficits*: The cerebellum is responsible for coordination and the accuracy of movements. Those with deficits in this part of the brain may present with the inability to coordinate their movements; they may seem clumsy or lacking in accuracy as they move (eg, like trying to touch something with a fingertip and missing the mark).

  Memory and cognition may interfere with correct motor-plan choices or may impair the ability to make choices that are safe.

- *Musculoskeletal deficits*: Muscle weaknesses or poor range of motion may impact the patient's ability to perform daily tasks, to walk, or even to perform simple transfers, such as getting out of a chair.

## Goals of the Balance System

The balance system has a number of jobs. It helps to regulate muscle tone, eye movements, and keep us upright. According to Shepard and Telian,[1] there are 3 goals of the balance system, as follows:

1. To correct any inadvertent displacement of the center of mass from its equilibrium position over the base of support and thus to prevent a fall (eg, if someone nudges you off center, you can control yourself without falling and bring yourself back to a balanced position).

2.  To provide accurate perception of the body's position in the environment along with perceptions of direction and speed of movement.

3.  To control eye movements so as to maintain a clear image of the environment while the individual, the environment, or both are in motion.

## Balance Basics

There are numerous descriptions and definitions of the word *balance*. The definition you will see most, at least within the medical community, is probably the following: "Balance is the ability to control the center of gravity over the base of support."

To understand this definition, you need to also understand the concepts of *center of gravity* (COG) and *base of support* (BOS). The COG is the average location of an object's weight. For example, consider a piece of high-density balance foam, such as used by therapists to test and train balance. These foam pads are rectangular, in one solid piece, and made up of the same material throughout. If you wanted to balance the foam on top of a point (like the top of a pyramid), it would make sense to place the point in the center of the pad. Intuitively, you understand that the pad's center is the spot where you will have the best chance of getting the pad to balance without falling, because there are equal amounts of weight on each side of the center, which is resting on the point.

Now imagine that you have a box that you need to balance on a point. The box is rectangular like the balance pad, but unlike the balance pad, it is not made up of the same material throughout. It may hold a variety of objects, each with a different weight and density. In this example, the left side of the box holds a 50-lb weight while the right side of the box holds a feather. If you were to try balancing the box on the pyramid point by placing the point in the center of the box's bottom, the box would quickly tilt and fall toward the side of the 50-lb weight. The COG of the box is clearly *not* going to be in the center of the box, since one side of the box is heavier than the other. This box's COG is located well toward the end with the 50-lb weight. In order to balance the box on top of the point, you would need to place the point of the pyramid well toward the side of the box holding the most weight; otherwise it would tilt and fall. The COG of a human body (in the anatomical position) is located just below the umbilicus and inside the body. As you move, the COG moves as well. Its location depends on your position, activity, clothing, and even heartbeat! It is not static. If your patient has had a limb amputation, his or her COG will shift toward the side of the body that has the intact limb, since that side of the body will weigh more.

Having constant awareness of the COG helps in the decision-making process that keeps a person balanced. Being able to sense the COG makes it easier to plan strategies to stay balanced and make decisions about movement. As in the case of the box and balance pad already described, you must support your COG to avoid falling. To balance well, you must know where your COG is located, have control of it, and support it. Whatever is being used to support the COG to maintain a stable position is known as the *base of support* (BOS). The BOS may change depending on a person's activity, posture, or choice. In standing, the BOS includes the feet and the area between the feet. In sitting, whatever is in contact with the chair is the BOS (usually the buttocks, but may also be the back). Basically whatever is in contact with a supporting surface and the area between points of contact is the BOS.

The next concept needed for further discussion of balance is that of the *limit of stability* (LOS). The LOS is the area of movement (or excursion) while standing or sitting, within which you have balance control without needing to take a step or adding external sources of stability, as by touching or leaning on something. You can move your COG within your BOS without falling or needing to create a new or additional BOS. If you move past this invisible boundary of control (the limit of stability), you begin to fall.

---

### Activity 1—Limit of Stability

While guarded, perform the following either without shoes or in shoes that do not have a raised heel. If you wanted to find your LOS in standing, you could do the following:

Stand with your feet together and hands at your sides. When moving, do not bend at the waist in any direction. Keeping your back straight, shift all your weight as far as you can in the direction indicated as long as you maintain control.

First, lean toward your toes without letting your heels lift off of the ground. Keeping yourself forward, shift your weight toward your right pinky toe. Again, go as far as you can without allowing your heels to rise from the floor. Keeping to the right, shift back to your right heel as far as you can. Keep your weight on your heels, and then shift to your left heel. Finally, shift to your left pinky toe and then return to center front. Finally, return to a comfortable stance. You have just found your limit of stability!

---

When you balance, you do so under variable conditions. Sometimes you are at rest, as you probably are right now, sitting in a chair. At other times, however, you are in motion, as when you are walking. The task of walking typically requires you to move your COG outside of your limit of stability. As you walk, you shift your weight from one leg to the other. That is, you transition your COG from one BOS (say your left foot) to another BOS (your right foot as it steps forward). Taking a step is an example of creating a new BOS to maintain dynamic standing balance. As you step, your COG moves outside an area of support or control. To avoid falling, you quickly move a leg and take a step in the direction in which you are falling and transition the COG to this foot, which becomes the new BOS. A person who does not move his or her COG outside of the BOS while ambulating appears to shuffle or take extremely small steps, where one foot does not pass the other.

The following are other examples of creating bases of support:

- In static standing, if you tilt or lean too much in any direction, you will fall. Sometimes, however, you choose to do this as when you lean against a wall. The act of leaning against a wall is an example of adding an additional point of contact in the BOS. The area of the body that is in contact with the wall is now an additional support, which you use along with your feet to support the COG.

**Figure 1-3.** Stacked boxes.

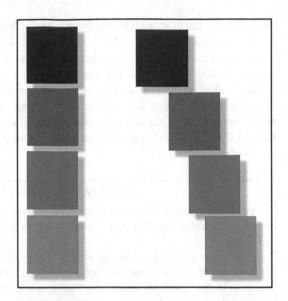

- In sitting, if you lean too far to one side or the other, you will fall when the COG moves past the limit of stability. Sometimes you may choose to do this, but you would likely place an extended arm out to the side and position your hand to accept the weight of your upper body as an additional point of support.

When there is a stable BOS, generally the person, object, or objects (eg, a stack of boxes) will be stable and will not fall. When the weight of the object or objects (or the COG) is outside of the base, a fall is more likely. Use the images of the stack of boxes (Figures 1-3 and 1-4) to assist with this concept. When stacked directly on top of each other, the COG of each box will be directly on top of the one below. The COG of each box is supported. Now imagine that you are stacking boxes, but as you place each new box on the stack, you position it a few inches off center of the box below. Each box has a COG, and if the COGs are located past the support of the box beneath, the boxes are more likely to fall. Figures 1-3 and 1-4 help to illustrate this concept.

Using the concepts discussed up to this point, review the 3 basic steps of balancing, which include (1) getting information, (2) processing the information, and (3) carrying out the plan.

## STEP 1: GETTING INFORMATION

As discussed, your body uses 3 main *input* systems to get the information needed to balance/move in the desired manner: visual, vestibular, and somatosensory.

The brain actually places importance on each of these inputs differently, based on activity. For example, in quiet standing, the brain places more importance on information received from the proprioceptors. When a person is moving, however,

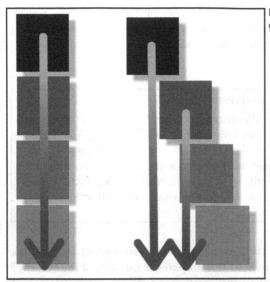

**Figure 1-4.** Stacked boxes with center of gravity.

the importance shifts to the vestibular system. It is hypothesized that the vestibular system contributes to 65% of dynamic body stability.[2]

## Vision

*Nystagmus* refers to an involuntary rhythmic motion of the eye. Scientific literature uses the singular form of the word *nystagmus* to indicate both singular and plural forms of the word. So this term may refer to one nystagmus beat or many. There are various types of nystagmus, and unless otherwise stated in this book *nystagmus* will refer to the "jerk nystagmus" type. Jerk nystagmus moves the eye quickly in one direction and slowly in the reverse direction. Nystagmus occur under different conditions and can occur throughout the day as needed to help keep the eyes on objects of interest or to help a moving person see more clearly.

We use our eyes to see the world. When moving, people use visual information to check their body positions as well as to help plan motor strategies based on what is in the desired path. For example, using visual information, you may check if you are standing straight, tilting, or swaying. Assuming that they have no visual deficits, people see out of both eyes. Since we have 2 eyes, their angles of view (when looking at the same object) are slightly different. Light enters the eye and the lens focuses it onto the back of the eye. To see an object clearly, people intuitively try to position each eye so that the image of the object falls on the *fovea*, which is the part of the retina that has the sharpest vision. The fovea is located in the macula of the eye, which is the central region of the retina.[3]

The retina contains photoreceptors called *rods* and *cones*, named for their shapes. These receptors have different functions regarding vision. The rods are extremely sensitive to light but have low resolution. That is, they do not detect very sharp images but help you see in darker environments. In contrast, the cones are not as sensitive to light but have very high resolution, so that they *do* provide very sharp vision. Further, the cones also allow us to see color. One way to remember the functions of the cones is to think of the cones as coming to a "sharp" point, like a colored pencil.

## Eye Movement

---

### Activity 2—Foveal Vision

Do the following to illustrate the differences between foveal "sharp" vision versus using the less sharp peripheral vision. This will help demonstrate the difference between the sharp foveal field dominated by cones and the less sharp areas of vision detected by the rods: Pick out an object in the room and stare at it. You will notice that the image of the object you are looking at is sharp. Without taking your eyes off of the target, pay attention to the peripheral areas of vision. You will notice they are somewhat blurred.

---

As already mentioned, people use their eyes to see the environment and to track moving objects within it. If there are deficits that impair the motions of the eye, they may contribute to balance deficits, difficulty reading, headaches, or sensations of dizziness and nausea. Different types of motion or muscle activity are used to move or steady the eyes in order to see clearly.

### Fixation

Fixation is the ability to keep the eyes stationary on an object. For example, you might ask a person to stare at the point of your pen as you hold it in front of his or her eyes. If the patient can keep the eyes still and focused on the pen point, this is *maintaining fixation*. This term also describes a patient who is looking at an object during certain tests. For example, if you observe nystagmus while you ask the patient to look at the pen tip, you would document that "nystagmus with fixation" occurred. The phrase *gaze holding* is also used to describe holding the eyes in a certain position. Reactions to trying to fixate sometimes offer clues indicating pathology. For example, if a patient develops nystagmus when trying to fixate on a target, this is suggestive of a central pathology. If a patient has nystagmus that stops while he or she is visually fixating, this is suggestive of a peripheral (outside of the brain) pathology. If the patient is unable to visually fixate, you will observe the eyes moving around the visual target instead of remaining still. This is another sign suggestive of central pathology.

### Smooth Pursuit

*Smooth pursuit* is a continuous tracking motion of the eyes, which varies with age. It is generally developed and close to an adult level of function by the age of 6 months[4] and continues to "fine-tune" through the preschool period. It degrades with age in some patients around the sixth decade. Smooth pursuit allows for clear vision of objects that are moving slowly within the visual environment, with the stimulus for smooth pursuit being the relative velocity of the object being watched. An example would be watching a person walk across the room while you are sitting still. As the person walks across the room, you "follow" by moving your eyes in the direction in which he or she is walking. You are able to do this if the object you are watching is moving within 0 to 0.5 Hz (1 Hz = 360 degrees of motion per second).[5] This is a very slow-moving object. Another example of smooth pursuit is when you are holding a pen in front of a person's eyes, and asking him or her to follow the pen (eyes only) while you slowly move it left and right of his or her center.

We also use smooth pursuit for keeping a stationary target on the fovea during self-motion—for example, if you want to keep your eyes on the television screen as you walk across the room. You are moving but the TV set is not.

Many things impact smooth pursuit, including age, alertness, medications, intoxicants, and degenerative disorders of the cerebellum or extrapyramidal systems.

---

### Activity 3 —Smooth Pursuit

Observe a colleague's eyes under 2 conditions while his or her head is still:
1. As the colleague watches someone walk across the room (and the visual field).
2. Instruct the colleague to try performing smooth pursuit while nothing is moving in the room. For example, "Imagine that you are watching someone walk across the room and move your eyes to follow him or her."

What did you see? For item 1, you most likely saw a smooth tracking motion. For item 2, your colleague's eyes "jumped" as they moved, and the motion was not smooth. Why? Remember, the stimulus for smooth pursuit is relative motion of a visual target. You cannot perform smooth pursuit without a visual target.

---

### Saccades

A saccade is a ballistic (quick) movement of the eye in one direction to bring an object that is in your peripheral vision to the fovea in the shortest possible time. In fact, saccades are the quickest of all eye motions.[6] The intrinsic stimulus for the choice of this motion is positional error of the object of interest's image on the retina. We use saccades to quickly move the eye. There are a variety of circumstances in which we need this—for example, when the visual target's motion exceeds the upper limits of smooth pursuit speed. That is to say, saccades come into play when whatever you are watching begins to move faster than you can follow by using only smooth pursuit. Another example of saccades is when you hold your head still while looking back and forth between 2 objects that you can see within your visual field (without moving your head). You are not slowly moving your eye between the objects as you would if tracking a slowly moving object but are instead jumping your eyes from one target to the next. Typically older adults who lack smooth pursuit (which may be an age-normal loss) instead use a series of saccades as a method of tracking moving objects. We describe this as *saccadic smooth pursuit*. Finally, we use saccades to quickly move our eyes to see objects that enter our peripheral vision.

### Optokinetics

The optokinetic system, sometimes abbreviated OPK, works to provide clear visual images during sustained head movements, sustained environment movements, or a combination of both. These motions trigger a jerk-type of nystagmus that allows people to track objects moving across their visual fields. Nystagmus that is activated by the OPK system is called *OPK nystagmus* and may be abbreviated OKN. An example is trying to watch the side of the road while riding in a car as a passenger.

As you watch the side of the road, objects are continuously moving across your field of vision. In the examples just used, if you are in a country where you drive on the right side of the road, the images for a passenger would be moving across his or her visual field from left to right. The OPK system detects movement of an object beginning in the left peripheral visual field and across it. Imagine that you see a tree while riding in the car. As you look out the passenger window, the tree first appears at the far left edge of your visual field, drawing your eyes far left in their orbits. The image of the tree moves from far left to far right across your visual field, but too quickly for you to track using smooth pursuit (since smooth pursuit can only track objects that move slowly). You track the tree from left to right and very soon find that you are at the end range of motion with your eyes looking to the right. The tree leaves your visual field completely as the car continues to move, and your eyes quickly jerk back to the far left so that you can find a new object to view and start the process all over. The tracking motions you have made from left to right as you track the tree are slower than the quicker motions to return your eyes to the far left. If you were to watch someone's eyes while he or she looked out of the car window, you would observe OKN with rhythmic eye motions alternating between slower tracking motions in one direction and quicker "reset" motions in the opposite direction, returning the eyes to the starting point.

---

### Activity 4: Nystagmus

Have a colleague sit in a chair that swivels. With his or her eyes kept open, spin the chair rapidly in one direction for about 20 or 30 seconds, then suddenly stop the chair and observe the eyes. You will see nystagmus. While the colleague is spinning, he or she is using OPK nystagmus with the quick phases in the direction of spin. Once the chair is stopped, you will observe jerk nystagmus with quick phases in the opposite direction of the spin. (The mechanics behind this phenomenon are explained in a later part of this book.) For safety, wait for the colleague's dizziness to end before allowing him or her to stand.

---

In order to accurately move the eyes to see clearly, one must use the integration of OPKs, smooth pursuit, saccades, fixation, and the nystagmus reflex. As far as movement is concerned, the eyes by themselves do not provide enough information to tell you if you are moving or if the world is moving around you. An example of this is when you are sitting in a car at a stop light and the car next to you starts to drift forward. The OPK system detects the movement of the car drifting; however, you do not know if the car next to you is moving or if your car is moving. As a result, you quickly press harder on the brake pedal. After a moment, you realize that you were in fact sitting still the entire time. If the car next to you drifts again, you do not have the same reflexive reaction to slam on the brakes, as your brain now realizes that you are not moving. Your eyes are only one of the systems contributing to a sense of motion and balance. We need information from other systems besides vision to appropriately detect and plan useful and functional movements.

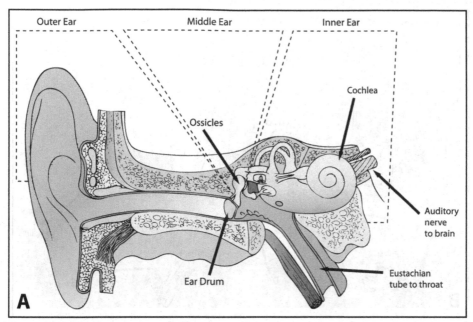

**Figure 1-5.** (A) Ear diagram. *(continued)*

## Vergence

When tracking an object that is moving toward or away from us, our eyes must move in opposite directions simultaneously. For example, if an object is moving toward us, each eye must rotate toward the midline as it tracks the object getting closer (called *convergence*). As the object moves away from us, each eye rotates outwardly (*divergence*) simultaneously. These motions allow each eye to center the image of the object we are tracking on the fovea, and we perceive one image.

## *Vestibular System Anatomy*

Figure 1-5A depicts a cross section (frontal plane) of the ear. The peripheral vestibular system includes the vestibular organs and the nerves, which are outside of the central nervous system, that conduct information to and from these organs. The vestibular organs are found in the inner ear between the eardrum and the cochlea (see Figure 1-5B, in which the vestibular organs are highlighted); their anatomy and physiology are well described in the literature.[1,7-11] The vestibular organs share cranial nerve VIII (the vestibulocochlear nerve) with the cochlea and has a number of jobs, including maintaining posture, regulating muscle tone, maintaining equilibrium, and stabilizing gaze when the head is in motion. Understanding how this system works will greatly improve your ability to understand the signs and symptoms of patients who complain of disequilibrium and/or dizziness.

The entire peripheral vestibular system (Figure 1-6) is about the size of your thumbnail, and you have a vestibular organ in each ear. A closer look at the

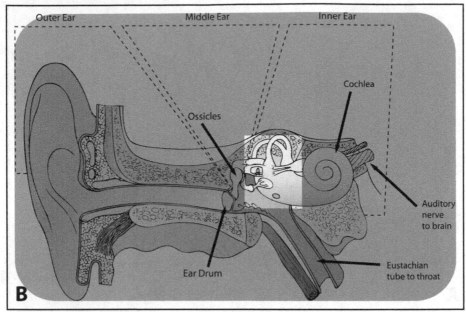

**Figure 1-5 (continued).** (B) Ear diagram with highlighted vestibular system.

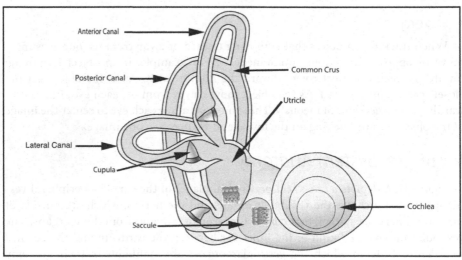

**Figure 1-6.** Vestibular system.

peripheral vestibular system allows us to see that there are 3 semicircular canals (also called *labyrinths*), and 2 chambers (collectively called the *otolith organs*) in each ear. The 3 semicircular canals—the *anterior* canal, *lateral* (or horizontal) canal, and *posterior* canal—are named for their orientation within the head. The otolith chambers are named the *utricle* and *saccule*. Each of the 3 canals begins and ends in the utricle.

The entire system floats in a fluid called *perilymph*, in a similar way as the brain floats in cerebrospinal fluid inside the skull. The canals and otoliths contain a fluid called *endolymph*, which has a high concentration of potassium. The endolymph of the saccule does not communicate with that of the other parts of the peripheral vestibular system.

The anterior and posterior canals are oriented closer to the vertical plane, while the lateral canal is oriented roughly with the horizontal plane. The canals are responsible for detecting *angular velocity changes of motion*, and do not normally detect the pull of gravity. The otolith organs are responsible for detecting *changes in linear velocity* (eg, up/down, front/back, and side to side), as well as the pull of gravity to detect tilting of the head. The system in the left ear is the mirror image of the system in the right. Between functions of the chambers and canals, you can be aware of any motion of your head.

The concept of neutral buoyancy is important to understanding the function of the inner ear. Before continuing to review vestibular anatomy and physiology, consider this concept. For a moment, imagine that you have a large glass of water sitting on a table. Above the glass you hold a rock. If you let go of the rock, it will fall through the air toward the glass of water. This happens because the rock is *heavier* than the air surrounding it. Once the rock hits the water, it will sink through it until it hits the bottom of the glass. This happens because the rock is *heavier* than the water surrounding it. Now imagine that you are holding a cube of ice. If you drop it while holding it over the glass of water, it will fall through the air until it hits the water. This happens because the ice cube is *heavier* than the air surrounding it. However, once it is in the water, the ice cube will float, not sink. If you were to reach down to the bottom of the glass while holding the ice cube and then let go of it, the ice would rise until it reached the surface of the water. This would occur because the ice cube is *lighter* than the water surrounding it. Finally, imagine that you had an object the size of the ice cube but it weighed *exactly the same as the water*. If you reached halfway down into the glass of water and let go, it would not rise, since it is not lighter than the water around it. It would not sink, since it is not heavier than the water around it. Instead, it would *stay* wherever you let go of it, since it is *neutrally buoyant,* weighing the same as the water around it. Parts of the inner ear that detect motion are neutrally buoyant and detect only movement velocity changes, while other parts are not neutrally buoyant and therefore may detect tilt due to the pull of gravity.

## Semicircular Canals

As mentioned, all 3 canals (anterior, lateral, and posterior) begin and end in the utricle. The anterior and posterior canals begin with a common canal (called the *common crus*), which divides to become these canals. They are sometimes referred to as the *vertical canals* since they are oriented (roughly) vertically to the ground and 45 degrees from the sagittal plane. The lateral canal is oriented roughly horizontal to the ground but with a 30-degree angle, angling upward (cephalad) as it moves anteriorly. All 3 canals leave the utricle and then bend back to reattach to it, forming a semicircle. Just before it reconnects to the utricle, the end of each canal widens into an area called an *ampulla*. Inside each ampulla are groups of hair cells contained in

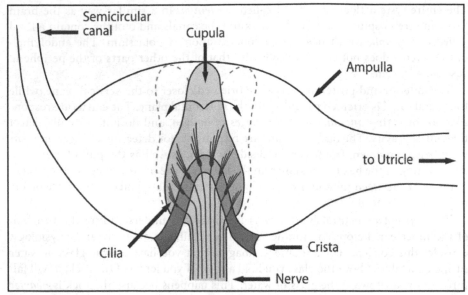

**Figure 1-7.** Cupula.

a gelatinous flaplike matrix structure called a *cupula* (Figure 1-7). The cupula in each of the canals completely blocks off the canal space, and endolymph cannot move past it. The hair cells inside the cupula connect to nerves leading to the brain. Movement of the cupula (and hair cells within it) changes the neural information (firing rates) of these nerves owing to angular head movements. The cupula is neutrally buoyant, weighing the same as the endolymph that surrounds it. Because of this, gravity does not affect the cupula. That is to say, if you tilt your head, the cupula will not sink or bend in the endolymph toward the ground. Being neutrally buoyant, the cupula of each canal cannot normally detect gravity; therefore you cannot use the information coming from the semicircular canals to tell you where the ground is or whether you are tilting. For example, if you move from sitting to lying, the cupula will not be "pulled down" by gravity. As you move your head, the fluid inside the system lags a bit behind the motion and the cupula will bend toward or away from the utricle, depending on the direction of fluid pressure due to this lag. These cupulae will detect the movement of the head's velocity, but not the ultimate position of your head with respect to gravity.

---

### Activity 5—Fluid Inertial Lag

To gain a better understanding of the inertial fluid lag, take a half-full clear bottle of water and hold it sideways (make sure the lid is tight!). If you quickly move the bottle to your left, you will see the water collect on the right side of the bottle. Why does this happen? Initially, as you move the bottle, it is moving faster than the water inside it. As a result, fluid builds on the right side of the bottle as it moves left. Eventually enough pressure is built up within the fluid that it too begins to move to the left.

As you quickly turn your head to the left, the motion of the endolymph inside the lateral canals of each ear lags behind the head motion—called *inertial lag*—and puts pressure on the cupula. Recall that the peripheral vestibular organs are mirror images of each other. So as you turn your head, the endolymph in the lateral canal of one ear will push the cupula inward toward the utricle, thus increasing the nerve firing rates, while in the other ear the endolymph will move away from and deflect the cupula of that ear away from the utricle, thus slowing the firing rates of that ear. This push-pull relationship holds true for each coplanar canal pair.

The nerves attached to the peripheral vestibular organs are constantly sending signals that change during velocity or position changes of the head. These nerves are always sending signals to the brain, even when you are still. At rest, the hairs of each group are standing up in a neutral position and the nerves fire at a certain rate, called the *resting rate*. However, if you move, the fluid presses or pulls against the cupula and makes the hairs bend. When the hairs bend, the nerves change their firing rates.

In each group of hair cells there are rows of hairs, with each row taller than the one preceding it in a stepwise fashion. We refer to these rows of hairs collectively as *stereocilia*. Ultimately you reach one very tall hair cell, called the *kinocilium*, which is the tallest in the group. The hair cells in each group connect to each other, and if one bends, they will all bend. If the group of hairs bends in the direction of the tall kinocilium, the associated nerve increases its firing rate. The farther the hairs bend toward the kinocilium, the faster the nerve will fire. Conversely, if the group of hairs bends toward the shortest row of hairs, the nerve will slow its firing rate. The farther the hairs bend toward the shorter rows, the more slowly the nerve will fire. The hairs return to their upright neutral position and nerve returns to the resting firing rate whenever the head is either still or moving at a constant velocity.

The resting-rate signal is between 70 and 100 spikes per second.[12,13] During angular head motions, the vestibular organ that is ipsilateral to the direction of motion can increase the firing rates up to 400 spikes per second.[14] The brain compares firing rates of the nerves in the cupulae of each canal as well as the firing-rate information from the otoliths to determine in which direction and how quickly the head is moving. It is the change from the resting firing rate that indicates how you are moving or turning, in which direction, and how quickly. The nerves attached to each group of hairs in the ampulla detect only changes in *velocity* of the head in angular motion, since the cupula is neutrally buoyant. Because the canals are semicircular, angular head motions will create endolymph flow, deflecting the cupulae.

Another common everyday analogy can help to clarify this process. Imagine you have a tire that you fill with water and then lay on the ground. How could you get the water inside the tire to move around the inside of it in a circular fashion? It you were to lift the tire up and down, the water would not move around in a circle. If you wanted to get the water flowing in a circular motion, you would have to move or spin the tire in a circle. Once you had it moving in a circle, the water inside the inner tube would begin to flow around either clockwise or counterclockwise, depending on which way you turned it. Now that you have this picture in mind, imagine that you are in an upright position and that each canal (anterior, lateral, and posterior), being almost a complete circle, is filled with fluid. The only way to get the cupulae to bend

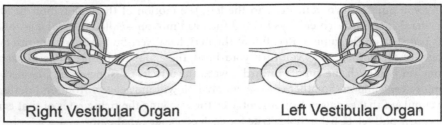

Right Vestibular Organ          Left Vestibular Organ

**Figure 1-8.** Vestibular organ of each ear.

(and thereby bend the groups of hairs within them) is to get the fluid moving in a circular fashion around the canal. If you simply moved up and down (as in an elevator), the fluid in the canals would not flow along them. However, if you were to turn or spin, the fluid would begin to flow. The direction of its motion would depend on the direction of your head's motion. The cupula will bend during angular motions, since angular motions will produce a lag or movement of the endolymph, which will push or pull the cupula.

Figure 1-8 shows the vestibular organ and cochlea of each ear. You can see that the vestibular organ of one ear is the mirror image of the other.

How do you know in which direction you are moving? The canals of one ear work in a push-pull system with those of the other ear. Canals that are in the same plane of motion work together; they are called *coplanar pairs*. The pairs that work together are as follows:

- Left anterior canal and right posterior canal: This pair is often referred to as the *LARP* (Figure 1-9A).
- Right anterior canal and left posterior canal: This pair is often referred to as the *RALP* (Figure 1-9B).
- Left lateral canal and right lateral canal (Figure 1-9C).

Taking a closer look at the lateral canals, you can see that each ear has groups of hairs in the lateral canal that are arranged from short to tall rows as you move in a lateral-to-medial direction (Figure 1-10).

If you turn your head to the right, there will be a lag in fluid that will push the groups of hairs in the lateral canals of each ear to the left. Recall the example of the bottle of water. If you move it left, the water will collect on the right side of the bottle due to inertial lag. In discussing the vestibular system, use anatomic referencing. You are not using your own perspective of left and right but instead that of the patient's left and right. If all of the hairs in each lateral canal bend in the same direction, you can see that in one ear they would all be bending toward the tall hairs (and making the nerves fire faster), while in the other ear they would all be bending toward the shortest hairs (making the nerves fire more slowly). This creates a sort of push-pull system. So whenever you turn in a new direction, the nerves of one ear fire faster while the contralateral ear's nerves slow their firing rates. The faster the turn, the farther the hairs bend and the more they change firing rates.

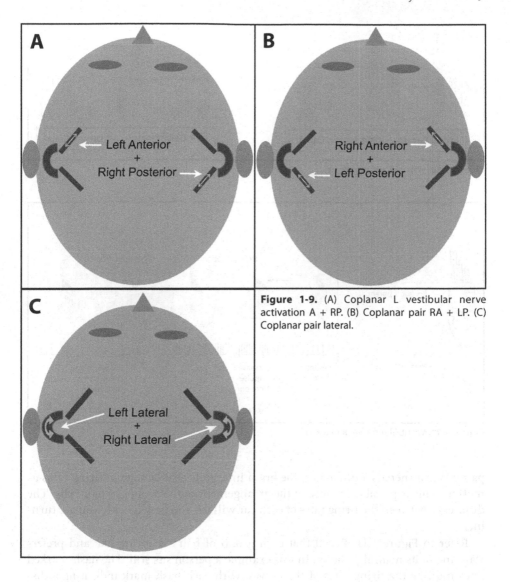

**Figure 1-9.** (A) Coplanar L vestibular nerve activation A + RP. (B) Coplanar pair RA + LP. (C) Coplanar pair lateral.

Just like a tug-o-war, each coplanar pair works as a push-pull system. If each ear is sending the same resting-rate signal, the brain senses no motion from the vestibular system. If you turn your head to the left, the left lateral canal will *increase* its firing rate while at the same time the right lateral canal will *decrease* its firing rate. If you were to rotate your head to the right, the right lateral canal would increase its firing rate while the coplanar pair (the left lateral canal) would at the same time decrease its firing rate. The hairs will bend only if there is a change of velocity. The brain compares the firing rate coming from each pair. So if you are turning continuously at constant velocity, the vestibular system would not detect the motion. Changes of velocity will produce a lag of endolymph causing different firing rates of the coplanar

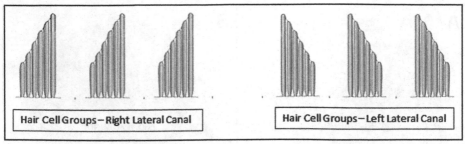

**Figure 1-10.** Hair cell arrangement.

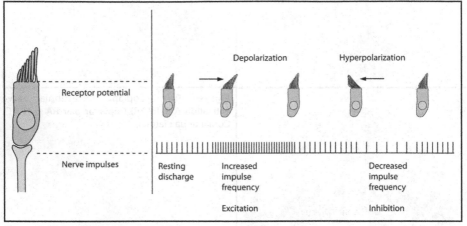

**Figure 1-11.** Vestibular nerve activation.

pairs. When there is a difference, the brain interprets that change in firing rates as motion. This is possible because of the arrangement of the groups of hair cells. The difference between the firing rates of each ear will tell you how quickly you are turning.

Refer to Figure 1-11. Recall that each group of hairs is spring-like and prefers standing in its neutral position. In this example a person sits still. The hash-marked lines indicate the firing rates of the nerves, with each hash mark indicating a discharge of the nerve. If you turn your head to the right, there is a lag in the fluid, which bends the hairs in the other direction. For the right lateral canal, this means you are bending the hairs toward the tall hair cell, and this increases the nerves' firing rate. If you stay still, the hair cells return to their preferred position, and the nerve returns to its resting firing rate. If you turn your head to the left, there is a lag of the fluid within the canal, and the hairs bend toward the small hair, slowing the nerves' firing rate. When you stop moving, the hairs once again return to their preferred resting position, and the nerve returns to its resting rate. Using Figure 1-11 as a reference, can you describe the firing rates of a nerve that is connected to a group of hairs in the contralateral lateral canal?

| TABLE 1-1 THE EFFECT OF LEFT POSTERIOR HEAD MOTION ON VESTIBULAR NERVE ACTIVITY | | |
|---|---|---|
| MOTION: LEFT POSTERIORLY | INCREASED NERVE FIRING RATE | DECREASED NERVE FIRING RATE |
| **Figure 1-12.** Left posterior motion. | Left posterior canal | Right anterior canal |

Using Figure 1-10, you can see that when all hair groups bend in the same direction owing to motion of the head, one ear would increase the nerve's firing rate while the other ear would slow its firing rate. Again, the brain compares the firing patterns of each coplanar pair. If there is a difference, you interpret that difference as movement. By comparing the firing rates, you know how fast and in which direction your head is moving. The following tables (Tables 1-1 through 1-6) and figures illustrate this point. The image is of the head as viewed from above. The canals are involved are also depicted.

## Otolith Organs

Like the groups of hair cells located in the cupulae of the canals, the otolith organs (utricle and saccule) each also have groups of hair cells on a kidney-shaped area called the *macula*. There are some differences between the arrangements of these groups of hairs compared with those at the end of the canals in the ampullae. As you have learned, the canals work as pairs during inertial lag owing to the push-pull system created by the mirror-image arrangements of the hair cells of each ear. This is not the case for the utricles and saccules of each ear. The hair cells in each otolith organ are not all arranged in the same orientation (such as each group arranged small to tall, laterally to medially). Instead, each macula has some groups arranged small to tall while others are tall to small. Imagine 2 armies facing each other on a battlefield. Each utricle and saccule has a macula that is roughly divided along the middle of the kidney shape—half of the macula having groups of hairs arranged small to tall while

| TABLE 1-2 | | |
|---|---|---|
| THE EFFECT OF RIGHT ANTERIOR HEAD MOTION ON VESTIBULAR NERVE ACTIVITY | | |
| MOTION: RIGHT ANTERIORLY | INCREASED NERVE FIRING RATE | DECREASED NERVE FIRING RATE |
| 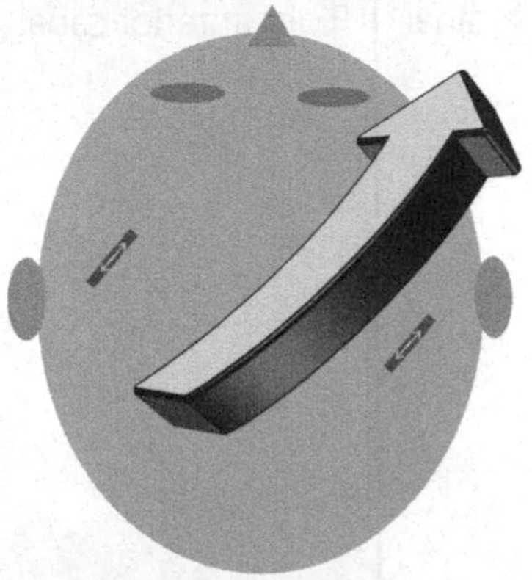  **Figure 1-13.** Right anterior motion. | Right anterior canal | Left posterior canal |

| TABLE 1-3 | | |
|---|---|---|
| THE EFFECT OF RIGHT POSTERIOR HEAD MOTION ON VESTIBULAR NEURAL ACTIVITY | | |
| MOTION: RIGHT POSTERIORLY | INCREASED NERVE FIRING RATE | DECREASED NERVE FIRING RATE |
| 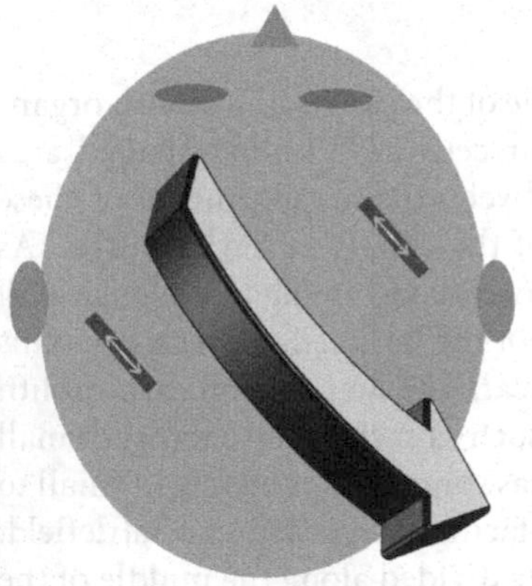  **Figure 1-14.** Right posterior motion. | Right posterior canal | Left anterior canal |

| TABLE 1-4 | | |
|---|---|---|
| **THE EFFECT OF LEFT ANTERIOR HEAD MOTION ON VESTIBULAR NERVE ACTIVITY** | | |
| MOTION: LEFT ANTERIORLY | INCREASED NERVE FIRING RATE | DECREASED NERVE FIRING RATE |
| 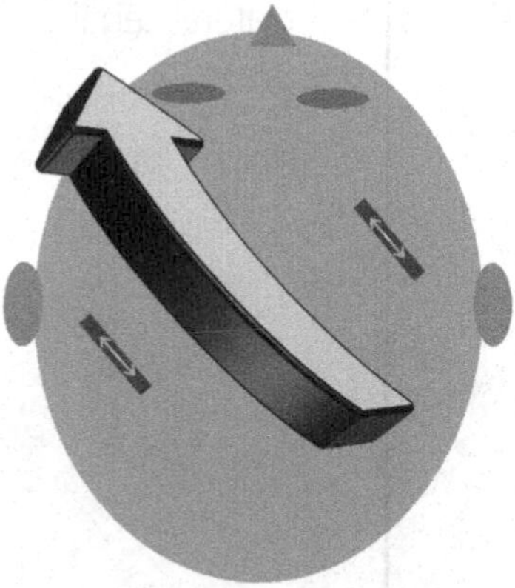  Figure 1-15. Left anterior motion. | Left anterior canal | Right posterior canal |

| TABLE 1-5 | | |
|---|---|---|
| **THE EFFECT OF RIGHT ROTATION HEAD MOTION ON VESTIBULAR NERVE ACTIVITY** | | |
| MOTION: RIGHT ROTATION | INCREASED NERVE FIRING RATE | DECREASED NERVE FIRING RATE |
| 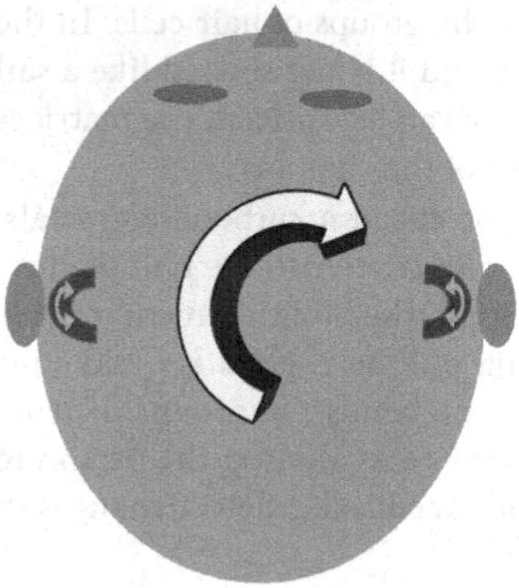  Figure 1-16. Right rotation motion. | Right lateral canal | Left lateral canal |

## TABLE 1-6

## THE EFFECT OF LEFT ROTATION HEAD MOTION ON VESTIBULAR NERVE ACTIVITY

| MOTION: LEFT ROTATION | INCREASED NERVE FIRING RATE | DECREASED NERVE FIRING RATE |
|---|---|---|
| 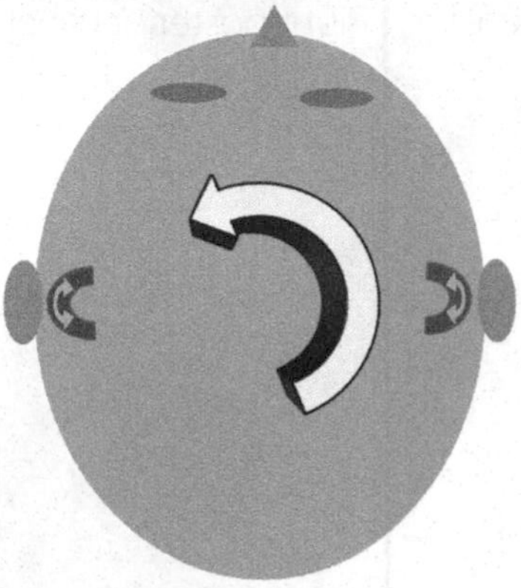 | Left lateral canal | Right lateral canal |

**Figure 1-17.** Left rotation motion.

the other half has groups arranged tall to small. When this one macula is moved, the nerves associated with it will not all send the same message, as is the case in the canals. Instead, it will send some nerve signals that are faster than the resting rate and some that are slower. When you compare the signals of the utricle or saccule of one ear with those of the other ear, you will not get a push-pull system. As a result, the otoliths do not work in pairs, since they are each sending the same types of information. Refer to Figure 1-18 for a cross section of an otolith organ (utricle or saccule).

Another difference between the maculae of the otolith organs and the cupulae of the canals is the shape of the matrix that contains the groups of hair cells. In the otolith organs, this matrix is the *otolithic membrane*, and it is not shaped like a sail or flap that blocks off an area, as the cupulae do in the canals. Instead, the matrices are like kidney-shaped pans and do not block off part of the chamber.

Finally, the utricles and saccules have *otoconia*, or calcium carbonate crystals, anchored on top of each otolithic membrane, making it sensitive to the pull of gravity. Since these crystals are heavier than the endolymph, the otolithic membrane is no longer neutrally buoyant. If you tilt, the otoconia pull on the matrix and shift it toward the ground. The shifting otolithic membrane bends the groups of hairs contained within, changing the firing rates of the nerves and alerting the person to head tilting. Besides detecting gravity, the utricle and saccule also detect changes in velocity, just as do the cupulae.

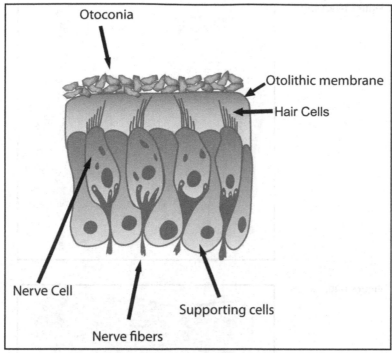

**Figure 1-18.** Utricle.

### Utricle

The macula of the utricle is oriented horizontally, with the groups of hairs coming up like grass growing from the ground. As you move front to back or side to side (any horizontal-plane movement), the hair cells bend and detect the motion. So when you press your foot on the gas pedal, you feel the acceleration of the car. When you see the police car waiting behind the billboard to catch speeders, you feel the sudden deceleration as you slam on your brakes! The utricle is responsible for these sensations. Since it also detects the pull of gravity, it can also detect tilt (Figure 1-19).

### Saccule

The macula of the saccule is located on its medial wall. This anatomy is similar to that of the utricle, but owing to the positioning within the chamber, its hairs come out laterally, as if growing out of a wall. When you move vertically, the force of this motion causes these hair cell groups to bend and give you sensations and information about these motions. When you are in an elevator, you can't see anything moving, but you feel yourself rising or falling. The saccule (Figure 1-20) is responsible for these sensations.

## Vestibular Neural Connections

The signals leaving the posterior semicircular canal and saccule travel along the inferior vestibular nerve. An easy way to remember this is to associate the vestibular

**Figure 1-19.** Utricle.

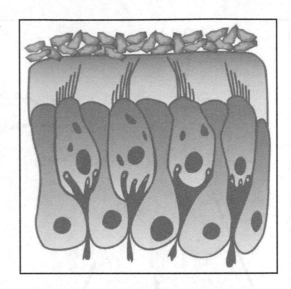

**Figure 1-20.** Saccule.

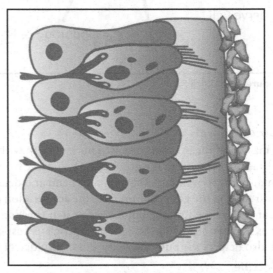

anatomical relationships of what is "in the back (posterior canal) and on the bottom (saccule)" as being "inferior." Signals from the anterior canal, lateral canal, and utricle travel along the superior vestibular nerve. These 2 nerves merge to form the vestibular nerve. The vestibular nerve merges with the auditory nerve to form the vestibulocochlear nerve (also known as the *eighth cranial nerve*). CN VIII (vestibular and auditory nerves) passes through the internal auditory canal, which is a tunnel passing through the skull that allows nerves and blood vessels to enter and exit the skull. Next, it travels through the cerebellopontine angle to finally arrive at the vestibular nuclei.

| TABLE 1-7 SUPERIOR VESTIBULAR NUCLEUS | | |
|---|---|---|
| **VESTIBULAR NUCLEUS** | **CONNECTIONS** | **JOB** |
| Superior | Afferent: The bulk of afferents that project to this nucleus come from the nerves at the ends of the semicircular canals. Another major group of afferent nerves comes from the cerebellum. There are also some connections from the otolith organs.<br><br>Efferent connection travel to oculomotor nuclei. | The superior nucleus is the major relay center for ocular reflexes that are triggered by information coming from the semicircular canals. |

| TABLE 1-8 LATERAL VESTIBULAR NUCLEUS | | |
|---|---|---|
| **VESTIBULAR NUCLEUS** | **CONNECTIONS** | **JOB** |
| Lateral (also known as *Deiters' nucleus*) | Afferent: Major afferent contributions are from the vestibular system and cerebellum, with some components from the spine and other areas.<br><br>Efferent: Most efferent fibers from this nucleus go to the spinal cord, although it also connects to oculomotor neurons. | It is important for the control of the vestibulospinal reflex. |

There are 4 main vestibular nuclei that process information.[15-17] They are the superior nucleus (Table 1-7), the lateral nucleus (Table 1-8), the medial nucleus (Table 1-9), and the inferior nucleus (Table 1-10).

## Vestibular Laws

There are a few "laws" governing the vestibular system. The first 3 are named after a German researcher named Arnold Ewald, who created them in 1882.

*Ewald's 3 laws* are as follows[18]:

1. A stimulation of the semicircular canal causes a movement of the eyes in the plane of the stimulated canal.

| TABLE 1-9 | | |
|---|---|---|
| **MEDIAL VESTIBULAR NUCLEUS** | | |
| **VESTIBULAR NUCLEUS** | **CONNECTIONS** | **JOB** |
| Medial (also known as the *triangular nucleus* or *nucleus of Schwalbe*) | Afferent connections: This nucleus receives afferent fibers from the contralateral medial vestibular nucleus and other areas of the brain. Specific sections of this nucleus contain different afferent connections.<br><br>• Superior section: contributing afferent fibers come from the semicircular canals and cerebellum.<br><br>• Middle section: contributing afferents from the utricle and saccule.<br><br>• Caudal section: contributing afferents come from the cerebellum.<br><br>Efferent connections run to the cervical and thoracic spinal levels, the oculomotor nerves, the cerebellum, and contralateral vestibular nuclei. | It is important for coordinating eye, head, and neck movements. |

| TABLE 1-10 | | |
|---|---|---|
| **INFERIOR VESTIBULAR NUCLEUS** | | |
| **VESTIBULAR NUCLEUS** | **CONNECTIONS** | **JOB** |
| Inferior (also known as the *descending* or *spinal nucleus*) | Afferent connections: from the semicircular canals and cerebellum.<br><br>Efferent connections: contralateral vestibular nuclei. | Integrates vestibular signals from each side (left and right ears and vestibular nuclei) with the cerebellum and reticular formation. |

For example, if you stimulated the right lateral vestibular canal, you would expect to see lateral eye motions.

2.    In the horizontal semicircular canals, an ampullopetal endolymph movement causes a greater stimulation than an ampullofugal one.

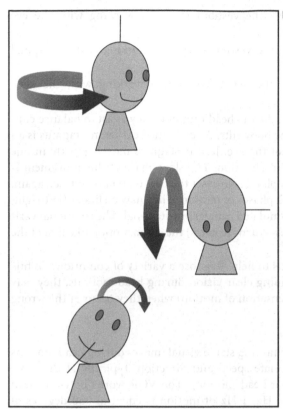

**Figure 1-21.** Vestibular reflexes.

The terms *ampullopetal* and *ampullofugal* describe the direction of endolymph flow within the canal. *Ampullo-* refers to the ampulla, while *–petal* indicates "moving toward." Therefore an ampullopetal motion is one that describes motion toward the ampulla. By contrast, *ampullofugal* indicates movement away from the ampulla. Ewald's second law tells us that the force of endolymph moving toward the ampulla will cause vestibular excitement. In the vertical semicircular canals, the reverse is true.

3.   The third law states that ampullopetal endolymph flow (movement toward the ampulla) causes less vestibular excitement than endolymph flow away from it.

Laws 2 and 3 are explained by the arrangements of hair cells within the lateral canals versus the vertical canals.

Another commonly referred-to law is *Alexander's law*. This law states that spontaneous nystagmus of a patient with a vestibular lesion is more intense when the patient looks in the direction of the quick phase than the slow phase.[19]

## How Is the Information From the Vestibular System Used?

The vestibular system mediates a number of reflexes whose names indicate the systems that are working together to produce the reflex. These include the VOR, VSR, and VCR (Figure 1-21):

- *VOR*: Vestibulo-ocular reflex (the vestibular system working with the eye motion)
- *VSR*: Vestibulospinal reflex (the vestibular system working with the spinal muscles)
- *VCR*: Vestibulocollic reflex (the vestibular system working with the neck muscles)

These reflexes keep vision stable during head motions: they assist in balance control and help to right the head if the body tilts. As explained earlier, nystagmus is an involuntary, rhythmic movement of the eye. Jerk nystagmus moves quickly in one direction and slowly in the opposite direction. The slow phase of this movement is for visual tracking, while the quick phase is to reset the eye to prepare to track again. Nystagmus are named for the quick phases of motion. They may be linear (left-right, up-down, or in the planes of the stimulated canals) or rotational. The rotational variety—*rotary* (or torsional) *nystagmus*—turns (rotates) the eye (a motion like that of the turning of a car's steering wheel).

You can use observed nystagmus to help diagnose a variety of conditions. While nystagmus are helpful for maintaining clear vision during head motions, they may also add to a feeling of vertigo (a sensation of motion) when they occur at the wrong times.

### The Vestibulo-ocular Reflex

The VOR is responsible for maintaining stable visual images during head motions by moving the eyes at the appropriate speed and direction (typically at the same speed but opposite the direction of head motion). The VOR works between head motions (frequencies) of 0.5 and 5 Hz; 1 Hz of motion is equal to 360 degrees of motion per second. Most head motions during the day are between 0.5 and 4 Hz, so you use the VOR throughout the day. The latency of the VOR is 5 to 7 ms.[20,21] This is much faster than eye motions generated by the smooth pursuit system, which are less than 60 degrees per second, with latencies up to 100 ms.[22,23]

The VOR works in 3 planes of motion: yaw, pitch, and roll. Yaw is the "no" motion of the head, pitch is the "yes" motion, and roll is the ear-to-shoulder motion. For example, pick out one letter on this page and keep your eyes on it while you shake your head "no" quickly. If your eyes do not move and instead move with the head as it turns, as you shake your head you will see whatever is in directly in front of you at each moment during the head turn and not on the letter on the page. In order to keep your eyes on a target while your head is in motion, the VOR turns your eyes in the *opposite direction* of your head motion and at *exactly the same speed*. In this way, your eyes always stay pointed at the target, even if your head moves. The VOR "turns on" to help you keep your eyes pointing at the visual target. As you shake your head, the inner ear detects the speed and direction of your head and relays the information to the oculomotor nuclei, which will activate the eye muscles to move the eyes so that they stay on the target. When everything is working correctly, you will be able to keep the image of your target clear (within the speeds of motion in which the reflex works).

### The Vestibulospinal Reflex

The VSR helps to maintain balance. If you tilt too far and are in danger of falling, the muscles on the side of the body ipsilateral to the tilt will go into extension and the arm and leg on that side will quickly come out to prevent you from falling. At the same time the muscles on the other side of the body will go into flexion or relax. This causes a righting reaction.

### The Vestibulocollic Reflex

The VCR is similar to the VSR, only it works on the neck muscles alone, not the entire body. It helps to right the head against gravity to maintain an "eyes level" posture. As your body tilts, this reflex rights your heads so that you see the world in a level fashion.

To summarize, the vestibular system provides information about your head motion as well as your position and allows you to use reflexes to move your eyes appropriately. It also adjusts muscle tone to keep you balanced and positioned upright against gravity.

# The Somatosensory System

The somatosensory system provides information about body movement and position as well as sensations of touch, pressure, and vibration.

## Somatosensory Receptors Types

There are 3 general types of somatosensory receptors:

1. *Mechanoreceptors*: Stimulated by mechanical displacement of body tissues, these receptors mediate tactile and proprioceptive sensations.
2. *Thermoreceptors*: These detect temperature.
3. *Nociceptors*: These detect pain.

Mechanoreceptors are the most numerous and transmit and process information from muscles, tendons, joints, and connective tissues of the musculoskeletal system. Information from these receptors allows for a sense of position of body parts, called *proprioception*, and also of body movement, called *kinesthesia*. Table 1-11 lists the various types of mechanoreceptors.[24] As you can see, the cutaneous mechanoreceptors detect tactile stimuli, while the musculoskeletal mechanoreceptors are all proprioceptive.

## Somatosensory Neural Pathways

Ascending pathways of the somatosensory receptors for fine touch, pressure, vibration, and position sense project into the dorsal column and terminate in the lower medulla. From there the medial lemniscus originates and projects to the ventral posterolateral nucleus (VPL) of the thalamus. VPL fibers connect to the primary sensory cortex and terminate topographically.[24] Descending fibers influence transmission and processing at each level to control input to the cerebral cortex and ensure that movements occur smoothly and accurately.

## TABLE 1-11
## SOMATOSENSORY RECEPTORS

| RECEPTOR TYPE | | STIMULUS | SENSATION |
|---|---|---|---|
| Cutaneous | Merkel cell | Skin distortion | Sustained pressure |
| | Ruffini ending | Skin distortion | Touch, shearing stress |
| | Meissner's corpuscle | Vibration | Flutter, contact |
| | Pacinian corpuscle | Vibration | High-frequency vibration |
| | Hair follicle | Hair movement | Contact, touch |
| | Free ending | Distortion | Mechanical deformation, intense heat, chemical irritants |
| Musculoskeletal | Muscle spindle 1 degree endings | Spindle stretch: length, rate of stretch | Proprioception |
| | Muscle spindle 2 degree endings | Spindle stretch: length | Proprioception |
| | Golgi tendon organ | Tendon tension | Proprioception— static limb position |
| | Joint receptors | Joint movement and pressure | Proprioception |

## Somatosensory Reflexes

The somatosensory input gives rise to the reflexes used in postural control. For example, during quiet standing, you use the proprioceptive information to detect body sway and local ankle reflexes to help reduce the sway (also known as the *ankle strategy*) by contracting your calves and tibialis anterior muscles. If you are nudged off balance or sway too far, the stretch receptors detect the quick change and initiate a reflex arc.

Table 1-12 lists some common somatosensory reflexes.

There are some cervical somatosensory reflexes that are mirrors of the vestibular reflexes. Just like the vestibular reflexes, they are named for the systems that are working together to form each reflex. They are as follows:

- *COR: Cervico-ocular reflex* (the proprioceptors of the neck working with the oculomotor system to move the eyes)

| TABLE 1-12 | |
|---|---|
| **SOMATOSENSORY REFLEXES** | |
| **REFLEX** | **IMPORTANCE** |
| Dynamic stretch reflex | Reacts to quick stretches. |
| Tonic stretch reflex | Reacts to slow, passive motions and helps to mediate muscle tone. |
| Inverse stretch reflex | When a muscle reaches a certain level of stretch, it will shut off to protect itself from damage. The contralateral muscle will be "excited" by the cross-component of this reflex. |
| Intersegmental reflexes | This reflex allows for the coordination of motor activity among limbs and axial trunk muscles. It helps limb-supporting reactions, righting responses, and rhythmic stepping. |

- *CCR: Cervicocollic reflex* (the proprioceptors of the neck working with the neck muscles to right the head)
- *CSR: Cervicospinal reflex* (the proprioceptors of the neck working with the spinal muscles to prevent a fall)

You initiate these reflexes by the bending or turning of the head relative to the body. Muscle spindles and joint receptors in the upper cervical spine provide the proprioceptive information needed for the reflex.

You will notice that if you were to replace *cervico-* with *vestibulo-*, you would have the vestibular reflexes. The vestibular and cervical reflexes act to accomplish the same things. While the vestibular reflexes use vestibular afferent information to drive the reflexes, the cervical reflexes use proprioceptive information. A big difference between these groups of reflexes is that the cervical reflexes are very weak. At best they are useful as a supplement to the vestibular reflexes, with the afferent somatosensory information acting to supplement that of the vestibular system. They may become more important if there is vestibular damage, because then the neck receptors will act as a source of information about head motion and position.

*Physical damage to the neck may sometimes help explain dizziness* (called *cervicogenic dizziness*). If the patient has a history of neck or head trauma, whiplash injury, or severe degenerative disease of the cervical spine, the clinician must carefully screen the neck to see if symptoms correlate with cervical motions or palpation.

# STEP 2: PROCESSING THE INFORMATION

Once the brain has the needed information, it has to choose which information is most important or relevant for the current circumstance in order to plan movements appropriately. Which muscles do you need? In what sequence do you need them? How much force is needed? How far will you need to move and how quickly? The cerebellum is the judge that will answer these questions. Using the information gained from the 3 input systems mentioned, the cerebellum, with the help of the basal ganglia, creates a plan of motion. The information you receive from the input systems (vision, vestibular, and somatosensory) are not used equally. How you use the gathered information depends on need. That is, whichever information is most useful for any given situation or environment gets top priority. For example, while you are in quiet standing (ie, not moving your feet), you use proprioception and cutaneous sensory information to plan and control maintenance of the desired posture and position. You also use this information while performing most ADLs.[25-27] The more complex the activity and the more challenging the environment, the more the brain will incorporate information from all inputs.[28] When movement is involved, the vestibular system's information suddenly becomes important. In fact, it is estimated that 65% of body stability during dynamic movement is due to vestibular contributions.[2]

## Cerebellum

In cases where the systems are in conflict (eg, your eyes and vestibular systems give conflicting information), the cerebellum decides which system it will pay attention to and use that information to help plan or alter movement. The cerebellum does not give equal weight to the information gathered by each input system. For example, when you are in quiet sitting or standing, the cerebellum uses more information from the somatosensory system, which provides information about pain, temperature, touch sensations, pressure sensations, joint position (proprioception), and joint movement (kinesthesia) than it does from the vision or vestibular systems. However, as you start to move, it puts more weight on vision and vestibular inputs. As the motion becomes more complex, the cerebellum adds more weight (importance) to information from these systems.

The cerebellum also acts to calibrate the input signals. In cases of pathology, the cerebellum may adapt signals in order to balance/move more efficiently. The brain makes a plan for balance and then activates the musculoskeletal system to carry it out. It compares what you intend to do (as far as a movement plan goes) to what you actually do and can make adjustments as you move. Your ability to balance and walk is a result of the collective function of these systems.

It is easy to think of the cerebellum as being responsible for functional motion, but many parts of the brain are involved in movement selection. This is especially true when you are performing automatic, repetitive motions such as walking or carefully thought out movements such as when you are learning a new complex task, like playing the piano. The lowest level of organization is at the level of the spinal cord, where the body creates local reflexes based on information from the afferent somatosensory receptors. The brainstem integrates the sensory information for posture and balance, regulates postural muscle tone, and contributes to anticipatory (feedforward) postural control. The cerebellum receives input information from the spinal cord, vestibular nuclei, and cerebral cortex. It compares the motor plan with the sensory data and makes adjustments as needed to keep your movements coordinated and to keep you balanced.

The thalamus processes most information coming into the cortex from the spinal cord and cerebellum. The basal ganglia are involved in motor control, planning, and strategy. It facilitates intended motor plans and motions while inhibiting all unwanted movements. The cerebral cortex chooses a course of action, programs movements, and identifies targets in space.

When there is damage to any of the brain's many parts, you may see different signs. For example, in the case of cerebellar damage, you may see ataxia, or signs of vestibular or oculomotor deficits. If there are problems in the basal ganglia, you may observe the generation of unintended movements, such as ticks or tremors. There may also be a limitation of wanted motions, manifesting, for example, as the freezing episodes that patients with Parkinson's disease experience. They say that the eyes are the window to the soul, but they are very useful windows into the vestibular system as well as the brain. Examination of eye motions sometimes leads to further examinations of the brain or vestibular systems, as issues with these areas may cause the eyes to move inappropriately.

Table 1-13 describes the areas of the brain involved with movement.[15,16]

# STEP 3: CARRYING OUT THE PLAN

Once the information is gathered (*step 1*) and a plan of action for movement and/or balance is created (*step 2*), the brain can send the information to the muscles to carry out the plan (*step 3*). Many things may affect balance. Some of the things adversely impacting balance stem from musculoskeletal issues, such as poor posture, insufficient strength, and poor joint range of motion due to deformity and/or muscle tightness.

To discuss how posture may affect a person's balance, compare a person to the stack of boxes used in discussing COG. As discussed then, in stacking boxes, you try to center each added box on the box below in order to prevent the stack from leaning or falling (Figures 1-22 and 1-23). In comparing the boxes in the figures (assuming that they are all of the same evenly distributed weight), I'm sure you would agree that the stack in which the boxes were placed neatly and straight would be more stable than a stack in which they were not placed directly on top of one another.

Why is this true? To answer that question, you need to consider the COG of each box. The same is true for humans. When you consider the entire person as an object, the COG is located just above the pubic bone and close to the center of the body's core. If you place your fist just below your umbilicus, you will have found the topical representation that corresponds to your COG. However, that is for the person who is standing straight and has all 4 limbs. Just as in the case of the stack of boxes, where you would consider the COG for each box, you can also consider the COG for your body parts (head, shoulders, hips, etc). If, like the boxes shown in the figures, someone did not "stack" these parts over a stable BOS (for example, the feet), he or

## TABLE 1-13

# AREAS OF RESPONSIBILITY OF THE CENTRAL NERVOUS SYSTEM

| AREA | BRAIN PROCESSING ACTION/RESPONSIBILITY |
|---|---|
| Spinal cord | • Lowest level of processing.<br>• Reception of afferent somatosensory information.<br>• Organization of reflexes and basic reflex/extension patterns of lower extremity muscles. |
| Brainstem | • Regulation of postural tone.<br>• Integration of sensory information for posture and balance.<br>• Contributes to anticipatory postural control. |
| Cerebellum | RECEIVES:<br>• Input from the spinal cord (movement information).<br>• Input from the cerebral cortex (movement planning).<br>• Input from the vestibular nuclei.<br>OUTPUT: To the brainstem<br>FUNCTION:<br>• Adjusts motor responses comparing plan and sensory data.<br>• Updates movement plan as needed.<br>• Modulates force and range of movements.<br>• Involved in motor learning. |
| Thalamus | • Processes most information coming into the cortex from the spinal cord and cerebellum. |
| Basal ganglia | • Higher-order cognitive aspects of motor control, such as planning motor strategy.<br>• Facilitates intended motions, inhibits all other unwanted motor plans. |
| Cerebral cortex | Involved in:<br>• Identifying targets in space.<br>• Choosing a course of action.<br>• Programming movements. |

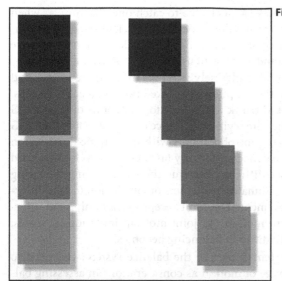

**Figure 1-22.** Stacked boxes.

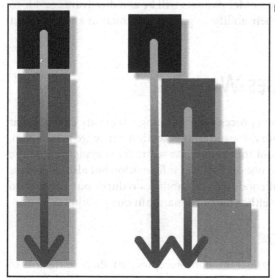

**Figure 1-23.** Stacked boxes with COG.

she would have less stable balance. The person might be able to maintain a less stable position given enough strength or external support, but it will take less force to push him or her past the limit of stability as compared with a person of equal strength who is standing straight.

Poor muscle strength causes disequilibrium in different ways. It may affect posture and place the COG closer to the limit of stability, or it may impair a person's ability to move as desired. For example, without enough strength, a person may not provide enough force needed to move a limb the correct distance to maintain balance while walking. If there is a need to make a quick step to catch one's balance, as when someone trips or is nudged off balance and does not have sufficient strength to generate the quick motion, he or she may fall. If the hips are weak, a person may have difficulty transferring from sit to stand and maintaining initial standing balance.

Joint range of motion deficits may also adversely affect balance. Limited trunk and postural joint motion may result in the adoption of a flexed posture (eg, bent knees, bent hips). Patients who have a flexed trunk will have a forward shift of their COG and may be prone to falling since they are trying to balance and move while the COG is located near the boundary of their control. Patients with poor ankle dorsiflexion may complain of frequently losing balance posteriorly (as their COG is being forced in that direction) and may also have difficulty clearing their toes during the swing phase of gait. Finally, recall that the somatosensory sensors in the joints send information regarding position and movement. The joint receptors can only send information regarding the available joint motion. As joint motion limitation increases, information decreases and the more difficult balancing becomes.

Because the musculoskeletal system is part of the balance system, you need to include strength, flexibility, and range of motion as considerations in assessing balance. Keep in mind that as people age, they become less flexible and lose muscle mass. Regarding the ability to balance, older patients will be at a disadvantage due to the age-related changes impacting their ability to gather information and carry out the desired motor plan.

# CHANGES WITH AGE

While we cannot consider the aging process as a pathology, there are changes that impact balance, which is why they are reviewed in this section. Once we have a plan, our musculoskeletal system carries out the plan. However, there is evidence that the aging process impacts our abilities to not only collect information but also to process it. Further, a decline in our physical condition and abilities reduces our capacity to carry out the plans we have made to either move or maintain our positions.

## Vision Changes With Age

Different types of conditions that affect the photoreceptors attribute to the loss of visual acuity. Loss of the cones (sharp vision receptors) will result in loss of visual acuity and legal blindness. Loss of rods will result in difficulty seeing in low levels of light, commonly referred to as *night blindness*.[3]

The normal function of the eye tissues decreases with age, and the best predictor of blindness and visual impairment is age.[29] According to T. L. Carter, there are normal visual changes that occur with age. Examples of these changes include presbyopia, decreased contrast sensitivity, decreased dark/light adaptation, and delayed glare recovery. There are also age-related ocular diseases that include macular degeneration, primary open-angle glaucoma, cataract, and diabetic retinopathy.[30]

### Macular Degeneration[3]

Central vision is critical for sight. Age-related macular degeneration is the most common cause of vision loss in people over the age of 55. This type of vision loss occurs due to degeneration of the cone photoreceptors. Loss of vision is gradual and usually noticed with blurred central foveal vision. These patients may benefit from a low vision program to provide strategies and equipment allowing for enhanced daily function.

### Drugs and Eye Movement

Many medications and drugs impair eye motion, even when used at therapeutic (nontoxic) levels. Smooth pursuit, eccentric gaze holding, and convergence are particularly susceptible to medications. Here are some examples, as described by Leigh and Zee[31]:

- *Drugs that impair smooth pursuit*—diazepam, methadone, phenytoin, barbiturates, chloral hydrate, and alcohol
- *Medications known to affect eye motion*—benzodiazepines, tricyclic antidepressants, phenytoin, carbamazepine, barbiturates, phenothiazines, lithium carbonate, amphetamines, alcohol, tobacco and nicotine, narcotics, baclofen, beta blockers, choral hydrate, nitrous oxide, risperidone, cocaine, and phencyclidine (PCP)

## Vestibular Changes With Age

According to Furman et al, age-associated changes in the vestibular system include degeneration of the otoconia (crystals), degeneration of hair cells, loss of vestibular afferents, and a reduction in the number of cells in the vestibular nuclei.[32]

Benign paroxysmal positional vertigo (BPPV) is more common with advancing age, which suggests there may be an age-related component. In a retrospective review of 53 patients diagnosed with BPPV, the incidence of BPPV increased 38% with each decade of life.[33] Further, vestibular function seems to decline with age. There has been one longitudinal study that looked at the vestibulo-ocular reflex (VOR) over a 5-year period ($n$ = 57, mean age 82). In this study, there was a significant amplitude-dependent decrease in gain and an increase in phase lead of the VOR. There was a decrease in gain of the visual-vestibular responses at low-frequency sinusoidal stimulation.[34]

The US National Health and Nutrition Examination Survey indicates that BPPV, or vestibular dysfunction, among those in their 60s, 70s, and 80s or older is 49.4%, 68.7%, and 84.8% respectively.[32,35]

## Somatosensory Changes With Age

First, let us discuss the changes to our input systems (those that collect information); a review of research by Shaffer and Harrison outlines the changes that occur with age.[28]

## Joint Receptors

For joint receptors, 2 studies have found a reduction in all mechanoreceptor types with increased age when looking at 23 subjects aging in range from 20 to 78.[36] An animal study examined the numbers of Ruffini's, Pacinian, and Golgi tendon-like ligament receptors in the anterior cruciate ligaments of rabbits and found a stepwise reduction in the numbers of these receptors in older rabbits.[37]

## Cutaneous Receptors

Shaffer and Harrison further reviewed studies that looked at cutaneous receptor changes with age. A decline in cutaneous vibration sense is associated with a reduction of Pacinian and Meissner's receptors with aging.[28] A different study compared 7 young adults (ages 23 to 26 years) with 95 older adults (ages 65 to 73 years), and found that the older adults had insensitivity to vibration and monofilament as compared with the younger subjects. This study also identified that in the early seventies the vibration perception threshold doubled. Finally, the monofilament test did not seem to be as sensitive in detecting changes in the older adults.[38]

There are numerous studies showing a decrease in 2-point discrimination in older subjects. One study found that the loss of 2-point sensation in the plantar toe surface, as well as an increase in mediolateral sway, was significantly greater in fallers than in nonfallers.[39]

## Proprioception (Joint Position Sense)

These receptors give us the information we need to control joint position and movement. Because nerves are needed to carry these messages, it stands to reason that the fewer intact nerves and receptors you have, the more limited your information-gathering ability will be. This was demonstrated in a study by Verschueren et al,[40] who found that adults in the oldest test category of their study (age 70 years) had the greatest performance variability and ability to identify the prescribed target angle when compared with young subjects (mean age 21.7 years). When vibration was applied to the tibialis anterior tendon, the older subjects (aged 60 to 70 years) had significant variance in their ability to identify the target angles. Vibration did not affect the younger subjects' ability to identify joint angles. Both younger and older subjects were able to improve their abilities with practice trials and knowledge of results.[40]

A reduction of proprioception is also strongly associated with a decline in single-leg stance time in older adults.[41] Distal joints, such as ankles, seem to be more affected by the loss of proprioception than proximal joints.[42]

# Nerve Conduction

Nerve conduction velocity parameters in adults seems to peak at age 40 and thereafter to decline.[43] Sensory fibers seem to be affected before motor fibers, and subjects older than age 80 years had global declines in both types of fibers.[44]

## Muscle Changes With Age

The word *sarcopenia* denotes age-related loss of muscle mass. As we age, we lose muscle mass, and this is believed to be a major factor in causing frailty and functional impairment. We lose not only muscle mass as we age but also some of the motor units that innervate our muscles.[45]

A study by Karaizou et al[46] compared the muscle fibers of 23 subjects within an age range of 26 to 93 years and found that individual muscle fibers (deltoid muscle, and extensor digitorum brevis muscle) had reduced spindle diameters as a function of age. No changes to quads or biceps were observed as a factor of age in this small sample.[28,46]

Based on these studies, the aging process has the following effects: Decreased visual acuity, vestibular organ degradation, increased likelihood of BPPV, decreased VOR gain and response, reduction in the number of mechanoreceptors, decline in vibration sense, decreased 2-point discrimination, increased variability in identifying joint angles, decreased nerve conduction velocity, and decreased muscle mass. As you can see from the research, loss of the supporting mechanisms for somatosensory information will limit the individual's ability to gather information. Assessment of the systems that gather the information used for balance should be a routine part of the assessment plan for any patient with poor balance or a history of falls.

# SUMMARY

There are many systems that contribute to balance. Some give us information, some process information and make a plan, and others carry out the plan. To balance and move as desired as well as to be able to see clearly while moving, these systems must work at peak efficiency. If there are problems in any of these systems, moving and balancing will be more challenging. The more deficits that exist, the more difficult maintaining balance and controlling movement will become.

The inputs (ingredients of balance) of visual, vestibular, and somatosensory functions provide information regarding the environment as well as a person's position within the environment. The brain, especially the coordinating actions of the cerebellum, provides a plan to balance and move as desired and actively fine-tunes needed movements to do these things accurately and efficiently. Finally, muscles, bones, and joints carry out the plan of action by using reflexes and volitional movements.

There is a learning curve when you are using tests that you are unfamiliar with. It takes time and practice to integrate new tests into your practice, and sometimes the effort required to do that seems overwhelming. How will you benefit from learning how to assess all of these systems? Knowing how the body systems interact to allow a person to balance will influence clinical evaluations, treatments, and interventions. If only a portion of these systems are examined or treated (for example, only focusing on the musculoskeletal system) but problems exist in other parts of the balance system, then patients will most likely not reach their maximum level of function. By understanding these systems, you will be prepared to perform a very thorough

| TABLE 1-14 | |
|---|---|
| **INFORMATION GAINED FROM AN EVALUATION OF SYSTEMS** | |
| SYSTEM | INFORMATION GAINED FROM EVALUATION |
| Information gathering from the visual, vestibular, and somatosensory systems | Are there deficits of information gathering that may be affecting the patient's functional ability or causing symptoms? |
| Cerebellar screen | Is there an information processing issue, or is the cerebellum affecting the other systems (eg, oculomotor, motor function)? |
| Musculoskeletal system | Do weaknesses, limited or excessive motion, or postural issues exist that may be impacting balance and function? |

examination, and be more likely to identify problems impairing the patient's function. Once you identify the problems, you can target each system that has a problem with interventions that make a difference. Refer to Table 1-14 to review the information to be gained by examining each system.

The patient's ability to perform the previous 3 steps reviewed (getting information, processing it, and carrying out the plan) is reflected in the ability to move and balance as desired. Quite often balance issues or functional motion problems are due to a combination of deficits in multiple systems. If there are problems at *any* step of this process, the outcome (desired motion or activity) may be affected, and the patient may not move appropriately or precisely enough for the given circumstances or environmental challenges.

It is a fact that aging often brings about changes to our bodies, impacting systems that affect balance and motion. Many elderly patients have poor eyesight, glaucoma, macular degeneration, decreased joint range of motion, neuropathies, arthritis, vestibular weakness, decreased muscle mass and flexibility, postural inadequacies, and memory/dementia deficits. Some of these elderly patients may not choose to move or walk often because of these issues; as a result they are "out of practice" with regard to walking or balance. So, with increasing age, people may have more things interfering with the balance process than they did when they were younger. The same holds true for aging athletes, who are less flexible or have decreased visual acuity and muscle mass as compared with their younger selves.

After reviewing the steps involved in the process of balance, you probably agree that it does not make sense for clinicians to give all of their balance patients the same exercises. If the patient has a visual or vestibular disorder, obviously "long arc quad" exercises should not be the first choice as a therapeutic intervention. If the patient is at high risk of falling, will walking him or her down a hallway yield the desired maximal therapeutic outcomes if the specific reasons the patient has balance issues are not assessed or addressed? In treating athletes, it does not make sense to give the same exercises and drills to players of different sports or even different team positions in the same sport. Customized drills, exercises, and activities will yield a better athlete. The same is true for the elderly patient. Someone with an inner ear problem will not need the same exercises as the patient who has weak hip abductors. A helpful analogy is that of getting your car repaired. Let us say, for example, that you take your car to the shop to have a cracked windshield replaced. After a wait of about 45 minutes, the mechanic tells you that the car is ready; however, you see that the windshield is still cracked. When you ask why this is, the mechanic tells you not to worry because the oil was changed. This was done, the mechanic explains, because "we do that for all our cars." In this situation, would you pay the mechanic? Besides not paying for the wrong service, you would probably have a few choice words to say! And your car would still have the problem—a cracked windshield. If the windshield was broken, should the mechanic not have fixed it?

Now let us apply this analogy to patients. If a patient has a "balance problem," you must first discover *why* that patient has such a problem. You can't simply "change the oil," providing the same interventions as for every other, similar patient. I'm sure you can agree that not everyone will need quad exercises or a dozen or so upper extremity strengthening exercises. With the information you gain in examining each system that contributes to balance and functional movement, you will discover the specific issues that are adding to the imbalance or dizziness. You will have the information you need to create a *specific* and *customized* plan of care that addresses these issues, and you will easily explain why each part of the plan of care is required and how it will help the patient.

You have now learned which systems are involved in the balance process. They include the vision, vestibular, somatosensory, cerebellum, and musculoskeletal systems. Further, you also know that practice and skill will affect ability.

The remaining chapters will help you to do the following:

- Identify the key points for performing a competent evaluation for these patients
- Give step-by-step instructions on how to perform the less common tests
- Demonstrate how to create a plan of care for the patient who has functional movement issues, complaints of dizziness, as well as gait and balance problems

The most effective plans of care, treatments, and therapeutic interventions will be those that address the specific deficits involved in each system and that also address function as a whole. Table 1-15 shows a typical evaluation sequence for a balance-impaired/dizzy individual.

To increase your success in treating balance/dizziness disorders and achieve the best possible outcomes, you must perform a thorough evaluation and refer to other members of the health care team when appropriate to gain further knowledge regarding the patient's complaints, signs, symptoms, and function.

A review of the body systems involved in the process of functional movement and balance will help you gain insight into how deficits in any system can impact function and how they relate to the patient's complaints. Once you have a basic

## TABLE 1-15
## TYPICAL EVALUATION SEQUENCE

| EVALUATION SEQUENCE | |
| --- | --- |
| System | Tests |
| Initial interview | ✓ Review previous medical history and tests results, medications, subjective complaints |
| Vision/oculomotor | ✓ Fixation, gaze, range of motion, smooth pursuit, saccades, vergence, cover tests |
| Vestibular | ✓ Function tests (Head Thrust, Head Shake) |
| | ✓ Pressure tests (eg, Tragal, Valsalva) |
| | ✓ Benign paroxysmal positional vertigo (Dix-Hallpike, Roll test) |
| Somatosensory | ✓ Light touch, proprioception, protective sensation testing (5.07 monofilament) |
| Cerebellum | ✓ Accuracy tests: finger-to-nose, point-to-point, heel-to-shin |
| | ✓ Coordination tests: diadochokinesia, hand clapping, foot tapping |
| Musculoskeletal | ✓ Strength and joint ranges of motion |
| Vital signs as needed | ✓ Heart rate and rhythm, blood pressures (supine, sit, stand) |
| Function | ✓ Standardized tests (balance, gait, fall risk, ADL, memory/cognition) |

understanding of these systems and deficits, you can choose applicable research to guide your choices of tests, measures, and interventions.

Body systems involved with balance include the following:

- Those that give us information—vision, vestibular, somatosensory
- Central processing—cerebellum
- Those that carry out the motor plan or reflex—musculoskeletal

Aside from the physical assessment, you must also assess function. Standardized tests are available to quantify function as well as risk. These tests not only assess function but also track patient progress and outcomes.

# REFERENCES

1. Shepard NT, Telian SA. *Practical Management of the Balance Disorder Patient*. San Diego, CA: Singular Publishing Group, 1996.
2. Allum HJ, Pfaltz CR. Visual and vestibular contributions to pitch sway stabilization in the ankle muscles of normals and patients with bilateral peripheral vestibular deficits. *Exp Brain Res*. 1985;58:82-94.
3. Purves D, Augustine GJ, Fitzpatrick D, et al. *Neuroscience*. 2nd ed. Sunderland, MA: Sinauer Associates; 2001.
4. Rine RM, Wiener-Vacher S. Evaluation and treatment of vestibular dysfunction in children. *NeuroRehabil*. 2013;32(3):507-518.
5. Martins AJ, Kowler E, Palmer C. Smooth pursuit of small-amplitude sinusoidal motion. *J Opt Soc Am A*. 1986;2(2):234-242.
6. Wong A. *Eye Movement Disorders*. Oxford, UK: Oxford University Press; 2008.
7. Alberstone CD, Benze, EC, Najm IM, Steinmetz MP. *Anatomic Basis of Neurologic Diagnosis*. New York: Thieme; 2009.
8. Herdman S. *Vestibular Rehabilitation*. 3rd ed. Philadelphia: FA Davis; 2007.
9. Baloh R, Honrubia V. *Clinical Neurophysiology of the Vestibular System*. 2nd ed. Philadelphia: FA Davis; 1979.
10. Greenberg D, Aminoff M, Simon R. *Clinical Neurology*. 8th ed. New York: McGraw Hill; 2012.
11. Albert M, McCaig LF, Ashman JJ. Emergency department visits by persons aged 65 and over: United States, 2009-2010. *NCHS Data Brief*. 2013;(130):1-8
12. Goldberg JM, Fernandez C. Physiology of peripheral neurons innervating semicircular canals of the squirrel monkey: I. Resting discharge and response to constant angular accelerations. *J Neurophysiol*. 1971;34:635-660.
13. Lysakowski A, Minor LB, Fernandez C, Goldberg JM. Physiological identification of morphologically distinct afferent classes innervating the cristae ampullares of the squirrel monkey. *J Neurophysiol*. 1995;73:1270-1281.
14. Fernandez C, Goldberg JM. Physiology of peripheral neurons innervating semicircular canals of the squirrel monkey: II. Response to sinusoidal stimulation and dynamics of peripheral vestibular system. *J Neurophysiol*. 1971;34:661-675.
15. Shumway-Cook A, Woollacott M. *Motor Control: Translating Research into Clinical Practice*. 3rd ed. Philadelphia: Williams & Wilkins; 2007.
16. Victor M, Ropper AH. *Principles of Neurology*. 9th ed. New York: McGraw-Hill; 2009.
17. Rutka JA. Physiology of the vestibular system. In: Roland PS, Rutka JA, ed. *Ototoxicity*. Hamilton, Ontario: BC Decker; 2004:20-27.
18. Hain T. History/Ewald. http://www.dizziness-and-balance.com/history/Ewald.html. Updated 2013. Accessed October 1, 2014.
19. Robinson DA, Zee DS, Hain TC, Holmes A, Rosenberg LF. Alexander's law: its behavior and origin in the human vestibulo-ocular reflex. *Ann Neurol*. 1984;16(6):714-722.
20. Huterer M, Cullen K. Vestibuloocular reflex dynamics during high-frequency and high-acceleration rotations of the head on body in rhesus monkey. *J Neurophysiol*. 2002;88:13-28.
21. Minor L, Lasker D, Bachous D, Hullar T. Horizontal vestibulo-ocular reflex evoked by high-acceleration rotations in the squirrel monkey: I. Normal responses. *Neurophysiology*. 1999;82:1254-1270.
22. Krauzlis R, Lisberger S. Temporal properties of visual motions signals for the initiation of smooth pursuit eye movements in monkeys. *J Neurophysiol*. 1994;72:150-162.
23. Krauzlis R, Miles F. Release of fixation for pusuit and saccades in humans: evidence for shared inputs acting on different neural substrates. *J Neurophysiol*. 1996;76:2822-2833.
24. Johnson EO, Soucacos PN. Proprioception. In: Stone JH, Blouin M, eds. *International Encyclopedia of Rehabilitation*. 2010. http://cirrie.buffalo.edu/encyclopedia/en/article/337/
25. Bacsi AM, Colebatch JG. Evidence for reflex and perceptual vestibular contributions to postural control. *Exp Brain Res*. 2005;160:22-28.
26. Kristinsdottir EK, Fransson PA, Magnusson M. Changes in posutral control in healthy elderly subjects are related to vibration sensation, vision and vestibular asymmetry. *Acta Otolaryngol*. 2001;121:700-706.

27. Lord SR, Clark RD, Webster IW. Postural stability and associated physiological factors in a population of aged persons. *J Gerontol.* 1991;46:M69-M76.
28. Shaffer SW, Harrison AL. Aging of the somatosensory system: a translational perspective. *Phys Ther.* 2007;87:193-207.
29. Loh K, Ogle J. Age related visual impairment in the elderly. *Med J Malaysia.* 2004;59(4):562-568.
30. Carter T. Age-related vision changes: A primary care guide. *Geriatrics.* 1994;49(9):46-47.
31. Leigh, RJ, Zee DS. *The Neurology of Eye Movements.* 4th ed. New York: Oxford University Press; 2006.
32. Furman J, Raz Y, Whitney S. Geriatric vestibulopathy assessment and management. *Curr Options Otolaryngol Head Neck Surg.* 2010;18:386-391.
33. Froehling D, Silverstein M, Mohr D, Beatty C, Offord K, Ballard D. Benign positional vertigo: incidence and prognosis in a population-based study in Olmsted County, Minnesota. *Mayo Clin Proc.* 1991;66(6):596-601.
34. Enrietto J, Jacobson K, Balow R. Aging effects on auditory and vestibular responses: a longitudinal study. *Am J Otolaryngol.* 1999;20(6):371-378.
35. Agrawal Y, Carey J, Della Santina C, et al. Disorders of balance and vestibular function in US adults: data from the national health and nutrition examination survey, 2001-2004. *Arch Intern Med.* 2009;169:938-944.
36. Morisawa Y. Morphological study of mechanoreceptors on the coracoacroial ligament afferents. *J Electromyogr Kinesiol.* 2002;12:167-176.
37. Aydog S, Korkusuz P, Doral M, et al. Decrease in the numbers of mechanoreceptors in rabbit ACL: the effects of aging. *Knee Surg Sports Traumatol Arthrosc.* 2006;14:325-329.
38. Perry SD. Evaluation of age-related plantar-surface insensitivity and onset age of advanced insensitivity in older adults using vibratory and touch sensation tests. *Neursci Lett.* 2006;392:62-67.
39. Melzer I, Benjuya N, Kaplanski J. Postural stability in the elderly: a comparison between fallers and non-fallers. *Age Ageing.* 2004;33:602-607.
40. Verschueren SMP, Brumagne S, Swinnen S, et al. The effect of aging on dynamic position sense at the ankle. *Behav Brain Res.* 2002;136:593-603.
41. Madhavean S, Shields R. Influence of age on dynamic posiiton sense: evidence using a sequential movement task. *Exp Brain Res.* 2005;164:18-28.
42. Pickard C, Sullivan P, Allison G, Singer K. Is there a difference in hip joint position sense between young and older groups? *J Gerontol A Bio Sci Med Sci.* 2003;58:631-635.
43. Taylor P. Non-linear effects of age on nerve conduction in adults. *J Neurol Sci.* 1984;66:223-234.
44. Bouche P, Cattelin F, Saint-Jean O, et al. Clinical and electrophysiological study of peripheral nervous system in the elderly. *J Neurol.* 1996;240:263-268.
45. Morley J, Baumgartner R, Roubenoff R, Mayer J, Mair K. Sarcopenia. *J Lab Clin Med.* 2001;137(4):231-243.
46. Karaizou E, Manta P, Lakfakis N, Vassilopoulos D. Morphometric study of the human muscle spindle. *Anal Quant Cytol Histol.* 2005;27:1-4.

# 2

# History

## CHAPTER GOALS

1. Explain the value of the patient history.
2. List history questions to ask.
3. Name a standardized questionnaire for balance.
4. Name a standardized questionnaire for dizziness.
5. Identify descriptors for the word *dizzy* and identify possible etiologies for each.

What makes a patient's history important? About 75% of the time, a diagnosis can be determined on the basis of a history alone.[1] You can get most of the information you need to begin your investigation by carefully questioning and listening to the patient during the history-taking process. The way you ask questions is critical if you want to get information that is helpful. At times this may require you to interrupt a patient and gently redirect the conversation to more quickly get to the relevant information. While there are a few questions that are unique to the dizzy patient, most questions for the patient complaining of dizziness/balance problems are the same as those you already use when questioning your orthopedic patients.

Plishka CM.
*A Clinician's Guide to Balance and Dizziness:*
*Evaluation and Treatment* (pp 47-57).
© 2015 Taylor & Francis Group.

The Vestibular Special Interest Group of the American Physical Therapy Association's (APTA) neurology section offers free podcasts on their website. (If you do an Internet search using the terms *APTA* and *vestibular* in the search box you will find it easily.) In one such podcast the commentators make an interesting comparison.[2] The podcast host suggests asking "any question you would of a patient regarding pain" but replacing the word *pain* with *dizzy*. This works equally as well in asking about disequilibrium. Review these common questions and fill in the blanks with *dizziness* and *disequilibrium*:

- When did the _____ start?
- Was onset sudden of _____ or gradual?
- Describe the _____.
- Rate your _____ using a scale.
- How long do sensations of _____ last (constant/intermittent, seconds, minutes, hours, days)?
- How does the _____ limit your function?
- Is the _____ better/worse at certain times of day?
- Is the _____ provoked by certain positions or activities?
- Have you had any tests for the _____? If yes, what were the results?
- Have you been treated for the _____ before? If yes, how, and what were the results of treatments/interventions?

While these questions gather most of the information regarding symptoms, there are some additional questions you should ask that are unique to dizziness. These questions include the following:

- Any recent added or changed prescription for eyeglasses?
- Are symptoms worse with head/body motions? Specific motions, or a particular motion?
- Worse in a specific body/head position? (This helps in deciding whether benign paroxysmal positional vertigo [BPPV] is a possible condition.)
- Worse in light or darkness? This question helps to differentiate between central (worse in the light) and peripheral vestibular (worse in the dark) issues.
- Provoked by visually stimulating environments?
  - While watching TV
  - Walking in grocery stores or shopping malls
  - When watching cross traffic while in a car
  - When seeing moving ceiling fans
- If dizzy, what does *dizzy* mean?
  - Vertigo (seeing or feeling the room move)
  - Disequilibrium (being off balance)
  - Light-headedness (presyncope)
  - Floating sensations
- Any recent head or neck trauma, falls, or car accidents?

- When did you last take any sedating medications such as antihistamines, benzodiazepines, or anticholinergics? (These drugs may skew test results by suppressing signs and symptoms.)
- Any recent changes to medications?
  - Some antidepressants and antipsychotic agents may impair oculomotor function, leading to positive findings that are caused by these medications.
  - Some medications have been associated with increased falls.
- Any previous history of dizziness? (This helps to differentiate various conditions, like BPPV or Ménière's syndrome.)
- Any recent hearing loss or changes in hearing?

It can be difficult to get a clear description of dizziness. You may ask, "What do you mean when you say you feel dizzy?" Often, the patient may provide other non-helpful descriptors, such as *woozy*. Or, worse, the patient may reply with nonessential information, offering a statement such as, "In 1964, when my husband had his hip replaced..." In these circumstances, it may be helpful to limit the patient's choices in discussing dizziness by providing descriptors from which to choose. Phrase your question in a similar way to the following:

"When you say you are dizzy, do you mean you feel light-headed, that you see or feel the room spin, that you are off balance, or something else, like floating?" This is discussed in more detail in the pages that follow.

If a fall is part of the history, make sure you find out the circumstances surrounding it. What activity was the patient doing when he or she fell? Describe the environment (light, dark, firm or unstable standing surface, inside/outside, etc). Was the patient standing still or moving when he or she fell? Has the patient fallen before, and if so, when? Have there been any recent changes in medications? What type of shoe was the patient wearing during the fall? Was the patient ascending/descending stairs or stepping over anything? Was the patient using an assistive device (walker, cane)?

Ask about the patient's ability to perform functional movements. Is the patient having trouble ambulating or performing activities of daily living (ADLs)? It is very common for elderly patients who have balance problems to deny any issues. When asked if they have any difficulties ambulating or performing ADLs, they report that they are doing just fine. If this is the case, it is often revealing to ask if the patient touches or holds onto things for balance when walking or performing ADLs. Patients tend to think that if they can function by holding onto furniture or walls while walking, they *can* function and must be OK. However, a positive answer to this question reveals an underlying balance problem. During your history taking, you want to be able to create a list of physical deficits as well as a list of functional ones.

# QUESTIONNAIRES

Another approach to gathering a history is to have patients fill out questionnaires while they are in the waiting room or mailing questionnaires to them prior to their appointments. Many questionnaires are available for specific types of complaints.

For example, there are multiple questionnaires that help quantify a patient's perception of his or her symptoms. All self-rating scales are limited by the fact that they are influenced by the patient's level of skill and literacy; also, not all questions necessarily apply to each patient.[3]

# Examples of Questionnaires for Balance and Vestibular Disorders

## The Activities-Specific Balance Confidence

The Activities-Specific Balance Confidence (ABC) questionnaire assesses self-perceived balance skill by asking patients to choose how confident they are while performing different functional tasks— feeling that they will not lose their balance or become unsteady. This is quick and easy to administer and may be self-administered or administered by another person in 10 or 20 minutes.[4] There is a list of 16 different tasks, for each of which the patient chooses 1 of 11 scores by rating the task from 0% to 100% (eg, 0%, 10%, 20%, etc), with higher percentages representing more confidence. The total possible score range is from 0 to 1600, which is then divided by 16 to get the ABC score. This questionnaire gives you a structured way to interview a patient about balance problems. It discriminates recent fallers from nonfallers[3]; however, it does not differentiate between skills that may be affected by vertigo versus other balance deficits.[5] It has been tested in the following populations: the elderly and patients with multiple sclerosis, Parkinson's disease, stroke, unilateral transtibial amputation, and vestibular disorders.[4]

## Modified Falls Efficacy Scale

This scale was developed by the National Ageing Research Institute[6] and was adapted from a falls efficacy scale developed by Tinetti et al.[7] It is a self-report measure of fear of falling and consists of 14 questions relating to activities. Administration time is between 5 and 15 minutes. Patients rate their perceived confidence in performing each activity without falling using a scale of 0 to 10. On this visual analog scale, 0 indicates "not confident/completely sure," 5 indicates "fairly confident/fairly sure," and 10 indicates "completely confident/completely sure."[8] Scores range from 0 to 140, with the total score being divided by 14.

## Vestibular Disorders Activities of Daily Living Scale

The Vestibular Disorders ADLs Scale was developed by an occupational therapist. It provides a thorough outline of ADLs but less so for instrumental ADLs (IADLs). Remember, ADLs are self-care things you typically do when you get out of bed (such as bathe, groom, dress, etc), while IADLs are things you do that are not direct self-care and often involve planning, such as planning a meal, shopping, or balancing the checkbook.[3] This scale has 3 subscales: functional, ambulation, and instrumental. The questionnaire has 28 questions and is self-administered. Administration time is between 5 and 10 minutes. It is useful for testing higher-functioning individuals and to document posttreatment changes.[3]

## Examples of Questionnaires for Dizziness

Vertigo and other forms of dizziness are common symptoms of an impaired vestibular system. Subjective perception of these symptoms may be influenced by the patient's personality, level of anxiety, and personal belief as to the cause of his or her symptoms. There are a number of questionnaires available to assess patients' self-reports of symptoms and the impact of these symptoms on their quality of life. However, the relevance and validity of these questionnaires have been questioned in a review of the literature by Duracinsky et al, who studied 29 such questionnaires between 1991 and 2004.[9] Even so, there have been other studies that have found these scales to be useful[10] in gauging change over the course of rehabilitation.[11-13]

### Dizziness Handicap Inventory

The Dizziness Handicap Inventory (DHI) is probably the most widely used questionnaire for dizziness. It is a "signs and symptoms" type of instrument that evaluates the self-perceived handicapping effects on daily life imposed by dizziness.[14] It is designed for ages 15 and above. Administration time is between 6 and 30 minutes. It has been tested in geriatric patients as well as others with vestibular disorders, benign paroxysmal positional vertigo, dizziness, multiple sclerosis, and brain injury.[15] There are 25 questions wherein the subject chooses 1 of 3 statements, "no (worth 0 points), sometimes (2 points), or yes (4 points)." Scores range from 0 to 100, with higher scores indicating a worse handicap.[14] Score interpretation is 0 to 30, mild handicap; 31 to 60, moderate handicap; and 61 to 100, severe handicap.

The results can also be broken down into 3 categories: functional (36 points), emotional (36 points), and physical (28 points). In assessing changes in a patient's self-reported condition, clinically relevant changes are indicated by at least a 10% change in score.[16] The DHI does not provide detailed information about actual functional limitations with regard to individual ADLs; therefore, its results cannot be used to create a plan of care.[3]

This questionnaire may help to identify patients who have BPPV, based on findings by Whitney et al, who found that using answers to 5 items within the DHI as a "subscale" could help predict the likelihood of BPPV. The 5 items used included looking up, difficulty getting out of bed, quick head movements, rolling over in bed, and bending. These 5 items have a combined possible score between 0 and 20 points (with 0 being the best possible score). Dividing this summed score by 20 and multiplying by 100 results in a BPPV subscore percentage. The estimated probability of BPPV based on this calculation is shown in Table 2-1.[10]

Whitney et al also found that the use of answers from only 2 questions (rolling over in bed and supine-to-sit) also served as a useful tool for predicting the likelihood of BPPV. By summing the scores for these 2 items, a score of 4 for this 2-item subscale indicated a 2.7 times increased likelihood of BPPV, while a patient who had a score of 8 was approximately 4.3 times more likely to have BPPV than one who scored 0.

| TABLE 2-1 | |
|---|---|
| DIZZINESS HANDICAP INVENTORY SUBSCORE INTERPRETATION | |
| BPP SUBSCORE (%) | ESTIMATED PROBABILITY OF BPPV (%) |
| 0 | 12% |
| 10 | 13% |
| 20 | 15% |
| 30 | 17% |
| 40 | 19% |
| 50 | 21% |
| 60 | 24% |
| 70 | 27% |
| 80 | 29% |
| 90 | 32% |
| 100 | 35% |

## Vertigo Handicap Questionnaire

The Vertigo Handicap Questionnaire (VHQ) is a psychological assessment tool that includes coping.[17] It assesses common beliefs, behaviors, and difficulties associated with vertigo. There is a long version comprising 26 questions and a short version of 14 questions. The VHQ has been shown not to be responsive to change after vestibular rehabilitation in at least one study.[3]

# DIZZINESS

You often hear patients say they are "dizzy," but what does this actually mean? It is a common complaint, and the description of what the patient means by the word *dizzy* may be extremely significant in the process of differential diagnosis. According to Hobeika[18]:

- Dizziness is the third most frequent reason people seek medical attention.
- It has been estimated that 65% of individuals older than 60 years of age experience dizziness or loss of balance, often on a daily basis.
- According to Ko et al, difficulty in performing one or more ADLs is highly prevalent among adults with chronic balance problems or dizziness: 11.5% with chronic dizziness and 33.4% with chronic balance problems.
- Dizziness is the most common complaint among patients above 75 years of age.[19]

## TABLE 2-2

## DIZZINESS DESCRIPTIONS AND POSSIBLE CAUSES

| DESCRIPTION | POSSIBLE CAUSES |
| --- | --- |
| Vertigo (illusion of movement) | Vestibular<br><br>• Vestibular loss/weakness<br>• BPPV<br>• Labyrinthitis<br>• Vestibular neuritis<br>Cerebellar involvement<br>Cervicogenic issues (neck problems) |
| Light-headedness | Orthostatic hypotension (blood pressure drop)<br>Cardiac arrhythmia<br>Hypoglycemia (low blood sugar)<br>Medication side effect<br>Cervicogenic issue<br>Sometimes vestibular loss/weakness |
| Disequilibrium | Multiple possible reasons |
| Floating out of body | CNS or psychiatric |

## What Does Dizzy Mean?

Patients very frequently complain of dizziness, but very often clinicians fail to ask the right questions to figure out what the patient means when saying, "I'm dizzy." As you know, there are many different causes of dizziness. When a patient says he or she feels dizzy, this may mean a variety of things, including a sensation of movement (vertigo), light-headedness (presyncope), lack of balance (disequilibrium), or a "floating out of the body" feeling. Each of these descriptors is very different from the others, yet they may all fall into the category of dizziness. If you know what dizziness means to the patient, it may help you to provide the correct intervention to address the underlying issue. Table 2-2 lists various descriptors of dizziness as well as common causes of these symptoms.

In questioning a patient regarding complaints of dizziness, this list may be very helpful in identifying the cause. During the evaluation process, give this list to patients and ask them to choose the descriptors that best fit their complaint. In trying to get patients to describe their dizziness sensations, ask them to choose one or more of the following:

When you say you are dizzy, do you mean that you:
- See or feel the room spin?
- Feel light-headed?
- Feel off balance?
- Or something else (floating)?

Patients may have multiple sensations occurring at different times. This short list will help you to decipher their descriptions, as most of these sensations are caused by different etiologies. For example, an impaired vestibular system often produces a sensation of vertigo (movement, usually spinning). In knowing this, if the patient complains of vertigo, you may suspect that the vestibular system is somehow involved. Feelings of light-headedness have multiple etiologies but commonly are caused by things like orthostatic hypotension, hypoglycemia, cardiac arrhythmias, or medication side effects. When a patient reports feeling off balance, the descriptor is not by itself enough to give you a hint of where to look for a problem. However, in the absence of the other descriptors, it might lead you to look at orthopedic issues, possible medication side effects, or perhaps a partially compensated unilateral vestibular problem.

The last descriptor is "Or something else?" Some patients report a feeling of floating out of their bodies. These sensations are usually caused by either psychiatric issues or central nervous system problems. Floating sensations have been reported by patients who are experiencing early symptoms of brain tumors.

By having the patient choose a descriptor for dizziness, you will have more information to guide your clinical thinking as well as the physical examination and test choices. In some cases, the time of symptom occurrence is itself a clue. For example, when a patient reports being dizzy upon getting up in the morning, it is helpful to ask what happens when he or she lies down or rolls in bed. This will help you differentiate between BPPV and orthostatic hypotension. If the patient is diabetic, you may consider assessing blood sugar at different times of the day. If the patient has a history of cardiac problems, you may wish to have his or her blood pressure recorded at different times of the day.

A study of 300 acutely dizzy patients presenting to the emergency room showed the type of dizziness to be an imprecise metric, with more than half of the patients unable to reliably report which symptom type most accurately reflected their complaint.[20] In fairness, is the patient with dizziness who presents to the ER really in a good frame of mind to give a good history? Many of the dizzy patients who go to the ER are vomiting and falling over. Anecdotally, some clinicians find using the "type of dizziness" list helpful in the outpatient and home health settings. The patient history can reveal very important data but may require skilled questioning to uncover the needed information. Open-ended questions asking someone to describe his or her symptoms can be very imprecise and of limited value with regard to dizziness. Further, as our "face time" with the patient is increasingly limited, asking open-ended questions may not be the best use that time. If the patient begins to stray from a direct answer, gently redirect him or her.

To demonstrate the usefulness of proving a list of descriptors to describe dizziness, review the following scenarios, which are real accounts of patient-clinician interactions.

Example 1 involves a male patient whose primary complaint was dizziness. The patient was given a sedating medication to treat the dizziness and was referred to a physical therapist. At the therapy office, he was asked to choose a descriptor from a list (light-headed, off balance, room spinning, or other) and chose light-headedness. Next, the patient was asked to explain when he became light-headed or dizzy. Was he light-headed at certain times of day or in certain circumstances? The response was that he typically woke dizzy but felt better after eating breakfast. Then he became dizzy again around lunchtime and again in the early evening. Eating seemed to resolve each episode. Further questioning revealed that this patient was diabetic, even though this fact was not reflected in his medication list. After reviewing this interaction, what type of issue do you suspect this patient may be having? What tests should be performed? Which members of the health care team would best assess the suspected issues? These symptoms are common for patients who have blood sugar irregularities.

Example 2 involves an elderly woman who told her doctor that she was dizzy. This patient was given a benzodiazepine to control the dizziness and sent to a physical therapist. When asked what *dizzy* meant, the patient said that she felt "off balance" and unable to walk a straight line. She denied any light-headedness or vertigo.

There are a variety of deficits that may cause disequilibrium, so this patient needs a very thorough evaluation of systems that contribute to balance. While a therapy evaluation was indicated, the choice of medication for this patient may not have been the best option. Classes of medications used to treat dizziness, such as benzodiazepines, and other medications that patients may be on, such as antidepressants, have been associated with increased falls.[21] This patient, who had a balance problem, was given a medication known to be statistically associated with falls because she used the word *dizzy* to describe her problem of disequilibrium. Obviously there *are* times when these medications are not only indicated but also very helpful. Good history-taking questions will guide the clinician toward the best treatment and intervention.

In each of these examples, a list of dizzy descriptors was used to more specifically identify patient needs. After using the dizzy descriptor list with a patient, you may decide to request further tests. You may begin therapy interventions to address the fall risk while arranging for additional testing to help rule in or out other possible etiologies.

Example 3 is that of a young woman in her late 20s who was dizzy and had sensations of movement, but these sensations did not seem to be provoked by motion or position. She was not taking any prescribed medications. The examination ruled out vestibular issues, but the patient had an abnormal oculomotor examination. Are there any red flags for this patient? The patient was young, female, and dizzy, with a central sign (due to the abnormal oculomotor sign). What tests would you recommend? This patient was referred to neurology, and a magnetic resonance imaging revealed neural plaque consistent with multiple sclerosis. Her age, gender, and positive central sign were initial clues that multiple sclerosis could be causing her dizziness.

To summarize, the patient history adds immense value to the clinical examination in the following ways:

- Providing clues based on the patient's subjective symptoms to help guide the examination
- Helping the examiner to form a hypothesis as to the etiology of the complaints and arrive at a diagnosis
- Identifying previously performed tests that the examiner may use
- Identifying any medications that may be additive to the patients' current complaints
- Identifying medications that may impede the examination or impair progress
- Alerting the clinician to patient conditions that require the expertise of other health professionals
- Uncovering the patient's goals for seeking treatment

# REFERENCES

1.  Lichstein PR. The medical interview. In: Walker HK, Hall WD, Hurst JW, eds. *Clinical Methods: The History, Physical, and Laboratory Examinations*. 3rd ed. Boston, MA: Butterworths; 1990. http://www.ncbi.nlm.nih.gov/books/NBK349/
2.  Kriekels W, Trommelen R. Podcasts. Available at http://www.neuropt.org/special-interest-groups/vestibular-rehabilitation/podcasts. Updated 2012. Accessed October 4, 2014.
3.  Cohen HS. Assessment of functional outcomes in patients with vestibular disorders after rehabilitation. *NeuroRehabilitation*. 2011;29(2):173-178.
4.  Rehabilitation Measures Database. Rehab measures: activities-specific balance confidence scale. Available at http://www.rehabmeasures.org/Lists/RehabMeasures/PrintView.aspx?ID=949;. Updated 2013. Accessed October 4, 2014.
5.  Powell LE, Myers MA. The activities-specific balance confidence (ABC) scale. *J Gerontol A Biol Sci Med Sci*. 1995;50(1):M28-M34.
6.  Hill KD, Schwarz JA, Kalogeropolous AJ,Gibson SJ. Fear of falling revisited. *Arch Phys Med Rehabil*. 1996;77:1025-1029.
7.  Tinetti M, Richmand D, Powell L. Falls efficacy as a measure of fear of falling. *J Gerontol*. 1990;45(6):P239-243.
8.  National Ageing Research Institute. *Modified Falls Efficacy Scale (MFES)*. Victoria, Australia: Department of Health; 2010. http://www.health.vic.gov.au/agedcare/maintaining/falls_dev/downloads/B1F2%281a%29%20Modified%20Falls%20Efficacy%20Scale%20%28MFES%29%20form.pdf
9.  Duracinsky M, Mosnier I, Bouccara, D, Sterkers O, Chassany O. Working Group of the Société Française d'Oto-Rhino-Laryngologie. Literature review of questionnaires assessing vertigo and dizziness, and their impact on patient's quality of life. *Value Health*. 2007;10(4):273-284.
10. Whitney S, Marchetti G, Morri, L. Usefulness of the dizziness handicap inventory in the screening for benign paroxysmal positional vertigo. *Otol Neurotol*. 2005;26(5):1027-1033.
11. Cowand JL,Wrisley DM, Walker M, Strasnick B, Jacobson JT. Efficacy of vestibular rehabilitation. *Otolaryngol Head Neck Surg*. 1998;118(1):49-54.
12. Johansson M, Akerlund D, Larsen H, et al. Randomized controlled trial of vestibular rehabilitation combined with cognitive behavioral therapy of diziness in older people. *Br J Surg*. 2001;125:151-156.
13. Brown KE, Whitney SL, Wrisley DM, et al. Physical therapy outcomes for persons with bilateral vestibular loss. *Larygoscope*. 2001;111:1812-1817.
14. Jacobson GP,Newman CW, Hunter L, et al. Balance function test correlates of the dizziness handicap inventory. *Am Acad Audiol*. 1991;2(4):253-260.

15. Rehabilitation Medicine Clinic. *Dizziness Handicap Inventory*. 2013. http://www.rehab.msu. edu/_files/_docs/Dizziness_Handicap_Inventory.pdf
16. Treleaven J. Dizziness handicap inventory (DHI). *Aust J Physiother*. 2006;52:52-37.
17. Yardley L, Putman J. Quantitative analysis of factors contributing to handicap and distress in vertiginous patients: a questionnaire study. *Clin Otolaryngol*. 1992;17:231-236.
18. Hobeika CP. Equilibrium and balance in the elderly. *Ear Nose Throat J*. 1999;78(8):558-562, 565-566.
19. Furman J, Raz Y, Whitney S. Geriatric vestibulopathy assessement and management. *Curr Opin Otolaryngol Head Neck Surg*. 2010;18:386-391.
20. Newman-Toker D, Cannon L, Stofferahn M, et al. Imprecision in patient reports of dizziness symptom quality: a cross-sectional study conducted in an acute care setting. *Mayo Clin Proc*. 2007;82:1329-1340.
21. Bronstein A, Lempert T. *Dizziness: A Practical Approach to Diagnosis and Management*. Cambridge, UK: Cambridge University Press; 2007.

# 3

# Equipment

Once you have taken a thorough history, you will begin your physical examination. Remember, there are systems that give us information; our brain processes that information and then chooses and activates motor programs, and our musculoskeletal system carries out the plan. To know why someone has a balance or dizziness issue, we need to examine the entirety of the systems that contribute to this process. We will examine the following:

- Vestibular function
- Vision/oculomotor function
- Somatosensory sensations
- Cerebellar function
- Musculoskeletal strength and range of motion
- Tests assessing function, skill, or fall risk

Plishka CM.
*A Clinician's Guide to Balance and Dizziness:*
*Evaluation and Treatment* (pp 59-68).
© 2015 Taylor & Francis Group.

After reviewing this list, identify which systems, if any, you are not currently assessing and incorporate them in your evaluation. When evaluations lack this information, you will invariably miss important clues as to etiologies that may be contributing to a patient's condition as well as opportunities to add interventions that may improve the patient's function and reduce symptomatology. Let us go through a typical evaluation system by system. In this book the term *bedside test* conveys situations in which clinicians do not have access to high-tech equipment. This may be in a physician's office, a therapy/nursing practice (acute, rehab, outpatient, or home health), or an emergency department where the clinician has basic tools available and can order further tests.

# EQUIPMENT

There is a wide range of equipment available to today's clinician, ranging from a simple pencil costing pennies to an automatic chair that is used to reposition loose inner-ear crystals and costs thousands of dollars. It is easy to perform a bedside examination with minimal equipment. If you frequently or routinely see patients who have balance deficits or dizziness complaints, you will most likely benefit from purchasing some special equipment. Review examples of commonly used equipment for the patient with balance/vestibular problems and then decide what you need depending on your practice setting. There are tools clinicians use that are fairly common to most disciplines, such as a watch with a second hand (or stopwatch), penlight, pen, tape measure, reflex hammer, and goniometer. While these items are common across different disciplines, some pieces of equipment are more specific to evaluating balance, eye motion, and dizziness. Tools that the audiologist; neurotologist; or ear, nose, and throat specialist often use, for example, may include machines such as caloric irrigators and electro- or videonystagmography equipment to evaluate vestibular and oculomotor function.

## Gait Belt or Transfer Belt

Therapists often use gait belts, but other disciplines do so less frequently. A gait belt is inexpensive and used as a safety device to prevent a patient from falling (early in the course of balance loss) or to help safely lower patients to the ground if they move past the point of fall prevention. The belt is placed snugly around the patient's waist near his or her center of gravity. In doing this, the clinician has more control over the patient's center of gravity. When placed on a patient who is sitting, it is important to realize that the belt will fit more loosely when the patient stands; you will likely need to adjust it when the patient changes position. In holding the belt, grab it in a palms-up grip. When held in a palms-down grip, the belt will more easily slip out of your hands. For obese patients, the belt can be placed higher on the body, or a bariatric-sized gait belt may be used. Where the patient's size or condition necessitates placement across the upper chest and under the axillae, the belt should never be allowed to pull on the patient's axillary regions, as this can cause injury to the brachial plexus. In training a patient's balance, use a gait belt. As the patient progresses, do not be lulled into a false sense of security. Remember you are placing your patient into balance-challenging situations designed to push the boundaries of control, and a fall is always possible. If you are not a therapist and are not familiar with the use of a gait belt, ask a therapist to visit your practice and give you in-service training. A gait belt is an inexpensive and simple safety tool that may prevent injury.

## Maddox Rod

A Maddox rod has a paddle at one end that is used to occlude (block) a patient's vision in one eye (Figure 3-1). The other end contains a red prism lens which, depending on how it is held to the patient's eye, will present the patient with either a vertical or horizontal line. The red lens has ridges that are parallel to each other. When the lens is placed in front of the patient's eye with the ridges running horizontally compared with the ground, the patient will see a vertical red line. When the lens is placed with the ridges running vertically (perpendicular to the ground), the patient will see a horizontal red line. You will often see the terms *OD* and *OS* in reference to the eyes. OD (oculus dexter) means "right eye" and OS (oculus sinister) means "left eye."

During the test of alignment, one eye is covered with the lens while both eyes fix on a penlight. The patient should see a red line (vertical or horizontal) and a white dot (penlight). When the eyes are properly aligned, these 2 visual images are superimposed on each other and remain so as the examiner moves the penlight. If they do not superimpose, the patient will see a space between the line and dot, indicating misalignment.[1] Keep in mind that the Maddox Rod test does not differentiate between tropias and phorias. Eye specialists may use prisms to measure ocular deviations in diopters. Therapists should not introduce prisms as an intervention without an eye specialist's examination and direction.

## Balance Foam

High-density foam is frequently used in testing of balance and also as a therapeutic intervention for patients with balance deficits.[2] It may also be used in the training of athletes (Figure 3-2). There are a variety of balance foams on the market, but there is currently no standardization to indicate which density of foam is best suited to balance testing. Generally most balance clinicians use high-density closed-cell foam. The benefit of the closed-cell foam is that it is easy to clean between uses. Clinicians use the foam as a tool to assess balance and also as an intervention. It is required by widely used balance tests—like the modified Clinical Test of Sensory Interaction and Balance, which has the patient stand on a firm surface and a foam surface.

If you work in the home health setting, keep the foam in the box between uses. During the summer months the foam gets hot while in the car and will deform when something is pressing against it, so that it permanently loses its shape. Keeping the foam in the box will protect it. Take care to guard anyone wearing a gait belt who is standing on the foam, and secure the foam so that it will not move or slide on a slippery floor.

**Figure 3-1.** Maddox rod.

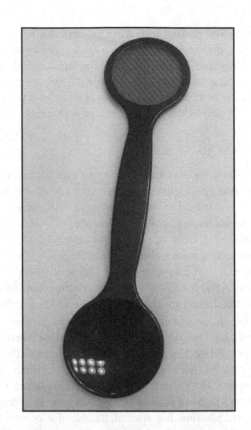

**Figure 3-2.** Balance foam.

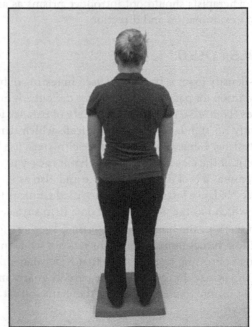

Currently there is no standardization of soft/compliant surfaces for balance testing. There are a number of companies that produce high-density closed-cell foam (you might want to perform a web search for *balance foam*). In the home health setting, you may even use a couch cushion as balance foam. The key to using soft surfaces for balance testing is that while the patient stands on the surface (foam or cushion), it does not compress enough to allow his or her feet to touch the floor through the material.

## Frenzel Goggles

Frenzel goggles (or optical Frenzel goggles) are another alternative to removing the patient's visual fixation as well as a way to observe patient eye movements. Looking much like a swimming mask, the Frenzel goggles have 2 magnifying lenses (+20 diopter) and have a light on the inside part of the mask, which is used to either light up the eyes or as a fixation light that the patient is asked to look at during a portion of the testing. The magnifying lenses take away the patient's ability to focus on any object, which can override nystagmus. These goggles may be used as a tool to differentially diagnose patients complaining of dizziness.[3]

The benefit to Frenzel goggles is the price, as they are significantly less expensive than infrared goggles and easily portable. The drawback to Frenzel goggles is that while the patient wears them, it is not always easy to observe eye motion. A good example is when the clinician positions the patient with the nose toward the ground. Another drawback to Frenzel goggles is that you cannot record eye motions to review later. Your only opportunity to observe the eye motion is while the patient is wearing the goggles.

## Infrared Video Goggles or Video Frenzel Goggles

The use of infrared goggles accomplish 2 things: (1) it removes visual fixation (ie, takes away a person's ability to look at and focus on an object) and (2) it allows the clinician to observe and record eye motions. Some goggles use one camera (monocular), while more expensive ones have a camera for each eye (binocular). These goggles connect to a monitor that allows the clinician to observe the patient's eye motion even while removing his or her vision (Figure 3-3). Eye motion is easy to observe, even with different patient body and head positions. You may review video recordings again later or share them with other health care professionals, as the case demands. There are software packages available that will actually track/detect nystagmus automatically.

## Caloric Irrigator

A caloric irrigator (Figure 3-4) blows air against the eardrum to change the temperature in the inner ear and thus induce nystagmus (older machines use sleeves filled with circulating water). The audiologist controls the temperature during testing and tests each ear independently. More detail on how the audiologist uses this test to assess vestibular function follows further on.

**Figure 3-3.** Infrared goggles.

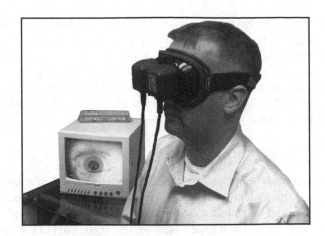

**Figure 3-4.** Caloric irrigator. (Reprinted with permission from Micromedical Technologies, Inc.)

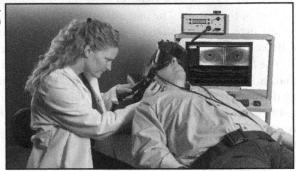

# Videonystagmography and Electronystagmography

Videonystagmography (VNG) is a test that uses computer software, a caloric irrigator, and infrared goggles. Older pieces of equipment do not use infrared video goggles to record eye movement but instead use electrodes placed around the patient's eyes to record the eye motions. Electronystagmography (ENG) and VNG are basically the same. The difference between these tests is how they record eye motions. The electronystagmograph uses the "electrode" type of equipment while the videonystagmograph uses an infrared goggle system and computer software to track eye motions. During this test, the audiologist uses a caloric irrigator to blow warm or cold air against one eardrum. After a few minutes, the temperature of the endolymph in the vestibular system changes and the endolymph flows. This *endolymphatic* flow moves the cupula, which will cause a difference in the vestibular firing rates of each ear, and nystagmus should be the result. The VNG/ENG records the nystagmus by tracking eye motions, and the clinician (or software) compares the results to established norms. This test is often used along with an audiogram to differentiate between a central and peripheral vestibular lesion.[4] The audiologist is the professional who most often performs and interprets this test, although there are many physicians who prefer to evaluate the test results and interpret them. Typically,

VNG/ENG tests are always accompanied by an audiogram (hearing test) and a battery of oculomotor tests. When a battery of tests is used, the audiologist can say whether there is a vestibular deficit and whether there are indications of peripheral (outside of the central nervous system) or central (within the central nervous system) signs that would point to the need for further examination or imaging.

## Rotational Chair

Vestibular function in both ears may be tested and recorded using a booth containing a chair that spins in each direction (left and right). The test is called the *Rotational Chair test* (or *Rotary Chair test*). The original chair was created by Dr. Róbert Bárány in 1907. He would spin the patient in the chair and then observe the nystagmus after a sudden stop. This test uses a recording device such as an infrared camera to capture the patient's eye motions during the spin. Because the camera is infrared, it captures the patient's eye in either light or dark environments, and the patient can be tested in either environment. VNG software will track eye motions occurring in response to the movements of the chair. When the patient is turning in the chair, both ears are stimulated, so this test is useful in simultaneous testing of vestibular function bilaterally. This is a high-tech test that balance clinics and neurotology offices commonly use. The rotational chair stimulates frequencies in a range between 0.01 and 1.28 Hz and is used to test vestibular function bilaterally, visual-vestibular interaction,[5] optokinetic after-nystagmus, high-velocity sinusoidal function, and off-vertical axis rotation.

## Treatment Plinth

If you are in a clinic setting, an adjustable high-low plinth, while not strictly necessary, will make your life easier and reduce your own physical requirements in administering position tests for dizziness. Whether or not the table is height-adjustable, you will need a place where you can have the patient lie down. In a hospital or institutional setting, if the headboard or footboard is removable, perform positional tests with the patient lying on the bed with his or her head toward the more accessible end. In any setting, when neither the headboard nor the footboard is removable, perform positional tests with the patient lying across the width of the bed (with assistance to raise the legs if needed). If you are using a massage table, make sure you know the weight limit of the table. (It is not a bad idea to write the weight limit on the underside of the table in permanent marker.)

## Space

Space requirements for balance treatment will be minimal in most cases. However, it is helpful to have a straight hallway or space to use for gait analysis and training. Outside spaces are convenient, but extreme weather sometimes hampers this as an option. At a minimum, you should have access to a covered straight path 15 to 20 feet long. If you are working with athletes, you will need larger spaces, as eventually you may have them running while performing their rehab tasks.

## Basic Equipment Needs

In examining each system that contributes to functional mobility and balance, there are a few things you will need to help you perform the evaluation. This would include some "bare essentials" as well as equipment that—if you plan to evaluate balance and dizziness routinely—would enable you to make a more ideal assessment. The bare essentials comprise the equipment you would need if you were stranded on a desert island and needed to evaluate someone's balance. Keep in mind that evaluating patients who have balance or dizziness issues using minimal equipment is by no means ideal; hence clinicians who routinely evaluate and treat patients with balance deficits or dizziness should try to obtain equipment that will provide more accurate measures or assessments. However, you may still gain a lot of information using bedside screening tests, then referring the patient for more testing if needed. Review the basic equipment needs below.

### Vision (Oculomotor)

- *Bare essentials:* Your finger or fingers may be used as visual targets in evaluating eye motions and control (eg, fixation, tracking, saccades, ranges of motion, gaze nystagmus, and vergence). Your hands may be used as visual occluders to test gross alignment of the eyes, phorias, and tropias. (If you don't know these terms, don't panic; you will learn them further on.)
- *More ideal:* Depending on your setting, you may want to have additional equipment. You may use a pen tip or penlight as a visual target and a paddle occluder or Maddox rod to check for phorias and tropias. The physician, nurse practitioner, physician's assistant, or more advanced therapist may use an ophthalmoscope. The audiologist will use oculomotor ENG/VNG equipment and software and audiometric computerized testing equipment.

### Vestibular

- *Vestibular function bare essentials:* Basic VOR testing at the bedside requires no special equipment. However, depending on the severity of the lesion, the patient may be able to suppress nystagmus if he or she uses vision to fixate. This will likely yield inaccurate results if the clinician examines the patient only in "vision-allowed" environments. Very gross examination of vestibular function requires only an attentive patient and a skilled examiner.
- *More ideal:* More telling and accurate examinations of vestibular function require some equipment. The level of sophistication (and expense) will vary depending on your practice setting and discipline. A common need for all settings is a way to examine the eyes for resting and gaze nystagmus with vision removed and also when vision is allowed and fixed on a target. You may do this by using either Frenzel or infrared goggles. A number of different companies manufacture these goggles. If you are looking for infrared goggles, there are a variety available, with some being attached to VCR machines and more portable ones that connect via USB ports to laptops and desk computers. A very detailed review of information on Frenzel and infrared goggles is available on

Dr. Timothy Hain's website, where he gives his personal opinions on the benefits of each (see http://www.dizziness-and-balance.com/practice/frenzels.htm).

The infrared video systems that allow you to record tests give you the opportunity to review or share the videos. This is extremely helpful when you are first starting, as you can repeatedly observe the eye motions you have recorded. Such a system can also be used as a teaching tool to show and explain symptoms and eye motions to patients, students, and other clinicians.

There are many manufacturers and vendors of balance, vestibular, and oculomotor examination equipment and software, including the following:

- Bausch + Lomb Instruments
- DIFRA Instrumentation
- GN Otometrics
- ICS Medical
- Interacoustics
- ISCAN, Inc
- Jintronix
- Micromedical Technologies
- Nagashima Medical Instruments Co., Ltd.
- Neurocom International
- Neuro Kinetics
- SensoMotoric Instruments
- Synapsis
- US Neurologicals

## Somatosensory

- *Bare essentials:* You do not need special equipment for touch and proprioception tests.
- *More ideal:* A 5.07 monofilament for pressure sensation testing of "protective sensations." For a more in-depth examination of touch sensations, there are a variety of monofilaments.

## Cerebellar

- *Bare essentials:* These tests require no equipment. Most cerebellar tests involve "return demonstration" of coordination and accuracy movements, while others involve passive limb movements performed by the examiner.
- *More ideal:* Note that some abnormal oculomotor findings may point to cerebellar dysfunction. The use of Frenzel or infrared goggles gives you a more definitive examination.

## Musculoskeletal

- *Bare essentials:* These tests require no equipment.
- *More ideal:* A goniometer to measure joint motion (in degrees). While most clinicians use manual muscle tests for strength assessment, there are

computerized dynamometers that can be used to measure "force" more objectively. While hydraulic dynamometers to gauge pinch and grip strength are fairly common in practice, electric push/pull dynamometers to test larger muscle groups typically cost over $600, and many clinicians rely on manual muscle testing.

## Standardized Tests of Function, Balance, or Fall Risk

- Different tests require the use of specific pieces of equipment. The clinician times or scores these tests. Timed tests will require a watch with a second hand or a stopwatch. Many common standardized tests of balance require the use of a chair, balance foam, or a way to record distance (eg, to measure ambulation or reach).

## Other Tests

Have a blood pressure cuff on hand for use in measuring orthostatic blood pressures. At times a glucometer may be helpful in checking blood sugar. Also a tuning fork is needed to perform a Weber test for the assessment of a unilateral hearing loss or to check for vibration-induced nystagmus.

There are many ways in which to assess patients. Some screening techniques are extremely valuable in identifying the need for more advanced testing. Having basic equipment will enhance your ability to identify a patient's needs, establish baselines, and identify signs that require further investigation.

# REFERENCES

1.  Hansen S. The Maddox rod test. *J Ophthal Med Technol.* 2006;2(2).
2.  Cohen HS, Mulavara AP, Peters BT, Sangi-Haghpeykar H, Bloomberg JJ. Standing balance tests for screening people with vestibular impairments. *Laryngoscope.* 2014;124(2):545-550.
3.  Ozono Y, Kitahara T, Fukushima M, et al. Differential diagnosis of vertigo and dizziness in the emergency department. *Otoneurology.* 2014;134(2):140-145.
4.  Mekki S. The role of videonystagmography (VNG) in assessment of dizzy patient. *Egypt J Otolaryngol.* 2014;30(2):69-72.
5.  Amin MS. Rotatry chair testing. http://emedicine.medscape.com/article/1832765-overview. Updated 2012. Accessed October 4, 2014.

# 4

# Vestibular Examination and Intervention

---

## CHAPTER GOALS

1. Identify medications that may affect vestibular test results.
2. Name 2 bedside tests of vestibular function.
3. Describe symptoms of acute and chronic vestibular loss.
4. List 2 diseases or conditions known to cause vestibular loss.
5. Describe interventions for vestibular loss.

---

## VESTIBULAR FUNCTION—BEDSIDE EXAMINATION

Clearly document any sedating medications the patient is taking or has taken within the prior 48 hours. If possible, have sedating medications held with a medical order at least 24 to 48 hours prior to testing. Some medications require a weaning schedule (eg, antipsychotics); this needs to be planned in advance. Note that you may *not* instruct a patient to withhold *any* medication without a physician's order, even when the medication orders are "as needed."

As discussed previously, there are high-tech options to test the vestibular system, and a physician or audiologist typically administers these. However, for clinicians who do not have access to these high-tech tests, there are some options to check gross vestibular function.

Plishka CM.
*A Clinician's Guide to Balance and Dizziness:*
*Evaluation and Treatment* (pp 69-110).
© 2015 Taylor & Francis Group.

The primary test of vestibular function checks if the vestibulo-ocular reflex (VOR) is intact. Most often, clinicians do this by stimulating the *lateral* vestibular canals to elicit a VOR; however, you can check this reflex by testing *any* of the vestibular canals. Using the typical test protocols, we check only the lateral vestibular canals and use the resulting VOR function to give an indication of the general function of the vestibular system. In reality these bedside tests of vestibular function do not truly test the entire vestibular system. Remember, the superior vestibular nerve innervates the lateral canal (along with the anterior canal and utricle), while other parts of the vestibular system (the saccule and posterior canal) are innervated by the inferior vestibular nerve. If you incorporate VOR testing of the posterior canals along with the lateral canals, you will get a more complete picture of the function of the vestibular canal system.

The VOR is relatively easy to elicit, and there are a few testing options. Three bedside tests are commonly used to assess VOR function:

1.  The Head Thrust test (also known as the *Head Impulse test*)
2.  The Head Shake test
3.  The Dynamic Visual Acuity (DVA) test

None of these tests localize lesions. That is, if there is pathology interfering with the VOR, these tests do not tell you exactly where the pathology is located. They do grossly indicate a left- vs right-sided vestibular problem, but you cannot tell from these tests if a lesion is *peripheral* (in the ear or outside the brain) or *central* (within the brain or central nervous system). If, in using one of these bedside tests, you determine that there is a unilateral vestibular deficit, all you can really say is that the vestibular system is somehow involved. There are some signs and symptoms that point us in the direction of peripheral vs central pathologies, but without more specific clinical tests, these bedside tests may only *suggest* which is involved. As this is the case, any time a clinician finds a positive bedside test, indicating a vestibular weakness, he or she should recommend further clinical testing. Usually, this means ordering videonystagmography (VNG) and an audiogram (hearing test). Using the VNG test, the audiologist can tell more specifically how much the vestibular apparatus of the ear is involved. Because some patterns of hearing loss indicate possible central pathology, the hearing test will help point to possible brain or nerve issues that would require further investigation, as with computed tomography or magnetic resonance imaging. When both a VNG and audiogram are ordered, the battery of tests used by the audiologist usually also includes a gross balance screen as well as an oculomotor examination. This battery of tests is extremely helpful in gaining information of vestibular function as well as to screen out more serious central pathologies.

While there are now some more portable electronics for vestibular and oculomotor testing, most bedside tests do not use computerized equipment to stimulate or record vestibular function, and they are limited in sensitivity. This means a negative test does not always mean the patient has "normal" vestibular function but that he or she does not have a deficit that is bad enough to be detected with a gross screen. If the patient has signs or symptoms that lead you to think that there may be a vestibular problem (eg, vertigo, loss of balance during head turns, nausea in busy visual environments), it is important to request more in-depth vestibular testing. Manual tests of the vestibular system require the clinician to move the patient's head passively and in some cases quickly. Therefore, prior to testing, the clinician should gauge the patient's active cervical range of motion and also check the integrity of the transverse and alar ligaments. This is especially true if there is a history of trauma. Many leaders in the vestibular research realm no longer recommend using the vertebral artery screen.

#  Head Thrust Test

The Head Thrust test, also known as the *Head Impulse test*, is a passive test on the patient's part that tells you which vestibular apparatus (left vs right) is working well enough to turn on the VOR for the canal that is being tested. The patient should be wearing his or her usual eyeglasses for this test, as the VOR calibration changes when he or she is wearing them.[1]

In using the most common testing method, you will be stimulating the lateral vestibular canals. You perform the head thrust test by quickly turning the patient's passive head in the yaw plane while instructing him or her to keep visual fixation on a target. A near visual target is usually the examiner's nose. The examiner quickly rotates the patient's head into left or right rotation of 5 to 10 degrees (note the small range used), with head flexion of 30 degrees to increase the sensitivity of the test.[2] This test may be repeated using both near and far visual targets.

Remember, lateral canals are not exactly parallel to the horizontal plane but are actually angled about 30 degrees from the horizontal plane, with the anterior portions being more cephalad. By positioning the patient in 30 degrees of head/neck flexion, the lateral canals will roughly be level with the ground. While in this test position, when you turn the patient's head in the yaw plane, you will better stimulate the lateral canals, as more force acts directly to move the endolymph in these canals.

You test each side (left and right) by turning the patient's head quickly and unpredictably toward the side you wish to test. For this test, *unpredictably* indicates that while prior to the test we instruct the patient that we will be turning his or her head, the patient does not know in which direction (left or right) we will turn it or exactly when. We *do not* say, "On three... 1, 2..." etc. By moving the head unpredictably, we can be sure that the patient is not anticipating the motion and using that information for motor planning. The side to which you rotate the patient's head is the side you are testing. For example, if you rotate the patient's head to his or her left, you are testing left vestibular apparatus. If you rotate the head to his or her right, you are testing right vestibular apparatus.

In performing this test, do not turn the patient's head while holding the jaw. Remember, the jaw has joints holding it to the skull (the temporomandibular joints [TMJs]); these move, and you may inadvertently strain them by turning the head rapidly while applying force to them. While you are performing the test, be sure to keep your hands high on the patient's head (ear level or higher). Refer to Tables 4-1 through 4-3 for test directions and interpretation.

*Discussion*: A common error that clinicians who are new to this test make while performing it is to turn the head away from midline and then immediately bring it

## TABLE 4-1
# HEAD THRUST TEST, STEP 1

**Instruction:** "Drop your chin slightly. I want you to look at the tip of my nose. While you are looking at my nose, I'm going to turn your head. Your job is to keep your eyes on my nose."

**Clinician:** The patient is in a seated position and the examiner is facing him. Hold the patient's head at ear level or higher and correct the head position if needed. If the patient has a hearing aid, you will need to hold his head above his ears to avoid creating feedback noise from the hearing aid.

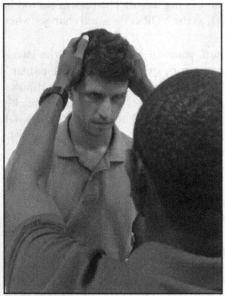

**Figure 4-1.** Head Thrust test beginning position.

back to center. Remember, turn the head and *stop it in the turned position.* Do not immediately bring it back to midline. If the patient is unable to keep his or her eyes on your nose while the head is being turned, he or she will have to make a corrective saccade (by moving his or her eyes) to look for your nose after the head is turned. If you observe a corrective eye motion, the test is positive. A positive test indicates a likely vestibular weakness (loss) on the side in the direction of head turn. For example, if you turn the patient's head to his or her right (as if trying to look over the right shoulder) and the patient's eyes move with his or her head, the eyes will no longer be looking at your nose when you stop turning the head. Instead, the patient will be looking off into the distance to his or her right. The patient will have to move his or her eyes to the left using a corrective saccade to find your nose again. It is this observed saccade that indicates vestibular weakness on this patient's right side. If the patient is able to keep his or her eyes on your nose, the test is negative. Test each side.

## TABLE 4-2
# HEAD THRUST TEST, STEP 2

**Instruction:** "Stay relaxed as I move your head, and keep your eyes on the tip of my nose."

**Clinician:** Quickly turn (rotate) the patient's head to either the left or the right, keeping within the patient's normal cervical range of motion. Stop and hold his head in the turned position. Do his eyes come off the target (your nose)? Repeat this test on each side.

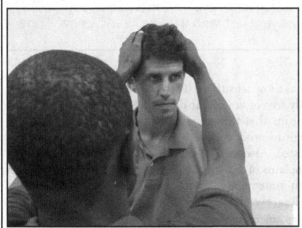

**Figure 4-2.** Head Thrust test end position, example 1.

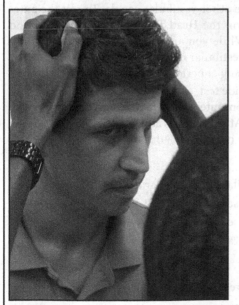

**Figure 4-3.** Head Thrust test end position, example 2.

## TABLE 4-3
# INTERPRETATION OF THE HEAD THRUST TEST

*Interpretation*

If the patient is able to keep his eyes on your nose while you turn his head, the test is negative and the vestibular system is working well enough to generate a VOR. (This does not mean that it is working at 100%.) If the patient is unable to keep his eyes on your nose while you turn his head, then when you stop turning his head, he will realize that he is no longer looking at your nose and you will see a corrective eye motion (saccade) as he looks to find you. This would be a positive test, with the "weak ear" being the one in the direction of head turn.

Keep in mind that this test has a low sensitivity. This means that a patient who has a negative test is not necessarily free of vestibular deficits. A negative Head Thrust test (in the yaw plane) just means that the lateral canals and superior vestibular nerves are working well enough to produce and transmit information needed for the VOR of the canal being tested. Always take the patient's subjective complaints into account. If the patient complains of dizziness, especially while turning, while in darkness, or in busy visual environments such as grocery stores or shopping malls, a VNG/audiogram may be revealing, even if the Head Thrust test is negative.

The superior vestibular nerves innervate the lateral vestibular canals. If the patient has a neuritis (nerve inflammation) of the *inferior* vestibular nerve (which innervates the saccule and posterior canal), the Head Thrust test may still be normal. You may also use the Head Thrust test to assess the other vestibular canals. To test the anterior or posterior canals, you would perform the Head Thrust test in the plane and direction of the canal you wish to test. While you are testing the posterior canals, information will travel along the inferior vestibular nerves. If you choose to test both lateral and posterior canals, you will be using superior *and* inferior nerve pathways.

There is a high-tech version of this bedside test, called the *Video Head Impulse test* (vHIT), which uses infrared goggles and computer software to record eye movements and then compares them with "norms." At least one study showed the vHIT to be highly sensitive and specific in testing any of the vestibular canals.

## Specificity and Sensitivity

- Bedside test—100% for complete unilateral vestibular loss (UVL)
- Bedside test—various UVL: average sensitivity, 36%; average specificity, 97%[3]
- Bedside test—various UVL: average sensitivity, 46%; average specificity, 75%[1]
- vHIT—specificity 95%, sensitivity 95%[4]

## Key Things to Remember

- Pitch the subject's head down 30 degrees while testing to increase sensitivity for testing of the lateral canals.[5]

- Do not hold the patient's head near the TMJs or jaw but instead hold it at ear level or higher.
- The timing and direction of head turn should be unpredictable so as to increase test sensitivity.[5]
- Passive head turning yields more accurate results than active or active-assisted motions. The direction of the head turn indicates the side being tested.
- If you see corrective saccades to find the visual target after the head turn, the test is positive and indicates a *likely weak side*.
- You can also check the anterior or posterior canals by thrusting the head in the plane and direction of the canal you wish to test.

#  Head Shake Test

The Head Shake test is also a test of the VOR. The results indicate whether one vestibular organ (left vs right) is stronger than the other. The clinician rapidly and passively rotates the patient's head back and forth in the yaw plane for about 20 to 30 seconds and then stops the head in a neutral position. The clinician then observes any post-head shake eye motion that may occur. Clinicians us the word *symmetry* in discussing the relative strength or weakness of the left and right portions of the vestibular system. If one side is grossly deficient, we expect to see asymmetrical vestibular function.

How does this test work? While the clinician is shaking the patient's head, the vestibular system is stimulated. Part of the cerebellum that deals with vestibular information, called the *velocity storage system*, gathers information about this repetitive head motion and buffers energy to help activate the nystagmus needed for the patient to see clearly while his or her head is in motion. A negative test (ie, all is working well enough to produce a VOR) is indicated by *not* observing nystagmus after the head shake. That is, when you stop shaking the patient's head, his or her eyes are still and there are no nystagmus. Refer to Tables 4-4 through 4-7 for test directions and interpretation.

*Discussion*: While this test is typically done with passive head shaking, you may allow active-assist if it facilitates the patient's willingness to allow head shaking, although this may introduce error into your test.

You will most often hear instructions to first stop shaking the patient's head, and to *then* ask the patient to open his or her eyes (with the head still in 30 degrees of flexion). If you wait until you stop shaking the head before you ask the patient to open his or her eyes, you may miss observing the nystagmus that may be occurring behind the patient's closed eyelids. This is especially true if the patient becomes dizzy during the test, as he or she will want to keep the eyes closed. It is a common occurrence in a vestibular clinic to hear the clinicians shouting, "Open your eyes!" To avoid this, when you are ready to look at the patient's eyes, keep shaking the head while you ask the patient to open his or her eyes. Once the eyes are open, stop shaking the patient's head.

## TABLE 4-4
# HEAD SHAKE TEST, STEP 1

**Instruction:** "Drop your chin slightly. I'm going to ask you to close your eyes while I shake your head 'no' for about 20 seconds."

**Clinician:** The patient is in a seated position and the examiner sits facing her. After the patient drops her chin to place her head in 30 degrees of flexion, the examiner corrects the head position. The patient is then asked to close her eyes so that she cannot visually fixate on anything and override any nystagmus that the testing may cause. Firmly hold the patient's head (ear-level or higher) with the head tipped down 30 degrees.

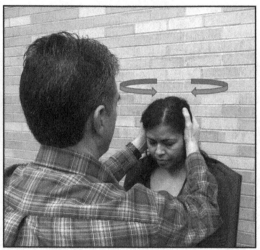

**Figure 4-4.** Passively shakes (rotates) head in the directions of the arrows in the yaw plane.

As for the 30 degrees of flexion, we place the patient in this position to get the lateral canals roughly level with the ground to more easily stimulate them during the head motion. However, it is the stored energy in the vestibulocerebellum that will drive the nystagmus for this test. At the end of the test, there really is no need to maintain a 30-degree flexed head posture. Further, it is natural for the patient to look at you when opening his or her eyes at the end of this test. While sitting with his or her head flexed—unless you place yourself in the patient's line of sight—the patient will look up in order to see you. This muddies your examination findings a bit. Did the patient look up or did he or she have an upbeat nystagmus? An experienced clinician may be able to tell the difference, but the novice clinician will not. For this reason, you may wish to slowly bring the patient's head out of 30 degrees of flexion (while still shaking the head) about 3 cycles before the end of the test. That is, as you are nearing the end of the shaking, bring the patient's head out of flexion with each turn of the head left and right. Once the head is out of flexion, instruct the patient to open his or her eyes. Now, when the patient opens his or her eyes, you will

## TABLE 4-5
# HEAD SHAKE TEST, STEP 2

**Instruction:** "Keep your eyes closed, and stay relaxed as I move your head. Don't try to help me. When I tell you to, open your eyes as quickly as you can, even if you feel dizzy."

**Clinician:** Rapidly shake the patient's head in the yaw plane left and right (as if making a "no" head motion) at a rate of about 2 Hz for 20 cycles (1 cycle = one complete motion of left head rotation to right rotation, and then back again to the starting position of left rotation [L-R-L]). Try to keep a pace of 2 cycles per second, with 1 second including motions L-R-L-R-L.

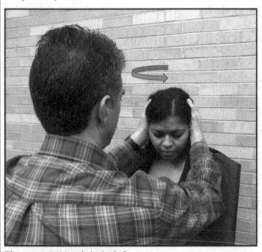

**Figure 4-5.** Head shake left.

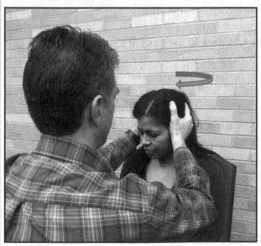

**Figure 4-6.** Head shake right.

---

TABLE 4-6

# HEAD SHAKE TEST, STEP 3

**Instruction:** "Open your eyes."

**Clinician:** When nearing the end of your 20 cycles, slowly bring the patient's head out of the 30 degrees of flexion (while still shaking and with the patient's eyes still closed). *While still shaking the patient's head, ask her to open her eyes.* Stop turning her head when her eyes are open, and observe if any nystagmus are present.

---

TABLE 4-7

# INTERPRETATION OF THE HEAD SHAKE TEST

*Interpretation*

Observation of quick-phase nystagmus laterally (left or right) indicates a vestibular weakness, with the likely stronger vestibular side in the direction of the quick phases of the nystagmus.

Vertical nystagmus on this test indicate central pathology.

Positive tests should be followed by more in-depth examinations (such as VNG/audiography) to help confirm vestibulopathy and rule out central pathologies.

---

be directly in front of him or her. You do not ask the patient to visually fixate on you, but the patient will naturally tend to look at you. Since you are now at eye level with the patient, if you see his or her eyes move up, it will be easier to distinguish this as an upbeat nystagmus vs the patient looking up to find you.

An alternative to bringing the head out of 30 degrees of flexion is for the examiner to stay lower than the patient during the test and in the patient's line of sight, so when the patient opens his or her eyes, he or she is already looking directly at the examiner. Two easy options for the clinician are to have the patient seated (1) on a high examination table or (2) in a chair while you are kneeling on the floor. These options are strictly a matter of personal preference on the part of the examiner.

If you observe nystagmus after shaking the patient's head, it is an indication of vestibular imbalance.[6] When you observe laterally beating nystagmus (left or right) after stopping the head, the quick phases will usually indicate the *more active side*. For example, if nystagmus is observed and the eyes are beating with quick phases to the left, it indicates that the left vestibular system is likely stronger than the right and the contralateral side is weak. Thus if you see left-beating quick phases, the right side is likely weak. If you see right-beating quick phases, the left side is likely weak. Again, since this is a bedside test, we cannot say where the lesion is located (ie, brain vs ear), and the wise course is to request further testing (VNG/audiography) to verify vestibular loss or a need for further central testing. Central signs for this test include post-horizontal head shake nystagmus that is beating vertically, or is dysconjugate.[7]

## Sensitivity and Specificity

- Various UVL: average sensitivity, 46%; average specificity, 75%[1]

Here is a simple explanation of how this test works: The brain keeps track of head motions. Let's say you are sitting in a chair that swivels and are turning clockwise. As you turn, you need to use the VOR in order to see clearly. As you are turning and accelerating, the vestibulocerebellum buffers information about the direction and speed of turning and uses that information to drive the VOR. This makes it easier and more efficient to turn on and use this reflex. Think of it this way: Imagine that you have a watch spring in your right ear, which provides the power to turn on the nystagmus (VOR) that are needed for seeing while turning to the right, and another watch spring in the left ear to activate the VOR needed for seeing while turning left. As you spin clockwise (right), you are winding up the right spring, storing energy, and then using it to turn on the nystagmus needed to see clearly. If you were turning left, you would store energy to turn on the VOR with quick phases to the left. When you stopped turning, you would continue to expend this buffered energy in the form of nystagmus until the watch spring unwound—the vestibulocerebellum buffer would be empty.

If we spin to the right, while we are spinning and accelerating we will get quick-phase nystagmus to the right. The changes in velocity stimulate the lateral canals of the vestibular system, but we also get some optokinetic stimulation through the eyes owing to the constantly moving environment. If we spin to the left, while we are spinning we will get quick-phase nystagmus to the left. When we are spinning at a constant velocity, the endolymph and cupulae are relatively still, as they are moving at the same speed, but now the optokinetic system is driving the nystagmus. When we decelerate or stop moving, the nystagmus will change direction owing to the inertia of the endolymph pushing on the cupula. That is to say, we stop moving, but the liquid endolymph in our ears does not. It pushes against the cupula and the vestibular system is once again excited. In one ear the flow of endolymph will be toward the cupula, while in the other ear it will be away from the cupula. A simple way to imagine fluid motion once we stop is to use a bucket of water. Using full shoulder motion, swing the bucket in a circle. What happens if you stop swinging and suddenly stop the bucket? The water will continue moving and slosh over the sides of the bucket, even though the bucket has stopped moving.

Now take your understanding of stored energy and apply it to our Head Shake test. What would happen if you *repeatedly and alternately* turn the patient's head left and right at a velocity of about 2 Hz? While you are shaking the patient's head, the head is accelerating to 2 Hz and then suddenly stopping, then reversing direction and accelerating again to 2 Hz (over and over). The vestibular system is excited by the lag of endolymph pushing on the cupulae because of these repeated changes in velocity in each direction. Would nystagmus be present if you stopped shaking the head after turning it alternately left and right for 20 to30 seconds, as when shaking the head "no"? The vestibulocerebellum will still be buffering information (winding our watch springs) while the head is moving. If each ear is working (and therefore equally strong), the vestibulocerebellum will buffer information about the head shake for *each* direction. Would you see nystagmus after stopping the head shake? The answer is no; you should not see any nystagmus after stopping the head. There is still stored energy, but when both ears are working, there are *equal amounts* of stored energy regarding each direction of spin. This is different from nystagmus observed after having a subject spin in one direction while his or her eyes are open. When spun in only one direction, only one ear is excited. When the subject stops spinning, one ear has buffered energy to expend and nystagmus will beat toward that ear. During the Head Shake test, however, the clinician moves the head in both directions (left and right). It is like a tug-o-war with Team Left and Team Right each trying to elicit nystagmus in its own direction. In keeping with our tug-o-war analogy, if one ear is stronger than the other, it will be able to pull the flag (nystagmus) in its direction. If one ear's watch spring (vestibular system) is working and storing energy while the other ear's watch spring is not working, there will be an asymmetry between the systems. Once the head stops shaking, the vestibulocerebellum will discharge energy. If there is more information regarding a healthy ear vs a damaged one, you will see quick-phase nystagmus in the direction of the stronger (or more stimulated) ear. If both ears are working enough, you should not observe any nystagmus.

### Key Things to Remember

- Position the patient's head down 30 degrees while testing (easily done by asking the patient to drop his or her chin).
- Firmly hold the patient's head at or above ear level.
- Stay in the patient's line of sight by either bringing his or her head out of flexion near the end of the head shake or by positioning yourself to be in the patient's line of sight while his or her head is flexed.
- When you are ready, ask the patient to open his or her eyes just prior to stopping the head.
- If you note nystagmus after the head shake, the test is positive, with quick phases moving toward the *stronger* (or more stimulated) side.
- Post–head shake vertical or disconjugate nystagmus indicates central pathology.
- Patients with positive Head Shake tests should be referred for further investigation (such as a VNG/audiogram).

## Dynamic Visual Acuity Test

This test determines the patient's visual acuity (sharpness of vision) while the head is still (static) or moving (dynamic) to help determine whether the vestibular system is working properly. There are 2 types of Dynamic Visual Acuity tests: the Clinical DVA and the Computerized DVA (also known as *Instrumented DVA*). The *Clinical DVA* is the low-tech version, which uses an eye chart. It has face validity; that is, it *seems* to measure what it is supposed to measure. However, it lacks consistent evidence for criterion-related validity, and its reliability in the vestibular hypofunction patient population is unknown.[8] There is now a computerized version of this test, called the *Computerized DVA*, which is reliable and valid for both healthy patients and those with vestibular hypofunction.[9]

## Clinical Dynamic Visual Acuity

The patient is positioned sitting or standing, facing an eye chart at the distance indicated by the chart. With the head still, the patient reads the eye chart from top to bottom and left to right. When you look at an eye chart, there are either letters or symbols in rows. We call each letter or symbol on the chart an *optotype*. As you move from top to bottom, the font size of each line gets progressively smaller. There are different types of charts, from the classic "Big E" chart (also called a *Snellen chart*) to charts that have equal numbers of optotypes per line. Some charts have symbols instead of letters, so you can test patients who do not read (eg, illiterate patients or children). To the right of each line is a group of numbers. The first set of numbers is usually a line number. We refer to the second set of numbers as a *Snellen fraction*; it indicates the patient's visual acuity—how "sharply" the patient can see. Without getting too technical, a simple way to understand the fraction is to read it as "What the patient can see / (over) what *most* people can see." For example, if you see 20/20, this means that what *you* can see at 20 feet is the same as what *most* people can see at 20 feet. If your visual acuity is 20/40, this means that what *you* see at 20 feet is the same as what *most* people can see at 40 feet (farther away). So for you to see them compared with most everyone else, the characters have to be larger.

The use of the Snellen (Big E) chart for use with the Clinical DVA has been critiqued as having problems, such as having different numbers of optotypes on each line as well as not having uniform size ratios between lines.[8] For this reason, if you decide to do the Clinical DVA, using the Early Treatment of Diabetic Retinopathy Study chart will eliminate some of these issues.

Remember, the purpose of the test is to indicate whether vestibular deficits are likely. Like the Head Shake test, a portion of this test involves passively shaking the head in the yaw plane. However, with this test you are not looking for nystagmus but are instead testing the patient's visual acuity (how sharply someone sees) while the head is moving vs still. During this test there is no way to measure if the patient is reading the chart while the head is moving at the correct speed (in the VOR range). If the patient begins to have difficulty reading the chart while you shake his or her head, he or she will often actively resist the head motion in order to slow the movement and thus make reading easier. *There is no consistent method of interpreting the Clinical (noninstrumented) DVA*, and it has yet to be validated as a test for vestibular deficits. In some of the literature, if the patient has a difference of 2 or more lines from static to dynamic visual acuity, the test is "positive" and indicates a possible vestibular deficit. Other journal articles state that the test is positive if the patient misses 3 or more lines. Because of these issues, you may wish to avoid using the Clinical DVA as part of an assessment or measurement for progress. However, you may choose to use it as an intervention to challenge the patient.

### Steps in the Clinical Dynamic Visual Acuity Test

The patient is seated or standing in front of the chart at the distance from the chart that the chart indicates (usually printed near the bottom). The examiner stands behind the patient and passively shakes the patient's head at a frequency of about 2 Hz.

1.  For the bedside Clinical DVA (noncomputerized), ask the patient to read an eye chart while his or her head is still. The patient reads each line, starting with the top line and working down, reading each line from left to right. Allow the patient to miss one letter or symbol (called an *optotype*) and still continue to the next line. If the patient identifies 2 or more optotypes incorrectly, he or she fails that line, and the line directly above the failed line will indicate his or her visual acuity. You will document the last line the patient passes as his or her "static visual acuity," as the patient keeps his or her head still (static) for the test.

2.  The next part of the test determines "dynamic visual acuity," since the patient's head will be moving (dynamic). As before, the patient is seated or standing in front of the chart at the appropriate distance. During this part of the examination the clinician stands behind the patient and passively shakes the patient's head in a "no" (yaw plane) motion. Speed of passive head motions is 2 Hz.[1] You may use a metronome to help maintain the correct speed of head motion. Generally, if you complete 2 cycles of head motion (L-R-L-R-L) per second, you will be testing at a good speed. While the examiner shakes the patient's head, the patient is asked to read the chart from top to bottom and left to right. Again, the examiner records the line or Snellen fraction indicating the patient's visual acuity.

### Test Interpretation

A patient passes a line if he or she can read it and not misread more than one optotype. If the patient misses 2 or more optotypes, the line directly above would indicate his or her visual acuity. A test would be "positive" if there were a 2- or 3-line difference between static and dynamic visual acuity, indicating a possible vestibular deficit. Why? Because while the head is being turned left and right during the test and the head is moving at the correct speed, the patient must use the VOR to see clearly. If the VOR is working as it should, the patient will be able to see clearly and read the chart. If the VOR is not working properly, the patient will have at least a 2- or 3-line difference between static and dynamic visual acuity

As mentioned, there are many difficulties with using this test for clinical data. While performing this test, the clinician must passively shake the patient's head quickly enough (at about 2 Hz) to require use of the VOR to read. If a patient is having difficulty seeing, he or she will resist the head motion by stiffening his or her neck muscles in order to slow the head speed and thus see the chart more easily; that is, it will be easier because the patient will not need to use the damaged VOR. If this happens, the test will be inaccurate and invalid. There is no way to accurately measure the patient's head speed during the Clinical DVA, nor is there a way to lateralize a vestibular problem to say which side is involved. As mentioned, this test has not yet been validated in patients with balance/vestibular problems. While it seems to be a great test and is widely popular, it is simply not reliable as a clinical measure and has questionable accuracy.

### Sensitivity and Specificity—Clinical Dynamic Visual Acuity

- Sensitivity unknown
- Specificity unknown

## Computerized Dynamic Visual Acuity

The high-tech computerized version of the DVA test uses a headset accelerometer and a computer monitor. The accelerometer is a device mounted on top of a headset that detects the patient's head velocity and direction of motion. Using this information, the software will display an optotype on the screen only when the patient is shaking his or her head fast enough to be in the VOR range of speed. This computerized version can also test each ear individually by displaying an optotype only in the direction of head turn that the clinician wishes to test. Since the computer displays the optotype only when sufficient head speed is present, the patient cannot cheat by slowing his or her head. The computerized test is reliable not only while testing the lateral canals but also while testing vertical head movements in both healthy subjects and those with vestibular hypofunction.[10] The Computerized DVA is highly specific, valid, and accurate.

### Sensitivity and Specificity—Computerized Dynamic Visual Acuity

- Sensitivity,[8] 94.5%
- Specificity,[8,9] 95.2%

## Key Things to Remember

- During the Clinical DVA, the patient is asked to read the eye chart twice; once with the head still (static) and one with head shaking (dynamic).
- There is no standard method of interpreting the Clinical DVA test.
- The Clinical DVA has not been validated in patients with vestibular problems.
- The Computerized DVA is valid and reliable and has been studied in the vestibular hypofunction population.

#  *Vestibulo-ocular Reflex Cancellation Test*

Do not be fooled by the name of this test. It is not a test of the VOR but instead assesses the cerebellum's ability to suppress the VOR. Some clinicians refer to the VOR Cancellation (VOR-C) test as the *Visual-Vestibular-Fixation Suppression* test. Remember, the VOR causes the eyes to move in the *opposite direction* to that of the head motion. For example, if you turn your head to the right, your eyes will reflexively move to the left. However, there are times when we don't want our eyes to move in the opposite direction as our head. When we watch a plane or bird fly across the sky or watch a tennis match, we need to have our heads and eyes moving in the same direction in order to keep the image of those objects on our retinas (foveae). To do this, we need to suppress (cancel) the VOR.[11] Refer to Tables 4-8 and 4-9 for test directions and interpretation.

---

## TABLE 4-8
# VESTIBULO-OCULAR REFLEX CANCELLATION TEST

**Instruction:** "Turn your head to the left and right while keeping your eyes on the target. I will guide you."

**Clinician:** There are variations to the testing method. The speed at which you move the patient is within the VOR speeds of 0.5 to 5.0 Hz. Recall that smooth pursuit's working range of speed is 0 to 0.5 Hz. In other words, you need to have the patient move her head and target faster than smooth pursuit. Some clinicians—while holding the patient's head and guiding the rotation left and right—stay in front of the patient and ask her to use the clinician's nose as a visual target. Others ask the patient to hold a visual target (typically the clinician will instruct the patient to stare at her own thumb, which is held directly in front of her eyes with arm extended, and then guide the patient to rotate her head and target together to the left and right in long ranges of motion. The examiner has to move with the patient while she is turning, so that the examiner always remains directly in front of her eyes.

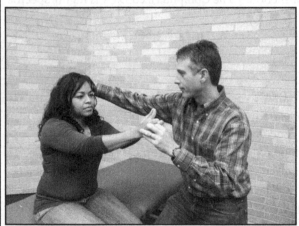

**Figure 4-7.** VOR-C.

---

## *Vestibulo-ocular Reflex Test Summary*

There are a variety of options to test vestibular function. You should use at least one bedside test of vestibular function (eg, Head Thrust, Head Shake, or Computerized DVA) along with the VOR-C in assessing a patient who complains of imbalance or dizziness unless you have more sophisticated equipment to do so (Table 4-10). You do not have to use all of these VOR function tests, but you may choose to use more than one if you suspect vestibular involvement but get a negative test on just one of them. Remember, if you find a positive test, the wise course is to recommend further

---

TABLE 4-9

# INTERPRETATION OF THE VESTIBULO-OCULAR REFLEX CANCELLATION TEST

*Interpretation*

During the test, the examiner observes the patient's eyes to see if they are able to maintain visual fixation on the target while they are moving. If the eyes drift off the target, the examiner will see the patient perform catch-up saccades. If the patient cannot keep her eyes on the target while her head is in motion, there is "failure of fixation suppression," which indicates cerebellar dysfunction.[11]

---

TABLE 4-10

# SUMMARY OF THE VESTIBULO-OCULAR REFLEX BEDSIDE TESTS OF FUNCTION

| TEST | POSITIVE WHEN |
|------|---------------|
| Head Thrust | Corrective saccades are noted post–head thrust to find the target. The deficient side is in the direction of the head turn. |
| Head Shake | • Post–head shake nystagmus are observed:<br>  ○ Quick phases of nystagmus indicate the stronger system (left or right).<br>  ○ Vertical nystagmus indicates central issues. |
| Dynamic Visual Acuity | • Clinical DVA (noncomputerized)<br>  ○ There is no standard guideline, with some advocating 2 or more lines difference while others advocate a 3-line change or greater between static visual acuity and dynamic visual acuity.<br>  ○ Does not lateralize deficits.<br>• Computerized DVA<br>  ○ Highly reliable and sensitive.<br>  ○ The software will provide test results.<br>  ○ The results are lateralized. |
| VOR-C | Corrective saccades occur when the patient is unable to keep his or her eyes on the target during head and target motions occurring in the same direction. A positive test indicates cerebellar dysfunction. |

testing, such as a VNG/audiogram. This may help to confirm a vestibular issue as well and to rule out central involvement.

Keep in mind that a negative bedside test does not necessarily indicate normal function. Take test results into consideration with current complaints as well as other signs and symptoms. Use more sophisticated tests to confirm or rule out pathology.

# PRESSURE TESTING OF THE EAR

Clinicians use pressure tests to detect possible perilymphatic fistulas and occasionally hypermobile stapes.[1] Pressure testing may also produce symptoms in patients with Arnold-Chiari malformations or canal dehiscence syndromes.[12] The various tests put either positive or negative pressure on the vestibular system or external auditory canal. If nystagmus or eye drifting is noted during testing, the test is considered positive. These pressure tests include Tragal Compression, the Valsalva maneuver, and pneumatic otoscopy. When possible, use Frenzel or infrared goggles during testing.

**Interpretation:** In tests of pressure, consistent eye deviation, or nystagmus implies abnormal coupling (connection) between either the outside atmosphere with the inner ear or the intracranial space and the inner ear. Likely locations of abnormalities include the following[7]:

- Oval window (fistula, excessive footplate movement)
- Round window (fistula)
- Lateral semicircular canal (dehiscence)
- Eye elevation and intorsion with loud sounds or during a nose-pinch Valsalva, suggesting superior canal dehiscence.[13]
- Vertical downbeating nystagmus with any maneuver that increases intracranial pressure, suggesting an abnormality of the craniocervical junction (eg, Arnold-Chiari malformation).

## Tragal Compression Test

During this test, the examiner changes intracranial pressure by pushing on the patient's tragus (part of the external ear). During the test, the patient is in a sitting position. Testing in other positions may change the intracranial pressure and affect the test results. See Tables 4-11 through 4-13 for test instructions and interpretation as described by Dr. Michael Schubert (oral communication, 2013).

## Valsalva Maneuver

The Valsalva maneuver is another test in which the clinician observes the patient's eyes for nystagmus or tonic deviation while pressure is placed on the inner ear (Tables 4-14 and 4-15).

## TABLE 4-11
## TRAGAL COMPRESSION TEST, STEP 1

**Instruction:** The patient is in a sitting position. The test is preferably performed with the patient's vision blocked by Frenzel or infrared goggles.

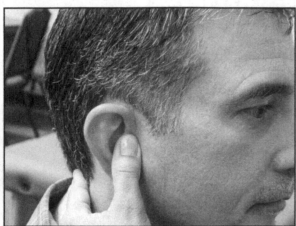

**Figure 4-8.** Tragal Compression test.

## TABLE 4-12
## TRAGAL COMPRESSION TEST, STEP 2

**Clinician:** With the patient sitting, the examiner firmly and steadily presses the tragus in toward the patient's external auditory canal for about 3 seconds while observing for tonic eye drift or nystagmus. During the test, sufficient pressure should be applied against the tragus (using fingers or thumb); this will be uncomfortable for the patient but not sharply painful. Each ear should be tested separately.

## TABLE 4-13
## INTERPRETATION OF THE TRAGAL COMPRESSION TEST

*Interpretation*
Observed nystagmus or tonic deviation of eye position during the test indicates possible deficits to the test side, such as perilymph fistulas and canal dehiscence.

## TABLE 4-14
## VALSALVA MANEUVER TEST

**Instruction:** The patient is in a sitting position. While keeping her eyes open, she is instructed to either pinch her nose closed or close her glottis while attempting to exhale with moderate force (performing a Valsalva maneuver).

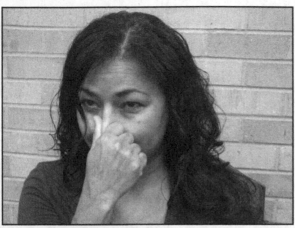

**Figure 4-9.** Valsalva maneuver.

## TABLE 4-15
## INTERPRETATION OF THE VALSALVA MANEUVER TEST

*Interpretation*

During the Valsalva maneuver, the examiner observes the patient's eyes for nystagmus or eye drifting. This test may produce signs and symptoms in patients with craniocervical abnormalities, perilymph fistula, or a canal dehiscence syndrome. A change in the direction of nystagmus during a nose-pinch Valsalva maneuver vs a closed glottis is characteristic of a superior canal dehiscence syndrome.[14]

## Pneumatic Otoscopy

While pneumatic otoscopy is frequently used for diagnosing otitis media with effusion,[15] it may also be a useful tool to screen for perilymphatic fistula and semicircular canal dehiscence syndrome.[16] Using a pneumatic otoscopic examination with a good seal, place positive and negative pressure on the tympanic membrane while asking the patient to look at a stationary target. This may be used as a subjective test, with the patient asked whether he or she perceives movement of the target or has symptoms of vertigo/disequilibrium. If the test is repeated with the same results, it is positive for an abnormal coupling between the external canal and the labyrinth, which is referred to as *Hennebert sign*.[17] Eye movements in Hennebert sign consist of 2 or 3 small-amplitude horizontal (not torsional) jerks that are away from the ear on positive pressure and toward the ear on negative pressure (which will elicit stronger responses). Other conditions that can cause Hennebert's sign include congenital syphilis, Ménière's disease, stapes surgery, footplate fractures, and sudden deafness.[18]

You may modify this test with the patient's vision blocked, using VNG monitoring to improve sensitivity of the test. Another variation of the test is to monitor postural sway using computerized dynamic platform posturography while applying pressure to the ear.[18]

# VESTIBULAR FINDINGS

We classify vestibular pathologies into 2 categories: *peripheral* and *central*. Peripheral pathologies are those outside of the central nervous system and include conditions like benign paroxysmal positional vertigo (BPPV), labyrinthitis, neuritis, and some tumors that are outside of the central nervous system. If the problem reduces vestibular function and is only on one side, the condition creates a UVL. The terms *vestibular loss, vestibular weakness,* and *vestibular hypofunction* all mean the same thing.

When there is weakness in bilateral vestibular function, the condition creates a *bilateral vestibular loss* (BVL). Don't be confused by the term *vestibular loss*. The word *loss* in this context does not imply 100% loss but instead indicates that the system *is not working at 100%*. Audiology testing using VNG/electronystagmography (ENG) can tell us what percentage of function has been lost (at least in the lateral canals).

As clinicians, when we discuss balance we typically think in terms of the geriatric patient. However, a Johns Hopkins survey shows that one-third of Americans over age 40 are up to 12 times more likely to have a serious fall because of an inner-ear dysfunction; people with diabetes were 70% more likely to suffer from vestibular problems; and 85% of people over the age of 80 had an imbalance problem.[19]

As we learned in Chapter 1, the nerves located in the peripheral vestibular system (inner ear) constantly send neural signals to the brain, even when we are sitting still. When there is a vestibular loss (weakness/hypofunction), one or both (left and right) vestibular organs stop either sending the correct signal (from the inner ears) or there is a central problem that is impairing the processing of the information in the vestibular nuclei or cerebellum. In some cases, impaired vestibular function is temporary, as in cases of some inflammations. However, when there is physical damage to the system or nerve pathways, loss may be permanent.

## *Vestibular Loss/Hypofunction*

### Unilateral Vestibular Loss

As mentioned, a UVL is also referred to as a *hypofunction* (*hypo* meaning less than normal) or *unilateral weakness*. The most common known cause of a UVL is an

**Figure 4-10.** Asymmetrical firing rates after damage to the right vestibular organ.

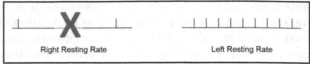

Right Resting Rate          Left Resting Rate

inflammation of the vestibular nerve (vestibular neuritis), commonly resulting from the herpes simplex virus.[20] The superior vestibular nerve is more likely to be involved than the inferior vestibular nerve.[21] There are many causes of unilateral vestibular weaknesses, including viral infections, inflammations, tumors, strokes, cerebellar problems, and diseases like Ménière's disease, multiple sclerosis, and Parkinson's disease. A bedside examination gives clues as to whether the issue is peripheral or central, but only diagnostic tests are definitive.

In the UVL case, one side stops sending or processing vestibular end-organ (inner ear) information. This creates an asymmetry between vestibular organ signals. Remember that when we are sitting still, each ear should be sending the same amount of neural signals. Just like a tug-o-war with evenly matched teams, each side acts to balance the other. There is a push-pull relationship between them. If we turn to the right, the right vestibular system increases its signal output while the left side would decrease its output. In the case of a UVL, however, one side is not sending the correct signal. Even when sitting still, there is no longer balance between systems and one ear is stronger, sending at a faster resting rate than the damaged side. Figure 4-10 demonstrates the differences in firing rates.

As you will recall, when there is a difference in firing rates, the brain interprets this as motion occurring in the direction of the ear that has the faster firing rate. In the case of a damaged right side, the left would be providing a normal signal output while the right would be sending a reduced signal. In such a situation, the brain would interpret this as the patient turning left.

Depending on the difference in function between each inner ear, and the level of compensation that has taken place (ie, how much the brain has learned to modify vestibular signals to restore balance between the ears), you may see any of the following when you are examining a patient with a UVL: spontaneous nystagmus, gaze nystagmus (at 45 degrees of lateral gaze), end-range nystagmus of greater than 3 beats, increased nystagmus with gaze toward the healthy ear, increased gaze with removal of fixation (closed eyelids, darkness, with Frenzel goggles or infrared goggles), falling or listing toward the lesion side, gaze-holding deficits,[14] and/or imbalance that is worse during turning motions. The patient may complain of balance problems, nausea, and/or dizziness. Patients with peripheral etiologies may have nystagmus that is suppressed when they are fixing on a visual target; they typically feel worse in the dark, when they cannot hold gaze on a visual target. Conversely, patients with central causes of dizziness often feel better in the dark and worse while fixing gaze.

## Acute Unilateral Visual Loss

Acute symptoms depend on how badly one side is damaged or inflamed and how asymmetrical the resting firing rates of the nerves are. If there is a huge difference, where one side is working normally while the other is barely working, the patient will complain of vertigo (spinning) and may vomit or fall in trying to walk. The patient will likely have resting nystagmus (nystagmus with quick phase in the direction of the stronger ear, even while sitting still), or gaze nystagmus at 45 degrees. These patients are often taken to the emergency room owing to the sudden onset and severity of symptoms. If the vestibular asymmetry is small, they may only have balance problems or dizziness when they turn quickly, but they have no resting nystagmus. The greater the asymmetry, the more signs and symptoms will be present. If the UVL is due to an infection or inflammation that is not doing any permanent damage, symptoms will eventually subside and function will return to normal while healing occurs.

Signs and symptoms of acute vestibular loss may include the following:

- Resting or gaze nystagmus
- Nausea
- Vomiting
- Disequilibrium
- Unidirectional resting nystagmus or gaze nystagmus that begins at 45 degrees of gaze, or greater than 3 beats near end ranges

## Chronic Unilateral Vestibular Loss

In cases of chronic UVL, there is permanent vestibular loss, leaving a hypofunctioning vestibular system. Patients with a chronic vestibular weakness may or may not complain of dizziness, depending on the level of compensation that has taken place. If they do, it is usually while turning quickly. They may also complain of balance deficits, nausea, or dizziness while in darkness or in a busy visual environment (such as a grocery store or shopping mall) and often report difficulty in concentrating and with short-term memory.

Over time, the brain may learn to alter vestibular signals to deal with this permanent loss, but this requires system stimulation, and the patient must be sufficiently active to drive the process. *Compensation* is the process whereby the cerebellum "corrects" signals for a weak ear. While the affected patient moves within his or her environment, the cerebellum will ultimately change the vestibular signals to improve balance and make normal functional movement possible again. This occurs because of the demand placed on the balance system by the patient's activity. If the patient spends most of his or her time sitting in a chair and not moving, there is not enough stimulus to induce change and compensation will be limited. If the patient is physically active, the cerebellum will compensate for the damaged side out of necessity and adjust the signals in order to have vestibular signal symmetry again. The cerebellum will boost the signals of the weaker ear and slow signals coming from the stronger, healthier ear in an attempt to get each side to produce the same resting firing rates. The closer the resting firing rates become, the less affected the patient will be by the damage. After compensation occurs, the patient usually does not have symptoms under most everyday conditions and activities. However, if such a patient turns very quickly, he or she may still experience slight disequilibrium and dizziness. Figure 4-11 demonstrates the process of compensation.

**Figure 4-11.** After damage, the brain attempts to compensate for the asymmetrical firing rates.

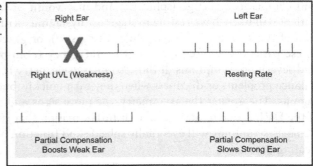

Vestibular therapy assists in the process of compensation and also helps patients learn to balance and perform activities of daily living (ADLs) again. The cerebellum maintains compensation when the patient is sufficiently active, whereas decompensation will occur if the patient becomes sedentary. This means that the patient will again experience dizziness and/or balance deficits if he or she does not provide enough challenges to the vestibular system.

Vestibular rehabilitation—as opposed to sham exercise, no vestibular rehabilitation, or usual care—improves subjective measures of dizziness, level of performance on the Dizziness Handicap Inventory, and gait performance as measured by the Dynamic Gait Index in people with chronic peripheral vestibulopathy,[22] as demonstrated by numerous studies.[23-28]

Signs and symptoms of chronic UVL may include the following:

- Dizziness while turning
- Disequilibrium while turning
- Nausea in busy visual environments (eg, grocery stores, highways, action movies, near ceiling fans)
- Unidirectional gaze nystagmus, sometimes elicited only at end ranges (more than 3 beats) or in darkness

## Bilateral Vestibular Loss

In cases of BVL, the vestibular end organ or the eighth cranial nerve is damaged on each side, with the most common cause being aminoglycoside antibiotic toxicity.[29-31] Other causes of BVL include vestibular neuritis, head injury, congenital or idiopathic loss, ototoxic chemotherapy, bilateral Ménière's disease, autoimmune ear disease, otosyphilis,[30,32] and diuretics.[31,33,34]

Patients with BVL typically experience disequilibrium, gait ataxia (including decreased arm swing, stiff trunk, and decreased head movement), and complain of oscillopsia (shaking visual environment) during head motions.[31] They will present with a wide-based gait pattern and positive tests of vestibular hypofunction (eg, Head Thrust tests) bilaterally. They do not complain of aural fullness, acute hearing loss, or tinnitus.[31] While patients with BVL often do not complain of dizziness, Telian and colleagues reported that 43% of their subjects with BVL had episodic vertigo.[35]

Even though the vestibular system is deficient bilaterally, vestibular therapy still helps patients with BVL; but recovery from bilateral deficits occurs more slowly than from unilateral lesions and not all patients improve.[36,37] Patients with BVL improve more with a customized exercise program than with a generalized strengthening program.[38,39] Goals for patients with BVL include enhancing gait stability by increasing function in whatever is left working in the vestibular systems and improving gait patterns by training them to substitute information from the vision and somatosensory systems for that of the missing vestibular input.[31,40]

Patients with BVL improve balance with vestibular rehabilitation but never return to their prior level of function, as ambulation never returns to normal. Further, they will continue to have difficulty in conditions of low light.[39]

Signs and symptoms of BVL may include the following:

- Oscillopsia
- Disequilibrium
- Abnormal gait pattern
- May or may not complain of dizziness
- Typically no resting or gaze nystagmus

# OTHER CONDITIONS AFFECTING THE VESTIBULAR SYSTEM

## *Vestibular Neuritis*

Strupp et al found that postural control measures improved more in a group of patients with vestibular neuritis who performed vestibular rehabilitation compared with no specific intervention other than encouragement to move.[22,41]

Teggi et al found that vestibular rehabilitation significantly reduced anxiety in people with acute neuritis compared with a control group.[22,24]

In the case of the vestibular system there is evidence of structural changes to the brain following bilateral vestibular loss[42] and vestibular neuritis.[43] Some evidence suggests structural cortical plasticity in multisensory vestibular cortex areas of the brain (measured by changes to gray matter volume) that may reflect central mechanisms of vestibular compensation.[44] What this means is that following damage or loss of vestibular function, the brain has made changes to cope with the loss of the vestibular information needed to balance and perform functional movement. Following a unilateral, irreversible peripheral vestibulocochlear lesion (after surgical removal of tumors), 15 patients were examined at 3 and 81 months postoperatively and compared with 15 controls. The patients in the surgical group had physical therapy during their acute care stay but not following discharge from the hospital. Looking at structural brain changes in these patients, Helmchen et al found an increase in gray matter volume in visual motion-sensitive areas, in the primary somatosensory cortex, and in regions of multisensory vestibular cortex areas that correlated with parameters of vestibulocochlear impairment. This suggests that substitution and compensation may take place following vestibular loss.[44]

## Acoustic Neuroma

An acoustic neuroma, also known as a *schwannoma*, is a nonmalignant tumor of the eighth cranial nerve (the vestibulocochlear nerve) that is most commonly seen on the inferior vestibular nerve. Incidence is 10 per 1 million persons. Symptoms may include one-sided slowly progressive hearing impairment, low-frequency hearing loss, a "cookie bite" pattern of hearing loss (referring to the audiogram pattern), vertigo, imbalance, facial sensory disturbances, headache, facial weakness, and facial twitching. Diagnosis may be made with ENG/audiography or an auditory brain response test, and magnetic resonance imaging with gadolinium enhancement.[45]

Physicians treat this tumor with surgery or radiation; symptoms are treated with medications and vestibular rehabilitation. Therapy goals are typically to decrease dizziness and oscillopsia and to improve balance.

## Benign Paroxysmal Positional Vertigo

BPPV is a condition of the peripheral vestibular organ when calcium carbonate crystals (otoconia) dislodge from their correct anatomical positions. The migration of these crystals into other parts of the vestibular organ or the effects of the new resting locations after the migration (as on the cupula) cause sensations of vertigo. BPPV has its own chapter in this book, as it requires a more in-depth discussion. Refer to Chapter 5 for further details.

## $B_{12}$ Deficiency

Vitamin $B_{12}$ deficiency affects about 10% of patients over 80 years of age. Symptoms may include gait ataxia and proprioception loss. Diagnosis is usually through measurement of serum $B_{12}$ levels. Treatment involves $B_{12}$ replacement via oral therapy, monthly injections, or a nasal spray.[46]

If gait ataxia is present, a referral to physical therapy may help to determine whether the patient is at risk of falling. Symptoms may resolve quickly once $B_{12}$ therapy is initiated if this is the cause of the patient's complaints. However, in the 80+ age group, it is not uncommon to find other premorbid conditions that still place the patient at risk of falling, even without the $B_{12}$ deficiency. A thorough evaluation can help to identify and improve issues that place the patient at risk of falling.

## Mal de Débarquement

Mal de débarquement is a condition causing vertigo and imbalance. It occurs after debarking from a long boat or airplane ride. Symptoms include a rocking sensation, as if one were still on the boat or plane, and it may persist for months or years. It occurs mostly in women between the ages of 40 and 50 who were recently on a cruise. The cause is unclear, but some experts believe it is a form of migraine.

Diagnosis is made by patient history and ruling out other conditions.[47] Treatment consists of medications to manage symptoms and vestibular therapy to hopefully hasten resolution.

## Ménière's Disease (Primary Endolymphatic Hydrops)

According to the US National Library of Medicine, Ménière's disease, also called *primary* (or *idiopathic*) *endolymphatic hydrops*, occurs when the pressure of the fluid in the inner ear rises too high. The exact cause of this disease is unknown. The pressure changes within the inner ear may affect both balance and hearing as well as causing symptoms such as vertigo.[48] The prevalence of Ménière's disease[49] is 190 cases per 100,000 persons, with a female-to-male ratio of 1.9:1.

The main symptoms include fluctuating hearing loss that gets worse over time, a sensation of pressure in the ear, tinnitus, and vertigo. Vertigo episodes may last from 20 minutes to a few hours and occur unpredictably.

There is no "gold standard" test to definitively diagnose Ménière's disease. Instead, the patient's history, along with clinical tests to help rule out other potential causes, are used.

There is no known cure for Ménière's disease. Current treatments focus on reducing symptoms. Vestibular therapy may offer some usefulness in between attacks to help the brain adapt to any vestibular loss that may have occurred and to help in the adaptation process after an attack, but it will not prevent future vertigo attacks. Medical management may include betahistine dihydrochloride, diuretics, and dietary changes such as following a low-salt diet and limiting caffeine and alcohol.

There is a device called the *Meniett Low-Pressure Pulse Generator*, available from Medtronic, that may help reduce symptoms. It is a computer-controlled device that delivers micro
pressure pulses of air through a tube held in the outer ear; the pulses travel through to the eardrum via a ventilation tube placed on the ear drum. These pressure pulses are believed to help redistribute the endolymph within the inner ear and thereby reducing symptoms.[50]

When other treatments fail, there are surgical options that permanently remove some or all of the vestibular function in the affected ear. Examples include cutting the vestibular nerve, injecting gentamicin in the middle ear, or removing part of the inner ear (called a *labyrinthectomy*).[48]

## Secondary Endolymphatic Hydrops

Like Ménière's disease, secondary endolymphatic hydrops is a condition due to excessive amounts of endolymph leading to damage to the inner ear. Causes include an existing underlying condition of allergies, diabetes, or autoimmune disease. Acquired causes include head injury or surgery. Treatment focuses on controlling symptoms and identifying/treating underlying causes.[51]

## Perilymphatic Fistula

Also known as *perilymph fistula*, this lesion is an opening between the inner and middle ear. Remember, the inner ear is full of fluid (perilymph). When a tear develops, the liquid perilymph can escape the inner ear, thereby changing the pressure within the inner ear. Head injury with a direct blow to the ear is the most common cause. Other causes include ear surgery, pressure trauma, congenital defect, and infection.[52]

Symptoms may include pressure sensitivity,[52] imbalance, positional vertigo, nystagmus, hearing loss, and the Tullio phenomenon (comprising a group of symptoms including vertigo, oscillopsia, nystagmus, ocular tilt reaction, and imbalance induced by auditory stimuli [eg, loud noise]).[53]

The bedside test to detect this condition is the nose-pinch Valsalva. Watch for downbeating nystagmus with a fast torsional phase toward the affected ear. Physical therapy is not offered for this condition; it is typically treated with rest, restriction of activity (such as lifting, bending, diving, and loud noises), and in some cases surgery.[52]

# VESTIBULAR INTERVENTIONS

As we have learned, underlying physical deficits may impact a patient's ability to perform functional movements with precision and skill. No one exercise program is effective for all patients.[39] It is critical that you customize each patient's interventions based on his or her underlying physical impairments, tolerance to treatment and interventions, as well as functional needs and personal desires. Vestibular rehab is indicated for a variety of conditions, including stable vestibular lesions, central lesions, mixed (peripheral and central) lesions, head injury, psychogenic vertigo, BPPV, and vertigo/dizziness of uncertain etiology (after diagnostic tests have ruled out other pathologies).[22,54] While most patients improve with vestibular rehabilitation, some do not improve or only make some improvements in certain areas.[55]

According to Herdman,[56] different "traditional" exercise approaches have been proposed to address the various symptoms experienced by patients with vestibular deficits, including the following:

- Habituation exercises[57-60]: These decrease symptoms by systematically provoking them in a controlled manner.
- Adaptation exercises[61]: These induce long-term changes in the neuronal response to retinal slip using head motions while looking at a visual target.
- Substitution exercises[61]: The patient performs exercises that teach him or her to use alternative strategies to replace vestibular deficits.

Improved function can be expected within 6 weeks,[54,62] but subjective improvement is often seen within 2 or 3 weeks following the initiation of vestibular exercises. Recovery will be slower for those who[54]:

- Are taking vestibular suppressant medications, antidepressants, tranquilizers, and anticonvulsants.[60,63,64]
- Are prevented from having the visuomotor experience.[65]
- Avoid movements and body positions that provoke vertigo.[63]
- Have a central or mixed lesion and have had a prolonged period of therapy, but where the final outcome does not vary with the location.[63,64,66]
- Have a cerebellar lesion.[67]
- Have had a head injury with an associated vestibular deficit. This combination has shown less improvement with treatment,[60] and these patients have significantly worse outcomes.[60]

Alghadir et al[68] identify other prognostic factors for negative outcomes:

- History of migraines
- Inability to move the head or body
- Distal sensory impairment
- Visual dysfunction
- Memory impairment
- Fear of falling
- Anxiety/psychiatric comorbidities

In a 2012 study,[55] Herdman et al found multiple factors accounted for significant percentages of recovery of some of the outcome measures:

- When looking at the subjective complaint of "Percentage of time symptoms interfered with activities" (%TSI), it was found that those who had anxiety and/or depression and had initially complained of a high %TSI were likely to have a high %TSI at discharge. These 2 factors accounted for 83.7% of this outcome.
- Disability: Patients who rated disability as "high" at discharge had the following at the initial visit: high %TSI reported, worse disability scores, and poor DVA scores. These 3 factors accounted for 47.8% of the disability score at discharge.
- Gait speed: Patients who walked more slowly at discharge were those who walked more slowly initially and were older. Some 55% of gait speed findings were accounted for by these 2 factors.
- Fall risk: Patients had poorer fall-risk scores—that is, lower Dynamic Gait Index (DGI) test scores—at discharge if they had a history of falls, had poor initial fall risk scores (based on the DGI), and were older. These 3 factors accounted for 42.5% of the DGI at discharge.

Using the results of this study will help clinicians develop expectations for recovery.[56]

How do vestibular exercises work? Like most therapy interventions, they challenge the body/central nervous system, and it must respond in order to facilitate the needed function. In the case of vestibular exercises, there are neuronal changes in the cerebellum and brain stem that result from the presented challenging exercises, which produce sensory conflicts due to the patient's vestibular pathology.[63]

A variety of vestibular protocols have been outlined by different authors. Most vestibular therapy protocols comprise balance and gait exercises, including vestibular exercises while walking or performing other activities.[56] Part of the art of vestibular rehab is knowing how much exercise or stimulation can be tolerated to sufficiently challenge the system but at the same time not make the patient overly symptomatic (eg, causing nausea, dizziness, or vomiting). Currently there is no standardized way to perform these exercises (ie, there is no standard way to progress exercises), and it is easy to inadvertently push the patient too far. Some clinicians tell patients to perform vestibular exercises longer than 1 minute. Others tell patients to use a nausea or dizziness scale, and to push into symptoms (eg, "go to 5 out of 10"). An important concept to remember for vestibular exercises is that frequent system stimulation that is *within the patient's tolerances* is sufficient to induce the needed changes in the brain. The more frequently the patient challenges the system, the better. However, there is no need to perform prolonged exercises that are outside of the patient's tolerance (eg, 5 minutes of continuous vestibular stimulation), which may lead to sickness. Research has shown that brief periods of stimulation are sufficient to improve patients' function and symptoms. For example, dynamic visual acuity was improved in patients with bilateral vestibular loss following vestibular exercises of 1 minute each or 1 to 2 minutes each.[69] It is likely that even brief periods of stimulation can induce recovery of vestibular function.[54] Patient participation and tolerance of interventions will improve with frequent interventions of short duration that do not create a situation that patients want to avoid. This does *not* mean you should do only 1 minute of vestibular exercises in your treatment sessions. What it *does* mean is that your patient does not need to perform each vestibular exercise or intervention all at once in order for them to work. Following interventions that stir patient symptoms, it is important to allow some time for recovery before proceeding to more exercises or interventions, even within the same treatment session.

How does a patient perform vestibular exercises? Two exercises in particular form the mainstay of vestibular stimulation exercises: VOR x1 and VOR x2. Just as we tell our orthopedic patients that interventions are not always "pain-free," vestibular exercises are likewise not completely benign with regard to symptoms of dizziness and nausea. Tell patients to expect some symptoms when they are performing these exercises. Patients should report any increase in dizziness or nausea while performing the exercises (these are completely normal and expected) but should avoid a level of exercise that induces symptoms that are more severe. A common rule of thumb is that if exercises induce symptoms that last longer than a few minutes, you may want to reduce the duration of the exercise.

## VOR x1, An Intervention for Hypofunction

Vestibular hypofunction intervention (VOR x1) is an exercise of the VOR where only one thing is moving: the patient's head. The patient chooses a stationary visual target which is either held in the hand or in the environment. The visual target is stationary while the patient shakes his or her head "yes" (pitch) for about 1 minute and then "no" (yaw) for up to 1 minute. Keep in mind that some symptom provocation is not only expected but normal. Instruct the patient to take a break if he or she becomes overly dizzy or nauseous.

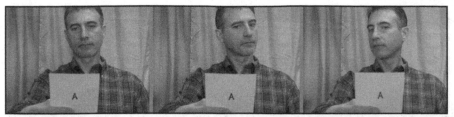

**Figure 4-12.** In performing VOR x1 yaw exercises, the visual target remains still while the head continuously rotates in the yaw plane (head shake "no" motion).

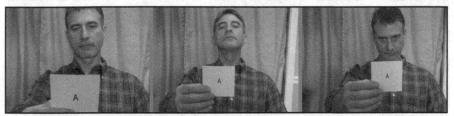

**Figure 4-13.** In performing VOR x1 pitch exercises, the visual target remains still while the head continuously rotates in the pitch plane (head shake "yes" motions).

When first giving VOR x1 as an intervention, begin using a stationary target with a solid background; later this may be progressed to a visual target with a busy background, such as a checkerboard. First patients are instructed to perform these exercises in a sitting position, but later they may progress to performing them standing or while moving (Figures 4-12 and 4-13).

## VOR x2, An Intervention for Hypofunction

VOR x2 is similar to VOR x1. The patient is looking at a visual target while shaking his or her head. What makes VOR x2 different from VOR x1 is that with VOR x2, two things are moving. The head shakes "yes" (pitch) or "no" (yaw), while the target moves in the *opposite direction* of head motion but at exactly the same speed. These exercises are repeated with vertical and horizontal motions (each x1 minute taking breaks as needed), and may be performed sitting or standing still. To go on to more advanced VOR exercises, have the patients perform these while walking or while standing on balance foam. Increase the duration of the exercise from 1 to 2 minutes as tolerated (Figures 4-14 and 4-15).

## VOR Exercise Variations

There are a number of ways to challenge the patient using VOR exercises by changing the conditions under which they are performed. For example, you may change the position in which the patient performs the exercise (sitting, standing, tandem standing), the visual target, speed of exercise, or add dual-task activities such as walking (or, for the athlete, running) while performing the VOR exercise. You may also change the visual stimulation of this exercise by using different visual

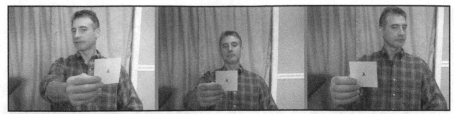

**Figure 4-14.** In performing VOR x2 yaw exercises, both the head and target move in the yaw (head shake "no" motion) plane, but in opposite directions.

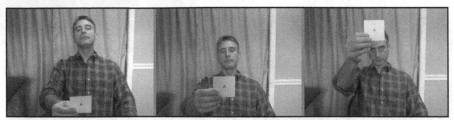

**Figure 4-15.** In performing VOR x2 pitch exercises, both the head and target move in the pitch (head shake "yes" motion) plane, but in opposite directions.

backgrounds. As mentioned, these exercises typically begin with the visual target on a solid-colored background. Later this may be progressed to a visual target with a busy background, such as a checkerboard. We honestly don't know if this makes a significant difference in the progression of the VOR gain, but it may help to increase patients' willingness to begin VOR exercises. When the vestibular system first begins to adapt, patients will more easily tolerate less challenging visual environments (and exercise target backgrounds). In general, when the vestibular system is uncompensated, busier backgrounds tend to make patients more nauseous owing to the added visual stimulation. Typical progressions include using a plain background and then moving to a busier background to increase visual stimulation during the exercise.

Here is an example of a beginning vestibular exercise: With the patient seated, perform VOR x1 up to 1 minute with a yaw head shake ("no" motion), followed by VOR x1 pitch motion up to 1 minute. Visual targets may include a single number or letter printed in the middle of a white piece of paper, junk mail with large letters, or playing cards with plain backgrounds. The patient picks a single letter or number as the visual target. The patient holds the target in his or her hand or has it placed on a wall or refrigerator. The patient takes breaks as needed based on exercise tolerance. For example, a patient might begin with VOR x1 yaw, but upon becoming nauseous after 30 seconds, he or she takes a break until the nausea subsides (usually within seconds or minutes). Once the patient feels better, he or she resumes the exercises until the prescribed "minute" is finished by picking up where he or she left off. In this example, once the exercise is resumed, the patient starts counting at "31." Next, the patient performs VOR x1 with pitch ("yes") motions, following the same guideline used in the yaw ("no") head shake example. Patients who often perform VOR x1 view exercises for 1 or 2 weeks in sitting and are progressed as soon as they tolerate more stimulation.

| TABLE 4-16<br>**EXAMPLE OF VESTIBULAR EXERCISE PROGRESSION** ||
| :-- | :-- |
| **THERAPY INTERVENTIONS** | **HOME EXERCISES** |
| Instruct and perform VOR x1.<br>Begin with VOR x1 view.<br>Position: Seated.<br>Visual background: plain background.<br>Timed: up to 1 minute pitch, then 1 minute yaw (taking breaks as needed to reduce nausea or dizziness). | VOR x1 seated x1 min pitch and yaw planes. Perform 3 or 4 times daily taking breaks as needed. |
| VOR x1.<br>Position: Standing on a solid surface (guarded at first for safety).<br>Visual background: Any as tolerated.<br>Timed: Multiple trials up to 1 minute pitch, then 1 minute yaw (taking breaks as needed to reduce nausea or dizziness). | VOR x1 with a plain visual background. Perform standing if safe to do so alone or continue seated VOR x1 if unsafe to stand without supervision. |
| VOR x1.<br>Position: Standing on a soft (compliant) surface like foam (guarded for safety).<br>Visual background: Any as tolerated.<br>Timed: Multiple trials up to 1 minute pitch, then 1 minute yaw (taking breaks as needed to reduce nausea or dizziness).<br>Variations: Speed, visual target distance and/or angle. | VOR x1 standing, with their back inches from the corner of a room and a chair back in front. This provides some amount of safety in case of loss of balance. If unsafe to perform standing alone, continue sitting VOR x1 as home exercise. |
| | *(continued)* |

How can we vary this exercise? Again, we use changes in position, environment, or task. To challenge the visual and vestibular systems, we can change exercise speed, exercise duration, visual targets, visual target angles (eg, the patient has to look up or down to see the target), distance to visual target, and background (eg, plain vs busy). To challenge balance while this exercise is being performed, we may have the patient stand on different surfaces or vary stance positions. For example, we may start by standing with feet shoulder-width apart on a firm surface but later progress to a more narrow stance, partial tandem stance, full tandem stance, or change the standing surface by having the patient stand on a piece of foam. Ultimately we want the patient to perform functional tasks while performing head turns (eg, walking). Take patients' abilities into account when advancing exercise difficulty and always make sure they are safe from falling. Use gait belts for VOR exercises that incorporate standing or walking. Table 4-16 presents an example of the progression of exercise.

| TABLE 4-16 (CONTINUED) |||
|---|---|
| **EXAMPLE OF VESTIBULAR EXERCISE PROGRESSION** |||
| **THERAPY INTERVENTIONS** | **HOME EXERCISES** |
| VOR x2.<br><br>Position: Standing on a soft (compliant) surface like foam (guarded for safety).<br><br>Visual background: Any as tolerated.<br><br>Timed: Multiple trials up to 1 minute pitch, then 1 minute yaw (taking breaks as needed to reduce nausea or dizziness). | VOR x1 with any tolerated background.<br><br>Perform standing if safe to do so alone, or continue seated VOR x1 if unsafe to stand without supervision.<br><br>Variations: Number of repetitions or time performed, visual angle or distance. |
| Ambulation while performing head turns at the discretion of the therapist.<br><br>• Randomize direction of head turns.<br><br>• Maintain head turn for 2 or 3 steps, then change. Simple left-center-right, and up-center-down patterns. | Ambulation with head turns every 3 or 4 steps using simple horizontal (eg, left-center-right-center-left), and vertical patterns (eg, up-center-down-center-up). |
| Ambulation while performing head turns at the discretion of the therapist.<br><br>• Randomize direction of head turns.<br><br>• Maintain head turn for 2 or 3 steps, then change.<br><br>• Head patterns now include looking up or down diagonally left or right.<br><br>• Variations: May include perturbations, or walking on different surface types. | Ambulation with head turns that now include diagonal patterns. |
| Athletes or healthier/active patients:<br><br>Quick walk or run forwards and backwards while performing VOR x1 with a fixed visual target. | Ambulation with head turns that now include diagonal patterns. |

## VOR Exercise Speed

The speed of the VOR exercises seems to make a difference. The head shake should be between 1 to 2 Hz. Recall that 1 Hz is equal to 360 degrees of motion per second. How do you estimate what 1 Hz of head motion for your patient would be? We typically do not have patients perform these exercises with large head rotations, but *imagine* a pace of head motion where the patient moves from full left cervical rotation to full right rotation and then back to full left again, doing this in 1 second. Now, keeping this speed of head motion in mind, imagine the patient performing the VOR exercises at that pace but without actually going to full rotation to each side. A simple instruction that helps convey this is to tell the patient to do the exercise "as fast as you can as long as the target is still visually clear." Generally this verbal cue is enough to get the patient to move at or above the 1-Hz mark. If it is not, you may wish to demonstrate a correct speed and use verbal or the auditory cues of a metronome to increase head speed as the patient performs the exercise. Many metronome phone and tablet apps are available. Using different frequencies (at or above 1 Hz) seems to be beneficial and should include some high-velocity stimulus.[70]

Cohen and Kimball, in a small sample size of subjects, reported no difference between rapidly performed vestibular exercises vs more slowly performed vestibular rehabilitation.[22,71] However, during head motions at frequencies less than 1 Hz, patients can use optokinetics and pursuit systems to stabilize eye gaze.[31] This would suggest that to effectively challenge the vestibular system, the pace (speed) of the exercise would have to be *at least* 1 Hz or faster to avoid the use of oculomotor and pursuit systems to accomplish the exercise task.

## VOR-C

If your examination reveals a deficient VOR-C, you may wish to try adding VOR-C as an exercise. There is currently no evidence directly supporting its use; however, if we use the general practice of challenging the deficient system to effect some kind of change, this intervention seems to have face validity. Remember, a deficient VOR-C indicates a central problem.

To perform VOR-C, instruct the patient to hold a visual target at arm's length and then move the target. As the target moves, the patient should move his or her head with the target so that it always remains directly in front of his or her nose (and view). You may have the patient perform these exercises for a set amount of time or repetitions (eg, 1 set of 20 movements).

## Cawthorne-Cooksey Exercises

These exercises were developed in the 1940s in London and were among the first interventions used for patients with vestibular problems who had undergone surgery of the labyrinth.[57,58] Table 4-17 offers a description of the Cawthorne-Cooksey exercises. The aim of the exercise plan was to do the following:

- Loosen up the muscle of the neck and shoulders to overcome the protective muscular spasm and tendency to move "in one piece."
- Train movement of the eyes independent of the head.
- Practice balancing under everyday conditions with special attention to developing the use of the eyes and muscle and joint sense.
- Practice head movements that cause giddiness and thus gradually overcome the disability.
- Become accustomed to moving about naturally in day light and in the dark.

---

**TABLE 4-17**
# CAWTHORNE-COOKSEY EXERCISES

The exercises as originally described are to be performed as follows[72]:

A. *In bed:*
1. Eye movements-at first slow, then quick
   a. Up and down
   b. Side to side
   c. Focusing on finger moving from 3 feet to 1 foot away from face
2. Head movements at first slow, then quick. Later with eyes closed.
   a. Bending forward and backward
   b. Turning from side to side

B. *Sitting* (in class):
1 and 2a
3. Shoulder shrugging and circling
4. Bending forward and picking up objects from the ground

C. *Standing* (in class):
1, 2, and 3,
4. Changing from sitting to standing position with eyes open and shut
5. Throwing a small ball from hand to hand (above eye level)
6. Throwing ball from hand to hand under knee
7. Change from sitting to standing and turning round in between

D. *Moving about* (in class):
1. Circle around center person who will throw a large ball and to whom it will be returned
2. Walk across room with eyes open and then closed
3. Walk up and down slope with eyes open and then closed
4. Walk up and down steps with eyes open and then closed
5. Any game involving stooping or stretching and aiming such as skittles, bowls, and basketball

A link to a copy of the original article detailing the exercises is available on Dr. Timothy Hain's website: www.diziness-and-balance.com/treatment/rehab/cawthorne/html

---

These exercises are still in use today, and many ENTs give them as home exercises. It is important to note, however, that supervision is recommended. If you read through the list of exercises, you can see that they do require the patient to perform a lot of dynamic movements, which may be challenging for a patient who is dizzy and/or whose balance is already compromised. Cawthorne-Cooksey exercises will stimulate the vestibular system, but there are no specific VOR exercises in the list. Does this make a difference? A study by Szturm et al compared Cawthorne-Cooksey exercises (given as home exercises) to a vestibular rehab program that was supervised (the frequency of treatments was 3 times a week for 12 weeks) and found a significant improvement in standing balance performance under dynamic conditions for patients in the rehab program but not for patients who performed the Cawthorne-Cooksey exercises.[73] In fairness, there was not a "supervised Cawthorne-Cooksey" exercise group with which to compare. How much of the improvement was due to supervision vs customizing the vestibular exercises is unknown.

## Efficacy of Vestibular Rehabilitation Therapy

Many research studies demonstrate efficacy of vestibular rehabilitation therapy[22,74]; it is now considered the standard of care for persons with peripheral vestibular dysfunction. In a 2011 Cochrane Review of 27 trials involving 1668 participants, individual and pooled data showed a statistically significant effect in favor of vestibular rehabilitation over controls or no intervention, without any adverse effects reported.[22]

Studies by Herdman,[74,75] Resende,[76] and Strupp[41] offer evidence for improvement in measures of balance, ADLs, and vision compared to no intervention or sham interventions.[23]

Other studies have found the following:

- Use of vestibular exercises is the main factor involved in recovery of dynamic visual acuity in patients with bilateral vestibular hypofunction.[69]

- In a study of 125 subjects, there was a fast recovery in the supervised vestibular rehabilitation exercise group.[77]

- A study of 37 patients in post-vestibular rehab observed a significant improvement in Dizziness Handicap Inventory scores.[78]

- There is evidence suggesting that an individualized exercise program is better than a generic exercise program.[39,63]

- Whitney et al compared the effects of age on outcomes following vestibular therapy. They found that age did not have a significant influence on the beneficial effects of therapy (using the Dizziness Handicap Inventory, Dynamic Gait Index) and reported number of falls as outcome measures. At discharge, there were no significant differences between older and younger subjects based on these measures. Herdman et al also found that age did affect which patients would improve; however, they did find that older patients walked more slowly and had poorer visual acuity during head motions as compared with younger patients, as would be expected based on the aging process. Older patients were also more likely to remain at risk for falls after treatment than were younger patients.[55]

# Effects of Vestibular Therapy on Balance and Fall Risk

- According to Alghadir et al,[68] vestibular exercises improve balance, decrease risk of falling, decrease dizziness, and improve quality of life.[22,38,41,73-75,79-82]
- Vestibular rehabilitation therapy plays an important preventative role in reducing falls in at-risk elderly patients. In a retrospective review of 70 patients older than 50 years of age, vestibular rehab therapy resulted in a statistically significant improvement in Berg balance scores.[83]
- In an observational study of customized programs of balance and vestibular habituation, Shepard et al report statistically significant changes before vs after therapy for both specific measures, and 80% to 85% of the patients showed reduction in symptoms and disability scores following therapy.[64]

## Bilateral Vestibular Loss

Even though the vestibular system is deficient bilaterally, vestibular therapy still helps patients with BVL; however, recovery from bilateral deficits occurs more slowly than from unilateral lesions and not all patients improve.[36,37] Patients with BVL improve more with a customized exercise program than with a generalized strengthening program.[38,39] Goals for patients with BVL include enhancing gait stability by increasing function in whatever is left working in the vestibular systems and improving gait patterns by training patients to substitute information from the vision and somatosensory systems for that of the missing vestibular input.[31,40]

## Chronic Vestibulopathy

Vestibular rehabilitation improves subjective measures of dizziness, level of performance on the Dizziness Handicap Inventory, and gait performance as measured by the Dynamic Gait Index in people with chronic peripheral vestibulopathy, as compared with sham exercise, no vestibular rehabilitation, or usual care.[22-24,27]

## Vestibular Neuritis

Strupp et al found that postural control measures improved more in a group of patients with vestibular neuritis who performed vestibular rehabilitation compared with no specific intervention other than encouragement to move.[22,41]

Teggi et al found that vestibular rehabilitation significantly reduced anxiety in people with acute neuritis compared with a control group.[22,24]

There is plenty of evidence to show that vestibular rehab is efficacious and safe and that it is applicable to many patient populations. The key for patient safety is to always refer patients with positive signs of vestibular function loss for further testing. These are not your patients with classic BPPV but those with either acute or chronic vestibular signs or symptoms. Vestibular therapy will most likely reduce or resolve symptoms, and there has to be a plan to rule out central findings to make sure that the therapy is not masking central signs and symptoms. Vestibular testing should be a part of any evaluation where the patient has difficulty balancing, has complaints of dizziness or nausea, or there is a recent history of a fall or head trauma.

# REFERENCES

1. Tusa R. History and clinical examination. In: Herdman S, ed. *Vestibular Rehabilitation*. 3rd ed. Philadelphia: FA Davis; 2000:107-124.
2. Schubert M, Tusa R, Grine L, Herdman S. Optimizing the sensitivity of the head thrust test for identifying vestibular hypofunction. *Phys Ther*. 2004;84(2):151-158.
3. Beynon G, Baguley DMA. Clinical evaluation of head impulse testing. *Clin Otolaryngol*. 1998;23:117-122.
4. Weber KP, Aw ST, Todd MJ, McGarvie LA, Curthoys IS, Halmagyi GM. Head impulse test in unilateral vestibular loss: vestibulo-ocular reflex and catch-up saccades. *Neurology*. 2008;70(6):454-463.
5. Grine E, Herdman S, Tusa R. Sensitivity and specificity of head thrust for peripheral vestibular patients. *Neurol Rep*. 2000;24:177.
6. Hain T, Fetter M, Zee D. Head-shaking nystagmus in patients with unilateral peripheral vestibular lesions. *Am J Otolaryngol*. 1987;8:36-47.
7. Department of Otolaryngology, Washington University School of Medicine. The ten-minute examination of the dizzy patient. Available at http://www.medscape.com/viewarticle/422863_3. Updated 2001. Accessed October 4, 2014.
8. Eggers S, Zee D. *Handbook of Clinical Neurophysiology*. Vol. 9. *Vertigo and Imbalance: Clinical Neurophysiology of the Vestibular System*. Amsterdam: Elsevier; 2010.
9. Herdman S, Tusa R, Blatt P, Suzuki A, Venuto P, Roberts D. Computerized dynamic visual acuity test in the assessment of vesitubular deficits. *Am J Otol*. 1998;19:790-796.
10. Schubert M, Herdman S, Tusa R. Vertical dynamic visual acuity in normal subjects and subjects with vestibular hypofunction. *Otol Neurotol*. 2002;23:372-377.
11. Slattery EL, Sinks BC, Goebel JA. Vestibular tests for rehabilitation: applications and interpretation. *NeuroRehabilitation*. 2011;29:143-151.
12. Rambold H, Deide W, Sprenger A, Haendler G, Helmchen C. Perilymph fistula associated with pulse-synchronous eye oscillations. *Neurology*. 2001;56:1769-1771.
13. Minor LB. Superior canal dehiscence syndrome. *Am J Otol*. 2000;21:9-19.
14. Leigh RJ, Zee D. *The Neurology of Eye Movements*. 4th ed. New York: Oxford University Press; 2006.
15. American Academy of Family Physicians; American Academy of Otolaryngology-Head and Neck Surgery; American Academy of Pediatrics Subcommittee on Otitis Media With Effusion. Otitis media with effusion. *Pediatrics*. 2004;113(5):1412-1429.
16. Goebel JA. *Practical Management of the Dizzy Patient*. 2nd ed. Philadelphia: Lippincott Williams & Wilkins; 2008.
17. Shepard N, Telian S. *Practical Management of the Balance Disorder Patient*. San Diego: Singular Publishing Group; 1996.
18. Merchant S, Nadol J. *Schuknecht's Pathology of the Ear*. 3rd ed. Middlesbrough, UK: McGraw-Hill Education; 2010.
19. Johns Hopkins. Survey suggests higher risk of falls due to dizziness in middle-aged and older adults. 2009.
20. Cooper C. Vestibular neuronitis: a review of common causes of vertigo in general practice. *Br J Gen Pract*. 1993;43:164-167.
21. Schubert M, Minor L. Vestibulo-ocular physiology underlying vesitbular hypofunction. *Phys Ther*. 2004;84:373-385.
22. Hillier S, McDonnell M. Vestibular rehabilitation for unilateral peripheral vestibular dysfunction. *Cochran Database Syst Rev*. 2011;16(2):CD005397.
23. Horak F, Jones-Rycewicz C, Black F, Shumway-Cook A. Effects of vestibular rehabilitation on dizziness and imbalance. *Otolaryngol Head Neck Surg*. 1992;106(2):175-180.
24. Teggi R, Cladirola D, Fabiano B, Pecanati P, Bussi M. Rehabilitation after acute vestibular disorders. *J Laryngol Otol*. 2009;123(4):397-402.

25. Giray M, Kirazli Y, Karapolat H, Celebisoy N, Bilgen C, Kirazli T. Short-term effects of vestibular rehabilitation in patients with chronic unilateral vestibular dysfunction: a randomised controlled study. *Arch Phys Med Rehabil.* 2009;90(8):1325-1331.

26. Vereeck L, Wuyts F, Truijen S, De Valck C, Vande Heyning P. The effect of early customised vestibular rehabilitationon balance after acoustic neuroma resection. *Clin Rehabil.* 2008;22:698-713.

27. Yardley L, Beech S, Zander L, Evans T, Weinman J. A randomised controlled trial of exercise therapy for dizziness and vertigo in primary care. *Br J Gen Pract.* 1998;48:1136-1140.

28. Yardley L, Donovan-Hal lM, Smith HE, Walsh BM, Mullee M, Bronstein AM. Effectiveness of primary care-based vestibular rehabilitation for chronic dizziness. *Ann Intern Med.* 2004;141:598-605

29. Gurr B, Moffat N. Psychological consequences of vertigo and effectiveness of vestibular rehabilitation for brain injury patients. *Brain Inj.* 2001;15:387-400.

30. Murray K, Carroll S, Hill K. Relationship between change in balance and self-reported handicap after vestibular rehabilitation therapy. *Physiother Res Int.* 2001;6:251-263.

31. Whitney S, France D. Bilateral vestibular disease: an overview. *NeuroReport.* 1996;20(3):41-45.

32. Furman J, Cass S. *Balance Disorders: A Case-Study Approach.* Philadelphia: FA Davis; 1996.

33. Hain TC. Chemotherapy. Available at http://www.dizziness-and-balance.com/disorders/bilat/chemotherapy.html. Updated 2013. Accessed October 1, 2014.

34. Hain TC. Causes of bilateral vestibulopathy. Available at http://www.dizziness-and-balance.com/disorders/bilat/bilat_cause.html. Updated 2013. Accessed October 1, 2014.

35. Telian S, Shephard N, Smith-Wheelock M, Hoberg M. Bilateral vestibular paresis: diagnosis and treatment. *Otol Head Neck Surg.* 1991;104:67-71.

36. Igarashi M, Ishikawa K, Ishii M, et al. Physical exercise and balance compensation after total ablation of vestibular organs. *Prog Brain Res.* 1988;76:395.

37. Krebs D, Gill-Body K, Parker S, et al. Vestibular rehabilitation: useful but not universally so. *Otolaryngol Head Neck Surg.* 2003;111:1812.

38. Krebs D, Gill-Body K, Riley P, Parker S. Double-blind placebo-controlled trial of rehabilitation for bilateral vestibular hypofunction—preliminary report. *Otol Head Neck Surg.* 1993;109:735-741.

39. Whitney S, Sparto P. Principles of vestibular physical therapy rehabilitation. *Neuro Rehabil.* 2011;29:157-166.

40. Herdman S, Clendaniel R. Assessment and interventions for the patient with complete vestibular loss. In: Herdman S, ed. *Vestibular Rehabilitation.* 3rd ed. Philadelphia: FA Davis; 2000:338-359.

41. Strupp M, Arbusow V, Dieterich M, et al. Perceptual and oculomotor effects of neck muscle vibration in vestibular neuritis. Ipsilateral somatosensory substitution of vestibular function. *Brain.* 1998;121:677-685.

42. Brandt T, Dieterich M, Strupp M. *Vertigo and Dizziness.* London: Springer; 2005.

43. Helmchen C, Klinkenstein J, Machner B, et al. Structural changes in the human brain following vestibular neuritis indicate central vestibular compensation. *Ann N Y Acad Sci.* 2009;1164:104-115.

44. Helmchen C, Klinkenstein JC, Krüger A, Gliemroth J, Mohr C, Sander T. Structural brain changes following peripheral vestibulo-cochlear lesion may indicate multisensory compensation. *J Neurol Psychiatry.* 2011;82:309-316.

45. Hain TC. Acoustic neuroma. Available at http://american-hearing.org/disorders/acoustic-neuroma/#whatis. Updated 2014. Accessed October 1, 2014.

46. American Hearing Research Foundation. B12 deficiency. Available at http://american-hearing.org/disorders/b12-deficiency/. Updated 2012. Accessed October 4, 2014.

47. Hain TC. Mal de debarquement (MDD). American Hearing Research Foundation Web site. http://american-hearing.org/disorders/mal-de-debarquement-mdd/. Updated 2012. Accessed 03/03, 2015.

48. Ménière's disease. *ADAM Medical Encyclopedia.* Available at http://www.ncbi.nlm.nih.gov/pubmedhealth/PMH0001721/. Updated 2013. Accessed October 4, 2014.

49. Harris J, Alexander T. Current-day prevalence of Ménière's syndrome. *Audiol Neurotol.* 2010;15:318-322.

50. Medtronic. Meiett device. Available at http://www.medtronic.com/for-healthcare-professionals/products-therapies/ear-nose-throat/menieres-disease-product/meniett-device-for-menieres-disease/index.htm#tab3. Updated 2013. Accessed October 4, 2014.

51. InnerEarProblems.net. Secondary endolymphatic hydrops. Available at http://www.innerearproblems.net/secondary-endolymphatic-hydrops-seh-general-information-common-symptoms-and-treatment-options/. Accessed October 4, 2014.

52. Hain TC. Perilymph fistula. Available at http://american-hearing.org/disorders/perilymph-fistula/#whatis. Updated 2012. Accessed October 4, 2014.

53. Fetter M. Vestibular system disorders. In: Herdman S, ed. *Vestibular Rehabilitation*. 3rd ed. Philadelphia: FA Davis; 2007:102-103.

54. Han BI, Song HS, Kim JS. Vestibular rehabilitation therapy: review of indications, mechanisms, and key exercises. *J Clin Neurol*. 2011;7:184-196.

55. Herdman SJ, Hall CD, Delaune W. Variables associated with outcomes in patients with unilateral vestibular hypofunction. *Neurorehabil Neural Repair*. 2012;26:151-162.

56. Herdman S. Vestibular rehabilitation. *Curr Opin Neurol*. 2013;26(1):96-101.

57. Cooksey F. Rehabilitation in vestibular injuries. *Proc Soc Med*. 1946;39:273-278.

58. Cawthorne T. Vestibular injuries. *Proc Roy Soc Med*. 1946;39:270-278.

59. Norris ME, De Weerdt W. Treatment of vertigo based on habituation: I. Physiopathological basis. *J Laryngol Otol*. 1980;94:689-696.

60. Shepard N, Telian S, Smith-Wheelock M. Habituation and balance retraining therapy: a retrospective review. *Neurol Clin*. 1990;8(2):459-475.

61. Herdman S. *Vestibular Rehabilitation*. 3rd ed. Philadelphia: FA Davis; 2007.

62. Herdman SJ, Whitney SL. Intervention for the patient with vestibular hypofunction. In: Herdman S, ed. *Vestibular Rehabilitation*. 3rd ed. Philadelphia: FA Davis; 1995:309-337.

63. Shepard N, Telian S. Programmatic vestibular rehabilitation. *Head and Neck Surgery*. 1995;112:173-182.

64. Shepard NT, Telian SA, Smith-Wheelock M, Raj A. Vestibular and balance rehabilitation therapy. *Ann Otol Rhinol Laryngol*. 1993;102(3 Pt 1):198-205.

65. Fetter M, Zee DS, Proctor LR. Effect of lack of vision and of occipital lobectomy upon recovery from unilateral labyrinthectomy in rhesus monkey. *J Neurophysiol*. 1988;59:383-389.

66. Keim RJ, Cook M, Martini D. Balance rehabilitation therapy. *Laryngoscope*. 1992;102:1302-1307.

67. Furman JM, Balaban CD, Pollack IF. Vestibular compensation in a patient with cerebellar infarction. *Neurology*. 1997;48:916-920.

68. Alghadir A, Iqbal Z, Whitney S. An update on vestibular physical therapy. *J Chin Med Assoc*. 2013;76(1):1-8.

69. Herdman SJ, Hall CD, Shubert MC, Das VE, Tusa RJ. Recovery of dynamic visual acuity in bilateral vestibular hypofunction. *Arch Oolaryngol Head Neck Surg*. 2007;133(4):383-389.

70. Clendaniel RA, Lasker DM, Minor LB. Differential adaptation of the linear and nonlinear components of the horizontal vestibuloocular reflex in squirrel monkeys. *J Neurophysiol*. 2002;88:3534-3534.

71. Cohen H, Kimball K. Increased independence and decreased vertigo after vestibular rehabilitation. *Otol Head Neck Surg*. 2003;128(1):60-70.

72. Fairley J, Fairley S. Cawthorn Cooksey historic source. Available at http://entkent.com/Cawthorne-Cooksey-Historical-Source.php. Updated 2014. Accessed October 4, 2014.

73. Szturm T, Ireland D, Lessing-Turner M. Comparison of different exercise programs in the rehabiitation of patients with chronic peripheral vestibular dysfunction. *J Vest Res*. 1994;4(6):461-479.

74. Herdman S, Clendaniel R, Mattox D, Holiday M, Niparko J. Vestibular adaptation exercises and recovery: acute stage after acoustic neuroma resection. *Otolaryngol Head Neck Surg*. 1995;113:77-87.

75. Herdman S, Schubert M, Das V, Tusa R. Recovery of dynamic visual acuity in unilateral vestibular hypofunction. *Arch Otolaryngol Head Neck*. 2003;129:819-824.

76. Resende C, Taguchi C, de Almeida J, Fujita R. Vestibular rehabilitation in elderly patients with benign paroxysmal positional vertigo. *Brazil J Otorhinolaryngol*. 2003;63:.

77. Topuz O, Topuz B, Ardic FN, Sarhus M, Ogmen G, Ardic F. Efficacy of vestibular rehabilitation on chronic unilateral vestibular dysfunction. *Clin Rehabil.* 2004;18(1):76-83.

78. Cowand JL, Wrisley DM, Walker M, Strasnick B, Jacobson JT. Efficacy of vestibular rehabilitation. *Otolaryngol Head Neck Surg.* 1998;118(1):49-54.

79. Pavlou M. The use of optokinetic stimulation in vestibular rehabilitation. *J Neurol Phys Ther.* 2010;34(2):105-110.

80. Helminski J, Zee D, Janssen I, Hain T. Effectiveness of particle repositioning maneuvers in the treatment of benign paroxysmal postional vertigo: a systematic review. *Phys Ther.* 2010;90(5):663-678.

81. El-Kashlan HK, Shpard NT, Arts HA, Telian SA. Disability from vestibular symptoms after acoustic neuroma resection. *Am J Otol.* 1998;19:104-111.

82. Jacob RG, Whitney SL, Detweiler-Shostak G, Furman JM. Vestibular rehabilitation for patients with agoraphobia and vestibular dysfunction: a pilot study. *J Anxiety Disord.* 2001;15:131-146.

83. Marcias J, Ellensohn A, Massingale S, Gerkin R. Vibration does not improve results of the canalith repositioning procedure. *Arch Otolaryngol Head Neck.* 2000;126(5):617-622.

# Benign Paroxysmal Positional Vertigo (BPPV)

## CHAPTER GOALS

1. Describe common symptoms of benign paroxysmal positional vertigo (BPPV).

2. Describe signs of canalithiasis and cupulolithiasis.

3. Name 2 tests of posterior canal BPPV.

4. Name one test of lateral canal BPPV.

5. Identify conditions requiring extra care during examination or treatment of BPPV.

6. Identify contraindications to testing/treating BPPV.

7. Name and describe a repositioning maneuver for BPPV of each canal.

BPPV is the most common vestibular disorder, accounting for one-third of vestibular diagnoses in the general population.[1,2] In BPPV, calcium carbonate otoconia have come loose from the otolithic membrane in the utricle and, when the patient changes head position or makes forceful head motions, move within the canals owing to the pull of gravity. This is a peripheral vestibular disorder. Within 7 days of posterior canal BPPV onset, 30% of patients will experience spontaneous remission.[2,3]

Make sure the patient does not have any contraindications to testing or treatment, such as the following[4]:

Plishka CM.
*A Clinician's Guide to Balance and Dizziness:*
*Evaluation and Treatment* (pp 111-189).
© 2015 Taylor & Francis Group.

- Acute fractures that prevent the patient from lying down quickly or rolling
- Recent neck fracture, surgery, or instability
- History of vertebral dissection or unstable carotid disease
- Recent retinal detachment

Patients with BPPV often experience delays in diagnosis and treatment, the mean delay being 92 weeks, and they are frequently treated inappropriately with vestibular suppressant medications.[2,5] The best treatment for BPPV is the use of canalith repositioning maneuvers, which resolve most cases. Reported recurrence rates after treatment[6-8] are between 22.6% and 30%, but the performance of repositioning maneuvers early after the onset of symptoms seems to decrease the rates of recurrence.[9]

During testing, the clinician observes the patient's eyes and pays attention to subjective patient complaints. The latency (how long it takes for symptoms and nystagmus to develop after the patient is placed into a test position), direction of nystagmus, and duration of nystagmus are used to classify the type of BPPV the patient has. It is possible to observe the nystagmus without special equipment, but the use of eye-magnifying Frenzel goggles or infrared goggles will enhance the clinician's ability to observe these eye motions, even subtle ones. Latency for the onset of signs and symptoms of posterior canal BPPV during testing ranges from 5 to 30 seconds and is usually not more than 15 seconds. Some patients may have latencies longer than 30 seconds.[10] The duration of the nystagmus typically is no longer than 1 minute for the loose type of "canalolithiasis" (or canalithiasis).[11]

# BENIGN PAROXYSMAL POSITIONAL VERTIGO SYMPTOMS

As the name implies, BPPV is a condition that creates sensations of motion (*vertigo*) that suddenly start and stop (*paroxysmal*) with *position* changes of the head with respect to gravity; it is nonlethal (*benign*). Patients usually describe experiencing a spinning sensation, with both seeing and feeling the room spin. This sensation may cause nausea and vomiting. The spinning vertigo typically lasts less than 20 seconds; it typically lasts less than 1 minute for the posterior canal but last longer when crystals are loose in the lateral (horizontal) canal.[12]

Patients often report that these symptoms first appeared while they were performing position changes, as while rolling in bed, getting out of bed, bending over to tie their shoes or pick up laundry, extending their heads while washing their hair, or while getting their hair washed/cut. While these are the typical symptoms, some patients report nonspecific dizziness, light-headedness, postural instability, and/or nausea without vertigo or nystagmus.[11,13-15] These patients may respond to canalith repositioning maneuvers.[11]

| TABLE 5-1 SIGNS OF BENIGN PAROXYSMAL POSITIONAL VERTIGO WHILE IN TEST POSITIONS | |
| --- | --- |
| **CANAL** | **OBSERVED EYE MOTIONS IN TEST POSITIONS** |
| Posterior | Upbeating with torsion |
| Lateral (horizontal) | Lateral beating either toward or away from the ground |
| Anterior | Downbeating with torsion |

# ▶ BENIGN PAROXYSMAL POSITIONAL VERTIGO SIGNS

In most cases clinicians observe nystagmus during testing. Crystals moving in different canals cause the eyes to move in different directions.[16] Table 5-1 provides a description of eye motions that occur with canal stimulation.

In anterior and posterior canal BPPV, vertigo and nystagmus occur when the head is in the provoking position and nystagmus reverse direction when the patient returns to sitting.

Let's take our understanding of the semicircular canals a bit further than we have done already. First, consider a semicircular canal. As described earlier, as the canal leaves the utricle it moves away from it and then at some point turns back and reattaches to it. The part of the canal *after* the bend, where it turns back, is shorter than the part of the canal before the bend, so we call it the short arm of the canal. The longer portion of the canal that is *before* the bend is the long arm.

Just before the canal reattaches to the utricle (after the bend, where it turns back) is a wide area called the *ampulla*. The area of the ampulla is wider than the rest of the canal; it houses the cupula, which completely blocks off the canal. During BPPV, the otoconia (crystals) that normally anchor to the otolithic matrix in the utricle are now loose and free-floating in the canal or ampulla, or stuck on the cupula. Either way, the crystals are where they do not belong.

We classify BPPV into 1 of 2 groups: loose or stuck. *Canalithiasis* is the term used to describe the loose variety. If we break this word down, we see *lith*, which is a derivation of *lithos*, or Greek for "stone"; we also see the word *canal*. So *canalithiasis* literally means "a stone that is loose in the canal." *Cupulolithiasis* describes the stuck variety of BPPV. Again, if we break the word down, we see that there is a stone (*lith*) and *cupulo*, referring to the cupula. The word *cupulolithiasis* therefore refers to a stone that is stuck on the cupula. In cupulolithiasis, the loose crystals move to the end of the canal and anchor to the cupula (remember that they are sticky). Now you have a weight attached to the cupula where there should be none. This added weight makes the cupula susceptible to gravity upon tilting, when normally it is only susceptible to velocity changes of the head. Some researchers dispute the concept of cupulolithiasis or argue that symptoms presenting as cupulolithiasis may have other causes. Some suggest that the crystals are not actually stuck on the cupula but instead are trapped in the short arm of the canal,[17] Since we can't get an image of moving or stuck crystals, we currently do not know who is right. However, what we do know is that some maneuvers work better than others, given a set of signs and symptoms. Whatever the reason behind the presentations of nystagmus, we will still classify them as either cupulolithiasis or canalithiasis, and we will choose from treatment interventions that have been shown to be effective for each type.

# BENIGN PAROXYSMAL POSITIONAL VERTIGO INCIDENCE

BPPV is the most common vestibular cause of dizziness in older patients[18] and the most common vestibular disorder in adults, with a lifetime prevalence[19] of 2.4%. Up to 90% of cases of positional vertigo/nystagmus are attributable to BPPV.[20] BPPV has different causes, but the largest group is *idiopathic*, meaning that we don't know what caused it.

Lee and Kim share the following facts about idiopathic BPPV[13]:
- It is more prevalent among the elderly and in women, with a peak age of onset in the sixth decade of life.[13,21,22]
- It is more likely to involve the right ear.[1]
- Nystagmus diminishes (fatigues) with repeated testing in the same session.

Fife et al share these facts about BPPV[23]:
- The term *BPPV* does not include vertigo caused by the central nervous system.
- Most cases of BPPV affect the posterior canal.
- Canalith repositioning is established as an effective and safe therapy that should be offered to patients of all ages with posterior BPPV.

*Secondary BPPV* results from some other event, illness, or injury. According to Riga et al, BPPV seems to be associated with inner-ear disease more often than was previously believed. The common conditions that cause secondary BPPV (and incidences based on a variety of studies) include head trauma (8.5% to 27%), vestibular neuritis (0.8% to 20%), Ménière's disease (0.5% to 30%), and surgical treatment (dental implants 3% and cochlear implants 0% to 28%).

BPPV secondary to head trauma occurs across all demographics; it is not uncommon to find young patients as well as old with a history of head trauma suffering from BPPV. There is a higher incidence of bilateral BPPV in patients with a history of head trauma vs the idiopathic type.[24]

In a study by Gross et al of 41 patients with a diagnosis of Ménière's disease, 18 patients had bilateral BPPV, 16 had BPPV of the same ear, and 7 had BPPV in the ear that was contralateral to that affected by Ménière's disease. In most patients who had BPPV in this patient population, onset began within a week following an attack, while 10% had simultaneous onset with the Ménière's attack.[25]

For BPPV in the patients with vestibular neuritis, onset of the BPPV occurred as late as 18 days after the onset of the neuritis.[26]

Migraines and sudden sensorineural hearing loss (0.2% to 5%) also play a role in the pathogenesis of BPPV.[24] In one study, the incidence of migraine in patients with BPPV was twice as high as in age- and sex-matched controls who did not suffer from migraines.[27]

A survey of female participants in one study ($n$ = 168) showed that 48.1% experienced their first episode of BPPV after menopause.[28] Other diseases associated with an increased incidence of BPPV include giant-cell arteritis, diabetes, and osteopenia/osteoporosis.[24]

# PATHOMECHANICS AND VARIATIONS OF BENIGN PAROXYSMAL POSITIONAL VERTIGO

In Chapter 1 we learned the anatomy of the vestibular system. Recall that there are otoconia (calcium-carbonate crystals) in the utricle and saccule that anchor on top of the otolithic membrane (the gel-like substance that contains the hair cells). The condition of BPPV occurs when bunches of these crystals break free of the otolithic membrane and move into one or more of the semicircular canals by virtue of the patient's head position or motion. Whenever the patient changes the position of his or her head with respect to the ground, the crystals will fall/sink toward the ground within the vestibular system. When the otoconia move into the canals, the patient may experience vertigo. This migration of crystals into the canals often happens during sleep, while the patient is rolling in bed. When the patient changes head positions and the crystals move, they push or pull fluid either toward or away from the cupula. This fluid motion causes the cupula to deflect (bend). When the cupula bends, the groups of hair cells that are contained within it bend and change the firing rates of the attached nerves. Depending on the direction in which the hair cells are bending, the nerves will either fire faster or slower, causing a difference (asymmetry) between the firing rates of each ear, and this asymmetry activates the vestibulo-ocular reflex (VOR). As a result, the patient complains of a "spinning" sensation and during the nystagmus may see the room spin. In most cases, this sensation lasts 1 minute or less, but it may occur again the next time the patient changes head position with respect to the ground (gravity).

Here is an easy way to understand the crystal movements. Imagine that you take a tire that is sitting on the ground (as if it were on a car) and drilled a hole in it, through which you dropped a bunch of pebbles. What happens? The pebbles would fall to wherever the ground was, but inside the tire. If you rolled the tire, the pebbles would move and roll inside the tire, again to lowest point closest to ground. This is what happens in BPPV with otoconia inside the vestibular system. You have a canal that is almost a complete circle and have a bunch of pebbles loose inside (otoconia) that will fall/roll to wherever the ground happens to be. Unlike the tire, the vestibular canals are full of endolymph fluid. As the otoconia roll, they push the fluid in front of them and pull (like a plunger) the fluid behind them. Depending on the direction of fluid motion, the cupula will bend either toward or away from the utricle. As the cupula

| TABLE 5-2 FREQUENCY OF BENIGN PAROXYSMAL POSITIONAL VERTIGO BY CANAL INVOLVEMENT[29] | |
| --- | --- |
| Posterior canal | 90% |
| Lateral (horizontal) canal | 3% to 12% |
| Anterior canal | 2% |
| Bilateral (both ears) BPPV[30,31] | 4.4% to 9.3% |

moves, the signals from that canal will either increase or decrease compared with the normal resting rate. The signal change depends on the canal that is being stimulated and in which direction the cupula of that canal deflects. Otoconia rolling in one ear will stimulate only that ear. Since both ears are now firing at different rates, the brain interprets the signal difference (asymmetry) as head motion and activates the VOR.

While it is in the anatomical position, the posterior canal sits the lowest (caudal) in the inner ear compared with the other canals. Most BPPV cases involve the posterior canals, as gravity pulls the crystals to the lowest point. However, you may see cases of BPPV in any canal, and sometimes in multiple canals simultaneously. Table 5-2 lists the frequency of BPPV by canal.

Common complaints from patients with BPPV are as follows:

- "I get dizzy when I get out of bed."
- "I get dizzy when I wash my hair"
- "I get dizzy when I bend over."
- And in our female patient group, "I get dizzy when I go to the hairdresser!"

The reported incidence of BPPV in each canal varies depending on the study, but by and large there is a common pattern, with posterior canal BPPV occurring most often, followed by lateral canal BPPV, and anterior canal BPPV occurring least frequently. Lateral canal BPPV (also called *horizontal canal BPPV*) may cause more severe symptoms of nausea and vertigo compared with BPPV of other canals.[32] Since the anterior canal is cephalad (closer to the top of the head) than the other canals, it has the lowest rate of BPPV incidence.

When patients say they get dizzy getting out of bed, you need to ask, "What happens when you lie down or roll over?" This will help to differentiate between symptoms of orthostatic hypotension and BPPV. With BPPV, the patient usually experiences vertigo, which is the illusion of movement (typically spinning) while either getting up or lying down. Symptoms of orthostatic hypotension occur when the patient moves from supine to sitting or sitting to standing, but typically not in the reverse direction.

Common causes of BPPV include viral infections of the ear and head trauma. There is also a significant correlation between the side on which a person sleeps and the side of posterior and lateral canal occurrences of BPPV.[33] Luckily this condition is typically easy to correct, with most cases resolved in only 1 or 2 treatments.

| TABLE 5-3 | | | |
| --- | --- | --- | --- |
| **SIGNS OF BENIGN PAROXYSMAL POSITIONAL VERTIGO BY CANAL** | | | |
| SIDE | ANTERIOR CANAL | LATERAL CANAL | POSTERIOR CANAL |
| Left | **Downbeating Left Rotational** <br><br> • Canalithiasis (loose): Latency up to 45 seconds, nystagmus < 1 minute <br><br> • Cupulolithiasis (stuck or near cupula): Immediate onset, nystagmus > 1 minute | **Lateral Beating Geotropic (loose)** <br><br> • Treat strong-symptom side <br><br> **Apogeotropic** (stuck or near cupula): <br><br> • Treat weak-symptom side | **Upbeating Left Rotational** <br><br> • Canalithiasis (loose): Latency up to 45 seconds, nystagmus < 1 minute <br><br> • Cupulolithiasis (stuck or near cupula): Immediate onset, nystagmus > 1 minute |
| Right | **Downbeating Right Rotational** <br><br> • Canalithiasis (loose): Latency up to 45 seconds, nystagmus < 1 minute <br><br> • Cupulolithiasis (stuck or near cupula): Immediate onset, nystagmus > 1 minute | **Lateral Beating Geotropic (loose)** <br><br> • Treat strong-symptom side <br><br> **Apogeotropic** (stuck or near cupula): <br><br> • Treat weak-symptom side | **Upbeating Right Rotational** <br><br> • Canalithiasis (loose): Latency up to 45 seconds, nystagmus < 1 minute <br><br> • Cupulolithiasis (stuck or near cupula): Immediate onset, nystagmus > 1 minute |

Otoconia, whether moving or stuck, in each canal will elicit specific eye motions. We use the eye motions that occur in response to changes in head position as a means of determining which canals are involved and which type of BPPV (stuck or loose) the patient has. When we document the findings of BPPV tests, we need to include the following:

- Which ear is involved (left or right)
- Which canal is involved (anterior, posterior, or lateral)
- Which variation is in question, canalithiasis (loose) or cupulolithiasis (stuck)

We choose which interventions to use based in a large part by these factors. In general we perform some type of "canalith repositioning" maneuver to move the crystals back into the utricle, where they will (hopefully) reattach to the otolithic matrix. Table 5-3 lists the expected eye motions that occur depending on the canal being stimulated.

For nystagmus stimulated by the crystals in the anterior and posterior canals, we expect to see both torsional nystagmus as well as an up- or down-beating nystagmus. These motions occur simultaneously and have quick and slow phases. The quick phase of the torsion will be toward the ear that is stimulated, while the up- or down-beating nystagmus tells you which canal is involved. The methods used to describe BPPV nystagmus can be confusing. Let's first describe them using the terms we have just defined.

First, imagine the patient in the anatomical position, facing you. When we reference anatomy on this person, we describe things from *the patient's* perspective. When we say "right," we mean what right is for the patient (not for you as you look at him or her). The same is true when we describe the direction of nystagmus beats or rotations (torsion). When we say "right-beating nystagmus," we mean that the patient's fast phases of nystagmus are beating toward *his or her* right ear. When we say that the patient has right torsion or right rotation, we mean that the superior pole of the patient's eye has fast-phase rotations toward *his or her* right side.

Now let's muddy the water a bit. There is also a convention to describe nystagmus using the terms *clockwise* and *counterclockwise*. The potential confusion is that when we use these terms, the perspective changes. We are *now* describing the patient from our own perspective! What is clockwise *for me* and not the patient? Let us use an example. If a patient has right torsional nystagmus, the eye has fast-phase rotation toward the patient's right side (from *his or her* perspective). We could describe this as either *right rotational* (or torsional) nystagmus, or we could say that the patient has *counterclockwise* nystagmus (from our perspective). Either convention is acceptable, although keeping things in the anatomical position convention may initially decrease confusion until you are more familiar with using these conventions.

Let's use some illustrations to describe observing eye motions. Note the blood vessels in the sclera. In examining eye motion, it is helpful to find a part of the eye to watch to help decide in which direction the eye is moving. In the case of light eyes (blue, green, hazel, etc), we can sometimes see darker flecks of color in the iris. These are more difficult to see in dark or brown eyes. If you cannot find anything in the iris to watch, look for either dark patches on the sclera (the white part of the eye) or blood vessels. In our example drawings, we use blood vessels and reference all motion from the starting position, which is eyes looking straight ahead. This is the "primary" position of the eye (Table 5-4).

We will use right-beating nystagmus as our example. With this type of nystagmus, the eyes will move quickly to the patient's right and have a slower, tracking motion to the patient's left. We describe the position or movement of the eyes by referencing their position compared with that of the primary position. Sometimes the patient's test position will change the way in which we describe or document the eye movements. Let's use the case of a lateral canal BPPV as an example. You would expect to see laterally beating nystagmus in cases of lateral canal involvement. If the patient is sitting, and the nystagmus is beating with quick phases to the patient's right, we document "right-beating resting nystagmus." However, if we have a patient with lateral canal BPPV and are seeing right beats while the patient is in the test position,

| TABLE 5-4 PRIMARY POSITION OF THE EYE | | |
|---|---|---|
| **PRIMARY POSITION** | **FAST PHASE** | **DESCRIBED AS** |
| 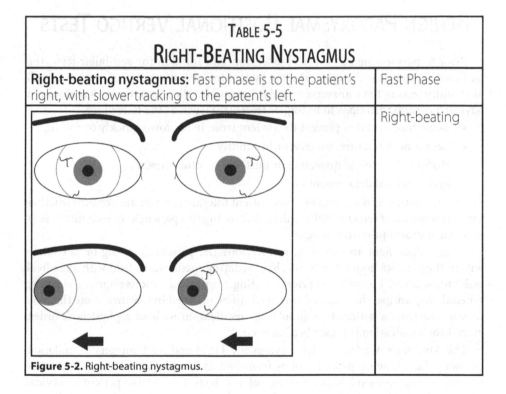  **Figure 5-1.** Primary position diagram. | None | Primary position (eyes are looking forward) |

| TABLE 5-5 RIGHT-BEATING NYSTAGMUS | |
|---|---|
| **Right-beating nystagmus:** Fast phase is to the patient's right, with slower tracking to the patent's left. | Fast Phase |
|  | Right-beating |
| **Figure 5-2.** Right-beating nystagmus. | |

the nystagmus would be described as either beating toward the ground (geotropic) or away from the ground (apogeotropic); these motions indicate lateral canal crystals.

In referencing nystagmus, we describe the direction of the fast phase. The eyes will move in one direction very quickly and then reverse direction and move slightly slower. For right-beating nystagmus, whether it is resting nystagmus or gaze nystagmus, the eyes will beat very quickly to the patient's right and slightly slower to his or her left. In the following illustration, the dark arrows indicate fast-phase motions (Table 5-5).

Rotational (torsional) nystagmus may also occur. This is an expected observation during episodes of BPPV of the anterior or posterior canals. In referencing torsion, use the superior pole of the eye as the reference point and describe the direction in which it is rotating more quickly (left or right). Keep in mind that in describing torsion (rotation), we use the patient's perspective of direction, not that of the observer. *Right torsion* describes eye rotation to the patient's right, not the observer's right.

Torsional nystagmus may occur at the same time as horizontal or vertical nystagmus (as in cases of anterior or posterior BPPV). If you wanted to describe these cases of nystagmus, you would describe each motion you observed. Using a commonly seen example of the right posterior canal, we could describe "right-torsional upbeating nystagmus" to designate the rotational and vertical components.

# Benign Paroxysmal Positional Vertigo Tests

Prior to performing any cervical extension and rotation for vestibular tests, the clinician should clear the cervical spine by looking at active range of motion as well as stability tests of the transverse and alar ligaments. Make sure the patient does not have any contraindications to testing or treatment, such as the following[4]:

- Acute fractures that prevent the patient from lying down quickly or rolling
- Recent neck fracture, surgery, or instability
- History of vertebral dissection or unstable carotid disease
- Recent retinal detachment

Modify testing as needed to improve patient tolerance. If you are not sure whether the performance of tests for BPPV will be safe owing to a patient's comorbidities, seek medical approval prior to testing.

Clearly document any sedating medications the patient is taking or has taken within the prior 48 hours. If possible, have sedating medications held with a medical order for at least 24 to 48 hours prior to testing. Some medications require a weaning schedule (eg, antipsychotics), and this needs to be planned in advance. Note that you may not instruct a patient to withhold *any* medication without a physician's order, even if the medication is prescribed "as needed."

The American Academy of Otolaryngology-Head and Neck Surgery Foundation excludes the following patient groups from bedside vestibular testing, while other researchers recommend "modification" of the tests for similar patients: cervical stenosis, severe kyphoscoliosis, limited cervical range of motion, Down's syndrome, severe rheumatoid arthritis, cervical radiculopathies, Paget's disease, ankylosing spondylitis, low back dysfunction, spinal cord injuries, and morbid obesity.

Because the Dix-Hallpike is a gravity-dependent positional test, the position of the head with respect to the ground is important, not whether or not the head is turned or extended on the body. The clinician may position the patient *en bloc*, with the neck kept in a neutral position to modify the test for special populations.

Much of the time clinicians' placement of hand position on the patient or verbal instructions are the result of their training. They may take on the testing methods they have learned, but it is important not to get wrapped up in the conventions of the test (eg, where they put their hands and verbal instructions) without thinking about the physiology behind what is meant to occur within the ear during testing or interventions. Remember that the key to assessing and treating BPPV is positioning the patient correctly and safely and then observing the resulting signs and symptoms. Whichever testing or intervention techniques you choose, try to keep in mind what is occurring within the patient's ears as you are performing the test or intervention.

BPPV most commonly affects the posterior canal. Because this canal sits anatomically more caudal than the other vestibular canals, it is easy to see why this is the case, since gravity pulls the crystals downward. Interestingly, BPPV in the right ear is more common, with the right side being 1.41 times more likely to have BPPV. It has been proposed that this is due to the fact that more people sleep on their right sides.[21]

## Anterior and Posterior Canals

In 2008 the American Academy Otolaryngology-Head and Neck Surgery Foundation convened a panel that made the following recommendations[19]:

1a. Diagnosis of Posterior Canal BPPV: Clinicians should diagnose posterior canal BPPV when vertigo associated with nystagmus is provoked by the Dix-Hallpike maneuver, performed by bringing the patient from an upright to supine position with the head turned 45 degrees to one side and neck extended 20 degrees.

1b. Diagnosis of Lateral Canal BPPV: If the patient has a history compatible with BPPV and the Dix-Hallpike test is negative, the clinician should perform a supine roll test to assess for lateral semicircular canal BPPV.

2a. Differential Diagnosis of BPPV: Clinicians should differentiate BPPV from other causes of imbalance, dizziness, and vertigo.

2b. Modifying Factors: Clinicians should question patients with BPPV for factors that modify management, including impaired mobility or balance, central nervous system disorders, a lack of home support, and increased risk for falling.

3a. Radiographic and Vestibular Testing: Clinicians should not obtain radiographic imaging, vestibular testing, or either in a patient diagnosed with BPPV unless the diagnosis is uncertain or there are additional symptoms or signs unrelated to BPPV that warrant testing.

3b. Audiometric Testing: No recommendation is made concerning audiometric testing in patients with BPPV.

4a. Repositioning Maneuvers as Initial Therapy: Clinicians should treat patients with posterior canal BPPV with a particle repositioning maneuver.

4b. Vestibular Rehabilitation as Initial Therapy: The clinician may offer vestibular rehabilitation, either self-administered or with a clinician, for the initial treatment of BPPV.

4c. Observation as Initial Therapy: Clinicians may offer observation as initial management for patients with BPPV and with assurance of follow-up.

5. Medical Therapy: Clinicians should not routinely treat BPPV with vestibular suppressant medications such as antihistamines or benzodiazepines.

6a. Reassessment of Treatment Response: Clinicians should reassess patients within 1 month after an initial period of observation or treatment to confirm symptom resolution.

6b. Evaluation of Treatment Failure: Clinicians should evaluate patients with BPPV who are initial treatment failures for persistent BPPV or underlying peripheral vestibular or central nervous system disorders.

7. Education: Clinicians should counsel patients regarding the impact of BPPV on their safety, the potential for disease recurrence, and the importance of follow-up.

While there are different tests of BPPV, the Dix-Hallpike test (used for anterior and posterior canal BPPV testing) has been described as the "gold standard" whereby to diagnose BPPV. It is performed by bringing the patient from a sitting to a supine position with the head turned 45 degrees toward the side being tested and the neck extended 20 to 30 degrees.[19] There is another test for the posterior canal called the *Side-Lying test*. As the name implies, instead of moving the patient into a supine position, the patient is placed into a side-lying position with the test ear as the one closer toward the ground. Observation of the patient's VOR will reveals which canals are being stimulated by loose debris.

##  Dix-Hallpike Test

The classic Dix-Hallpike test places the patient from long sitting into a supine position with cervical extension over the edge of the treatment table; then the head is rotated toward the side to be tested. Most clinicians today have the patient long-sit, turn the head 45 degrees toward the side being tested, extend the neck 30 degrees, and *then* have the patient lie down with the head hanging off the bed/table. Remember, the important thing is knowing the patient's restrictions and then safely placing the patient's head in the proper position with respect to the ground. The clinician's hand placement is really a matter of personal preference and patient safety. The head and face are very intimate areas for people; most do not like someone they don't know grabbing, twisting, and turning their heads. By limiting how much you touch the patient's head and face and by giving him or her more control over the test, the patient may be more comfortable and relaxed during the test. For example, we know that ultimately the patient's head is in 45 degrees of rotation to the testing side and extended 30 degrees. Many clinicians grab the patient's head and turn and extend it for them. However, aren't most patients capable of turning their own heads? Do they *really* need us to do that for them? The simple instruction to "turn your head halfway" while tapping the patient's shoulder on that side as a tactile cue will accomplish the goal of placing the patient's head in the correct position of rotation for testing. If needed, I touch a patient's head only long enough move it to the correct the position, and then ask the patient to maintain that position. When the patient moves into supine and naturally goes into cervical extension, then you may use one hand as a support and guide.

Make modifications to accommodate patients who are restricted from neck extension or rotation or can't tolerate it. For example, clinicians in a hospital setting can use a tilt table or hospital bed to position the patient's head down 30 degrees (with

## TABLE 5-6
# MODIFIED DIX-HALLPIKE TEST, STEP 1

**Instruction:** The patient is asked to "turn your head halfway" toward the side being tested and then lie back quickly.

**Clinician:** The clinician stands behind the patient, who is long-sitting on the table/bed. Give the patient a tap on the shoulder as a tactile cue to the side that is to be tested, meanwhile giving instructions to turn the head. Patients who have low back issues may wish to keep their knees bent to reduce discomfort.

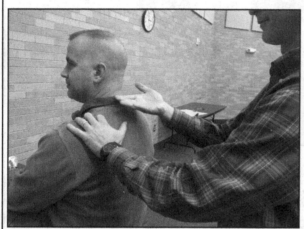

**Figure 5-3.** Dix-Hallpike 1.

the neck in neutral) instead of requiring cervical extension. In the home health or clinic setting, clinicians may have the patient move from sitting into a supine position without any cervical extension. In this position, you will likely still get a good response to elicit nystagmus, but without cervical extension, the likelihood of moving the crystals into a different canal during your test or treatment interventions increases. While this may necessitate more maneuvers, ultimately the clinician can still clear the canals of debris. If the patient cannot rotate his or her neck, position the head toward the side you wish to test while keeping the head and neck in neutral by positioning/rotating the entire body *en bloc*. Remember, it is the position of the head with respect to the ground that is important. You can achieve the same positions of the head with respect to the ground by moving and turning the neck, by keeping the head and neck in neutral and instead moving the entire body, or using a combination of head rotation and body positioning. Tables 5-6 through 5-9 provide the directions for the modified Dix-Hallpike test.

## Dix-Hallpike Sensitivity

Published estimates of the Dix-Hallpike test's sensitivity[11] range from 48% to 88%.

## TABLE 5-7
# MODIFIED DIX-HALLPIKE TEST, STEP 2

**Instruction:** "Keep your head turned and lie down quickly.'"

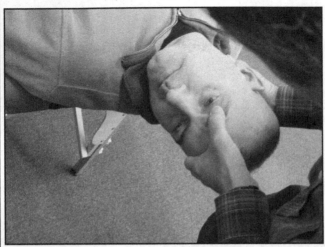

**Figure 5-4.** Dix-Hallpike 2.

**Clinician:** Position the patient such that when he is supine, the head will be off the edge of the table. With one hand gently resting on the scapula of the side to be tested (try not to grip the shoulder), and the other hand held near the occiput (palm up) in preparation to support/guide the patient's head, the patient is instructed to lie back quickly. Guide him into about 30 degrees of cervical extension (while maintaining 45 degrees of rotation toward the test side) and support the head with one hand. Keep your other hand free in case you need to use your fingers to gently open an eyelid (sometimes the patient will squeeze the eyelids shut during vertigo/nystagmus). Hold the test position for up to 45 seconds while observing the eyes for nystagmus. Document the duration of any observed nystagmus. Take the patient out of the test position when:

1. Nystagmus is seen and timed and lasts less than 1 minute.
2. Nystagmus is seen and timed and lasts longer than 1 minute.
3. No nystagmus is observed after 45 seconds.
4. The patient cannot tolerate the position.

---

### TABLE 5-8
## MODIFIED DIX-HALLPIKE TEST, STEP 3

**Clinician:** Observe nystagmus. If the patient has nystagmus, note the direction of the quick phases of nystagmus. There are typically vertical and rotational (torsional) components. You need to figure out if the quick phases are up or down and whether the quick rotational phases are left or right beating. For a diagnosis of BPPV, both torsional and vertical components are typically present. The rotational component may be difficult to see without having the patient wear goggles.

---

### TABLE 5-9
## INTERPRETATION OF THE MODIFIED DIX-HALLPIKE TEST

*Interpretation*

**Upbeating:** Posterior canal involvement with torsional component.

**Downbeating:** Anterior canal involvement with a slight torsional component. For anterior canalithiasis, the nystagmus is mainly downbeating (vs rotational) owing to the predominantly sagittal orientation of the canal, and the torsional component may not be readily seen.[34]

**Torsion:** Quick-phase rotation will be in the direction of the involved ear.

**Absence component:** In the absence of either vertical or rotational components, consider the possibility of a central pathology.

---

##  *Side-Lying Test*

The Side-Lying test is an alternative to the Dix-Hallpike test (Figures 5-5 and 5-6); it is useful for those who have limited active or passive ranges of motion. However, unless modifications are used, it still requires head rotation. It is a very helpful test for the therapists in the home health setting, or in the physician's office where there is insufficient space to perform a typical Dix-Hallpike test, which requires the patient's head to hang off a bed or exam table.

With the Side-Lying test, the patient does not lie supine but instead moves from sitting to side-lying in the direction of the ear to be tested, with the head turned 45 degrees and the nose toward the ceiling, so that the ear that is to be tested is closer to the floor when the patient is in the test position. Position hold times and observations of nystagmus are the same as described in the Dix-Hallpike instructions. This is a valid test as determined by a study of 61 subjects.[35] Figures 5-5 and 5-6 show the patient positioned for a test of the left side. The clinician would be near the patient's head, ready to correct the position and to observe for nystagmus.

**Figure 5-5.** Side-Lying test 1.

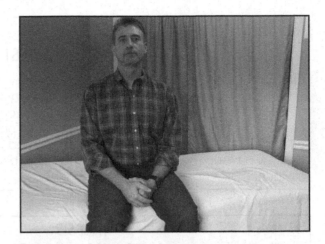

**Figure 5-6.** Side-Lying test 2.

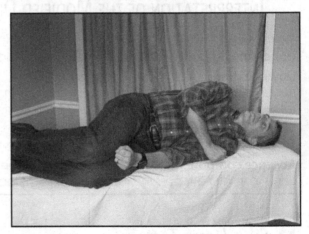

## *Lateral Canal Tests*

Like the tests of the anterior and posterior canals, there are different BPPV tests of the lateral canal. The Roll test is a test of lateral canal BPPV. Another test, the Bow-and-Lean test, is not for diagnosing BPPV but is useful to help lateralize the condition. That is, it will help you figure out which ear is involved once lateral canal involvement has been determined. When the patient has BPPV of a lateral canal, the test will be positive on either side, so that we need to distinguish the quick-phase direction of the nystagmus to determine which ear is involved.

Before we discuss the test procedure, we need to learn some new terminology that will describe the nystagmus that occurs in lateral canal BPPV. When the patient is in the roll-test position, one ear will be toward the ground and the other toward the ceiling. Nystagmus seen during BPPV of the lateral canal beats laterally, with quick phases either beating toward the ground or away from it. We use the following names to describe this:

| TABLE 5-10 CHARACTERISTICS OF NYSTAGMUS VARIANTS OF THE LATERAL CANAL | |
| --- | --- |
| **GEOTROPIC** | **APOGEOTROPIC** |
| Beating toward the ground | Beating away from the ground |
| Free-floating/moving | Either stuck to the cupula or trapped within the short arm of the canal |
| Usually easily resolved with canalith repositioning maneuvers | More involved interventions using liberatory maneuvers; then, if needed, other canalith repositioning maneuvers |

- Geotropic: Quick phases toward the ground (or earth)
  Remember, *Geo* means "earth" (as in the word *geo*graphy). This is theoretically a canalithiasis variant with loose crystals.

- Apogeotropic: Quick phases beating away from the ground
  This is theoretically a cupulolithiasis variant (ie, with stuck crystals) or crystals trapped in the short arm (closer to the cupula) of the canal.

For lateral canal BPPV, the quick phases of the nystagmus of each ear should present in the same way. That is, if they are geotropic when the right side is being tested, they should *also* be geotropic on testing the left. Another way to describe it this is to say that if they have quick phases beating toward the ground on the right side (geotropic), they should also have quick-phase beating toward the ground (geotropic) when testing the left.

The conventional theory is that when nystagmus are *geotropic*, the crystals are loose, and this represents the canalithiasis type of BPPV. When the nystagmus are apogeotropic, the crystals are either adherent to the cupula or somehow stuck in the short arm of the canal (Table 5-10). *Apogeotropic* nystagmus represents the cupulolithiasis type of BPPV. Remember, in cases of canalithiasis there are usually a few seconds between placing a patient into the test position and the onset of nystagmus. In cases of cupulolithiasis, onset is immediate when the patient is placed into the test position, with nystagmus lasting a minute or longer. Geotropic BPPV (loose crystals) is easier to correct using repositioning maneuvers. One way to remember the terminology is to equate *geotropic* (which begins with the letter "G") with *ground* and *good* (which both *also* begin with the letter "G"). Geotropic nystagmus has quick phases that beat toward the ground and are good because the crystals are loose and the BPPV will be easy to fix.

Apogeotropic nystagmus (which begins with the letter "A") beats away from the earth. The words *again* and *apologize* also begin with the letter "A." The crystals are either "stuck" on the cupula or otherwise trapped in the short arm of the canal. You will probably have to treat the patient more than once (again and again) and may feel that you want to apologize for the apogeotropic nystagmus.

## Roll Test (Pagnini-McClure Maneuver)

The lateral canals are pitched approximately 30 degrees from the horizontal plane, so the Dix-Hallpike maneuver will not sufficiently place them in a position to be tested for loose crystals. Therefore the clinician needs to place the head in a different position with respect to the ground, using the roll test to accomplish this. A couple variations exist in performing this test. The first variation is the starting supine position, where some clinicians have the patient's neck in neutral, while others start with the patient in supine and neck flexed 30 degrees to better position the lateral canals perpendicular to the ground. Because the flexed position better places the lateral canals vertically, anatomically speaking this should be ideal. However, studies have cited both methods, and either method is valid—neck flexed or in neutral. The other portion of the test that has variations in testing method is how the clinician moves the patient from position to position during testing. Some advocate having the clinician move the passive patient's head into the test positions in rapid thrusting motions. Given that this is a gravity-driven test (that is, gravity is pulling the crystals), quick head thrusting motions are not required. Tables 5-11 through 5-13 show instructions for the roll test.

If you observe *apogeotropic* nystagmus on one test side (quick-phase nystagmus *away* from the ground), you should *also* observe *apogeotropic* nystagmus in testing the contralateral side. If this is not the case, then a diagnosis of lateral canal BPPV is in question.

Sometimes, in testing the lateral canals, it is difficult to determine which ear has the stronger, more robust nystagmus. Because of this, the resolution rate after interventions with various maneuvers[36-38] is between 60% and 90%. At times it is difficult to tell whether one ear has more signs than the other. Luckily, there is an additional test you may use to help you decide which ear to treat. The *Bow-and-Lean test* is available to help you localize the cause of the BPPV.[39]

### Bow-and-Lean Test

The Bow-and-Lean test (also known as *Choung's test*) is useful when the patient presents with a lateral-canal BPPV and the involved side has not been determined. As explained in discussing the Roll test, it may be difficult to determine which ear is involved. This test will help you decide which side to treat. During the Bow-and-Lean test you compare the direction of the quick-phase nystagmus when the patient is sitting and in a head bow (flexion) or lean (extension). As the patient bows and leans, the crystals will move either toward or away from the cupula of each ear, making them deflect toward or away from the utricle. This migration of otoconia will activate nystagmus. Using the direction of the quick phases and the patient's test position, you can determine which ear is involved. Tables 5-14 through 5-17 give the directions for performing this test.[39]

## TABLE 5-11
# ROLL TEST, STEP 1

**Instruction:** (Once the patient is supine) "Turn your head as far as you can to this side." (Tap shoulder of patient's test side.)

**Clinician:** The patient is positioned supine with the head in neutral (some examiners flex the head to 30 degrees to place the lateral canals roughly perpendicular to the ground). Ask the patient to rotate his head to one side (to roughly 90 degrees). Allow the patient to turn his own head if possible, assisting only when needed. The clinician is directly behind the patient's head, supporting the head in one hand while keeping the other hand free in case of a need to gently open the patient's eyelid during testing to observe the eye motions. If the patient lacks cervical range of motion, he should be asked to roll his body to help place his head in the correct position. If the patient is restricted from cervical rotation, roll the patient *en bloc* (head neutral) until the head is rotated 90 degrees from the starting position. Remember, this is a gravity-driven test and there is no need to turn the head quickly.

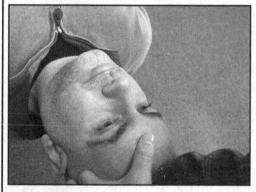

**Figure 5-7.** Roll test 1.

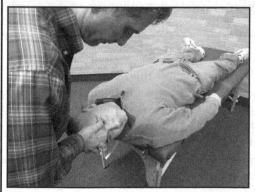

**Figure 5-8.** Roll test 2.

## TABLE 5-12
# ROLL TEST, STEP 2

**Instruction:** Observe the patient's eyes for 30 seconds for nystagmus. If nystagmus are seen, note the direction of the quick phases (geotropic or apogeotropic) and time the duration of nystagmus (eg, less or greater than 1 minute). If there is no observable nystagmus, have the patient return his head to neutral rotation. After 30 seconds, test the contralateral side.

## TABLE 5-13
# INTERPRETATION OF THE ROLL TEST

*Interpretation*

After testing each ear, you will want to document the test results, making sure to include the following information:

- If the test was positive (nystagmus were present) or negative (nystagmus were not present)
- If the test was subjectively positive, meaning that the patient complained of dizziness but was without nystagmus
- If nystagmus were geotropic or apogeotropic
- If the duration of nystagmus was greater or less than 1 minute
- Categorize the nystagmus as indicating canalithiasis or cupulolithiasis
    - *Canalithiasis*: Quick phases toward the ground (geotropic) on each side; treat the side with stronger nystagmus/symptoms (involved ear).
    - *Cupulolithiasis*: Quick phases toward the sky (apogeotropic) on each side; treat the side with weaker nystagmus/symptoms (involved ear).
    - The Bow-and-Lean test may help you to determine which ear is involved.

Let's use our "G" and "A" words to help us remember this test:
- During the Supine Roll test, if the patient has *geotropic* nystagmus; then, during the Bow-and-Lean test, while sitting and looking at the ground in the bow, the eyes will beat *toward the affected ear*.
- During the Supine Roll test, if the patient has apogeotropic nystagmus, then, during the Bow-and-Lean test, when the patient is sitting and looking at the ground in the bow, his or her eyes will beat away from the affected ear.

### TABLE 5-14
# BOW-AND-LEAN TEST, STEP 1

**Clinician:** Using the Roll test, confirm whether the nystagmus is geotropic (canalithiasis) or apogeotropic (cupulolithiasis) in the supine position.

---

### TABLE 5-15
# BOW-AND-LEAN TEST, STEP 2

**Instruction:** With the patient sitting on the side of the table/bed, instruct him or her to *flex* the head/neck to 90 degrees (this is the "bow" part of the test).

**Clinician:** Observe the quick-phase direction of nystagmus.

---

### TABLE 5-16
# BOW-AND-LEAN TEST, STEP 3

**Instruction:** With the patient still sitting on the side of the table/bed with his or her head back in the neutral position, ask the patient to *extend* the head/neck 45 degrees (this is the "lean" part of the test).

**Clinician:** Observe the quick-phase direction of nystagmus.

---

### TABLE 5-17
# INTERPRETATION OF THE BOW-AND-LEAN TEST[39]

| TYPE: CANALITHIASIS | TYPE: CUPULOLITHIASIS |
|---|---|
| **Nystagmus direction:** Geotropic while in the supine roll test. | **Nystagmus direction:** Apogeotropic while in the supine roll test. |
| **The affected ear** is determined as being the one that is in the same direction to that of bowing quick-phase nystagmus and in the opposite direction as that of the leaning nystagmus. | **The affected ear** is determined as being the one that is in the opposite direction to that of the bowing nystagmus and in the same direction as that of the leaning quick-phase nystagmus. |

# BENIGN PAROXYSMAL POSITIONAL VERTIGO INTERVENTIONS

Prior to performing any BPPV interventions, you must know your patient's physical limitations and restrictions (as was true in examining the patient for BPPV). Make sure that the patient does not have any contraindications to testing or treatment, such as the following[4]:

- Acute fractures that prevent the patient from lying down quickly or rolling
- Recent neck fracture, surgery, or instability
- History of vertebral dissection or unstable carotid disease
- Recent retinal detachment

There are a number of different maneuvers to move crystals back to the utricle. We refer to the process of moving crystals from the canal back to the utricle as *canalith repositioning.* This is the term you should use in your plan of care. Do not specify one repositioning maneuver, such as the Epley maneuver, as your plan. If you do, it will lock you into using only that maneuver unless you change your plan. However, if you use *canalith repositioning* as your plan, then you may use any repositioning maneuver, which you would specify in your treatment documentation.

Some repositioning maneuvers use patient positioning and gravity as a means of moving crystals. Others involve forcefully moving the patient's head to create a flow of the endolymph toward the utricle; imagine a river sweeping toward the utricle that carries the crystals along with it. In the case of crystals that are stuck, as in cupulolithiasis, forceful movements may be used to break the crystals free (or liberate them) from the cupula. As a group, we refer to these forceful interventions as *liberatory maneuvers.* At times simple positioning will accomplish the job of moving otoconia, as in cases where prolonged positioning uses gravity to liberate the crystals from the cupula.

As discussed earlier, in using gravity as a means of moving crystals for testing or repositioning, the position of the patient's head with respect to gravity is most important. If you need to restrict the patient's head or neck movements because of a medical condition or discomfort, keep the patient in a neck-neutral position and move the entire body to position the head. With respect to the ear and its position relative to the ground, there is no difference between lying supine with the head rotated 90 degrees to the right, on the one hand, and, on the other, keeping the neck in neutral and log-rolling (*en bloc*) the entire body to the right. In both instances, the ear is in exactly the same position. In the first example, the ear is positioned by rotating the neck; in the second, the ear is positioned by rolling the entire body. Both positioning methods accomplish the same task, positioning the right ear to the ground. Know your patient's physical restrictions prior to performing any type of canalith repositioning and make modifications as needed.

No matter which repositioning technique you use, keep in mind that most patients will have symptom resolution within just a few treatments. If signs and/or symptoms persist after a few treatment visits, consider referring the patient for further clinical testing to confirm BPPV and rule out other pathologies that may mimic BPPV.

# Resolution Rates for Canalith Repositioning

What kind of success should you expect from repositioning maneuvers? A recent study found the following resolution "cure" rates[40]:

- Posterior canal, 95%
- Lateral (horizontal) canal, 87%
- Anterior canal, 87%

This study also suggested that there is a poorer initial response to repositioning maneuvers for anterior canal BPPV and also a poorer response to maneuvers for recurrences of lateral canal BPPV.

# Pre-Maneuver Considerations

Before you begin a canalith repositioning procedure, there are a couple things to think about. Does the patient get sick or vomit from the BPPV? Are there any restrictions the patient needs to observe? Which maneuver or maneuvers do you want to use? How long do you hold each position during canalith repositioning? Are there any hints of possible central pathology that may be mimicking BPPV?

### Nausea

Often patients with BPPV become nauseous and occasionally vomit when they experience vertigo. It is always good practice to ask whether the patient's condition has previously made him or her vomit. If the patient has vomited from BPPV, chances are good that he or she will vomit while you are performing a test for BPPV or even during repositioning maneuvers. Have a plastic bag or bucket ready for this eventuality. Also, an ice-cold wet towel placed across the back of the neck does wonders to reduce nausea. If the patient becomes overly nauseous, ask the referring physician to prescribe some type of anti-nausea medication prior to performing repositioning maneuvers. This will help the patient tolerate the interventions and increase his or her willingness to participate.

### Maneuver Hold Times

Hold times for different repositioning maneuvers vary depending on the researcher. The hold times for gravity-driven maneuvers are basically just the time it takes for crystals to fall toward the ground inside the canal. You want to be sure to give the crystals enough time to move to the lowest possible position within the canal. For canalithiasis, latency times (the time it takes for signs and symptoms to begin) may range from 5 seconds to 1 minute.[19] Keeping this in mind, most hold times range from 30 seconds to 2 minutes. A common practice for testing (eg, with Dix-Hallpike) is to wait at least 45 seconds before calling a BPPV test negative. For repositioning techniques, a common practice is to wait for nystagmus/dizziness to end and then add another 30 seconds to the hold time. Remember, holding longer won't affect the outcome; but if you don't hold the position long enough, you may not allow enough time for the crystals to move before you move into the next position of any maneuver. If you proceed through the maneuvers too quickly, the crystals may move (or fall back) in the wrong direction, and the maneuver will need to be repeated. Take your time! Slower is better than faster for gravity-driven tests and maneuvers.

### Hand Position and Patient Instructions

As discussed earlier, during testing and repositioning maneuvers, the position of the vestibular system within the head with respect to the ground is key, and not so much the position of the rest of the body. As a general rule, if patients can move, turn, or position without assistance, *let them*. This gives them a sense of control. When you are performing repositioning maneuvers, the same holds true. We do not always need to grab someone's head and turn it. Most people have head and neck control, and it is much friendlier to simply ask someone to turn his or her head and then guide or make corrections only as needed. Keep this in mind during repositioning maneuvers. When instructions call for the head to be turned or rotated, can the patient do that without *you* touching or moving the head? In some cases, the position changes are quick, and the clinicians need a more hands-on approach. For gravity-driven maneuvers; however, it is easy to simply direct the patient to move into the desired position with as little "hands-on" help as possible unless safety, maneuver requirements, or patient confusion requires it.

### Which Maneuver Should I Use?

The choice of repositioning maneuver may change depending on your practice location, the size of your patient, which canal is involved, and clinician preference. The canal that is involved will limit your options, but there are still many personal preference choices available.

### Multiple-Canal Benign Paroxysmal Positional Vertigo

The incidence of multiple-canal BPPV varies depending on the research study and ranges from 4.4% to 9.3%.[30,31] Patients with multiple-canal involvement may have BPPV occurring in multiple canals of one ear or in both ears simultaneously. Which ear do you treat first? At least one study suggests treating the more symptomatic side first, since symptoms of bilateral involvement may be erroneous, possibly caused by incorrect head positioning during testing.[41] If bilateral symptoms disappear after treatment of the more symptomatic side, it is likely that the patient did not truly have bilateral BPPV. In cases of multicanal involvement, the sequence of which canal is treated first is not critical and should not affect the outcomes of interventions. However, if you treat the more symptomatically bothersome canal first (followed by the next most bothersome), the patient may have improved tolerance during your interventions.

## Posterior Canals—Repositioning Maneuvers

There are many canalith repositioning maneuvers, and the list seems to grow daily. A systematic review of studies between 1966 and September 2009 by Helminski et al[2] concluded that randomized controlled trials have provided strong evidence that canalith repositioning maneuvers (CRMs) resolve benign paroxysmal positional nystagmus of the posterior canal. Further, repositioning maneuvers done by a clinician in combination with self-administered repositioning is more effective than

| TABLE 5-18 |
|---|
| **RASHAD'S MODIFIED CANALITH REPOSITIONING STEPS** |

**INSTRUCTIONS**

**Equipment used:** Stiff cervical collar, treatment table with the head of the table lowered 30 degrees.

**Patient position:** The patient (wearing the collar) long-sits on the table and is in a position such that when lying down, the head is supported by the table.

**Hold times:** In the study, each position (sequence) was held 2 minutes, or 1 minute after subsidence of any nystagmus (whichever was longer).

**Patient instructions:** Instruct the patient to lie rapidly on the side of the involved ear without touching him or her.

Roll the patient onto the other side (neck position is neutral and prevented from rotating by the collar).

Instruct the patient to lie face-down.

Return the patient to an upright position and remove the collar, then instruct him or her to flex the neck, avoiding painful motions.

The patient's head/neck is returned to neutral, and the cervical collar is reapplied.

CRM performed by a clinician alone. For self-administered treatments, CRMs were more effective than liberatory maneuvers; the Brandt-Daroff was the least effective self-administered treatment.[42]

Clinicians new to vestibular interventions for BPPV commonly ask whether canalith repositioning is safe to perform with geriatric patients. If performed properly, this type of intervention is safe and well tolerated by most patients. Always remember to know your patients' physical limitations, medical precautions, and cervical ranges of motion. Most patients are able to perform testing and interventions for BPPV with very few modifications. If you are ever in doubt, get medical clearance from those specialists who can best address your concerns. Remember, you can always keep the patient in neutral and move/rotate the entire body to reposition crystals.

## Treatment of Patients With Cervical Pathology

There are cervical conditions that require caution in testing or treating BPPV. A study by Rashad of 40 patients who had neck conditions typically thought to preclude BPPV interventions found that these patients could be treated with canalith repositioning if the intervention was modified. For these patients, a diagnosis of BPPV was made using the patient's history of positional vertigo, but the use of the Dix-Hallpike test was avoided in this patient population for fear of inducing spinal fracture. Those with symptoms of cervical pathology—including cervical spondylosis, disc prolapse, previous cervical spine fracture, and cervical spine rheumatoid arthritis—had their conditions confirmed by radiology. Rashad's modified canalith repositioning maneuver[43] used the protocol shown in Table 5-18.

The subjects were given postmaneuver instructions and were reviewed after 2 weeks, 1 month, 3 months, and 6 months; 90% reported complete relief at the 1-week review. Of the 4 subjects who did not have complete resolution, 3 had major improvement and the fourth did not have resolution. This study demonstrates that with careful planning and modification, you can treat even those with significant cervical issues safely and effectively. Most of our patients will not require such drastic modifications, but it is good to know that there are options available for patients with more severe cervical comorbidities.

##  Modified Epley Maneuver

Dr. John Epley, the inventor of the Epley maneuver, designed the maneuver as a way of moving the otoconia out of the canals and back into the utricle.[44] This is the most widely used repositioning maneuver, although over the years modifications have been recommended by other researchers. While designed to treat BPPV of the posterior canals, this maneuver is also useful to treat canalithiasis of the anterior canal. The Epley maneuver is efficacious, with a high success rate of symptom resolution.[45] Review the original description of the maneuver given in Table 5-19, keeping in mind that many clinicians today modify it based on more recent research. Without a doubt, this maneuver revolutionized not only the treatment of BPPV but also the direction of research for BPPV interventions. The original article describes applying vibration to the ipsilateral mastoid, but studies since then have not supported this practice.[42,46,47] The original thinking was that the vibration helped the migration of the crystals. Another modification from the original instructions involves having the patient keep the head upright for 48 hours. Most studies today do not support postmaneuver restrictions such as this.

Table 5-19 shows how Epley originally described the maneuver sequence for a left posterior canal.[44]

Many researchers have suggested variations to this sequence. One interesting study by Herdman et al demonstrated better remission rates[48] when repositioning maneuvers were repeated several times versus only once (93% vs 83%). If you are testing and retesting multiple times within a treatment session, it is not uncommon to have signs of nystagmus diminish due to neural fatigue. That is, you get less response from the test because of neural fatigue, not necessarily because you have improved the condition by returning otoconia to the utricle. Following a treatment intervention session using canalith repositioning, it may be helpful to wait 24 hours or more before retesting so as to separate the effects of treatment vs a lack of signs and symptoms due to neural fatigue.[21]

Let's now outline a modified Epley maneuver. We will take the approach of having as much of a "hands-off" procedure as possible, allowing the patient to move from position to position with verbal instructions and minor tactile cues. Remember, this is a gravity-driven technique that does not require forceful motions. If the patient moves too slowly while changing test positions, you may not see nystagmus. Remember to keep verbal instructions as simple as possible. It is also extremely

| TABLE 5-19 CANALITH REPOSITIONING AS ORIGINALLY DESCRIBED BY EPLEY | | |
|---|---|---|
| SEQUENCE | PATIENT POSITION | CRYSTAL POSITION |
| 1 | Sitting | Near cupula |
| 2 | With the patient in sitting, position the head over the end of the table with the head (rotated) 45 degrees to the left | Center of posterior canal |
| 3 | The head is kept downward (extended); it is rotated 45 degrees to the right | Crystals reach common crus (where the anterior and posterior canals divide from one common canal) |
| 4 | Rotate the head and body (to the right) so that the head points down toward the ground at 135 degrees from supine | Crystals move past the common crus |
| 5 | With head maintaining its position, return the patient to sitting | Crystals enter utricle |
| 6 | Once in sitting, flex the head 20 degrees | No explanation is given for this position in the article |
| Hold each position until induced nystagmus "approaches termination," or latency + duration of nystagmus. Repeat until no nystagmus occurs in any position. | | |

helpful to first demonstrate the maneuver so that the patient can see what will occur during this intervention. Avoid using technical terms like *rotate, extend, degrees,* or *maintain.* Most people do not use these terms daily and may find them confusing. Try to use everyday words in your instructions.

Instructions for the modified Epley maneuver are given in Tables 5-20 through 5-25.

An easy way to remember the steps of the modified Epley maneuver is to say the phrase, *"Look away, roll away, and sit up."* For the modified Epley, we always start on the side to be tested and then have the patient *look* away from the test ear, *roll* away from the tested ear, and finally return to *sitting.*

Table 5-26 shows the sequence without the clinician.

## TABLE 5-20
# MODIFIED EPLEY MANEUVER, STEP 1

| PATIENT POSITION | PATIENT INSTRUCTIONS |
|---|---|
| Sitting | The patient is told to long-sit on the bed/table, bending the knees if needed for back comfort. |

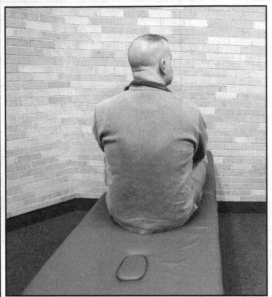

**Figure 5-9.** Modified Epley 1.

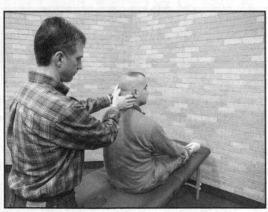

**Figure 5-10.** Modified Epley 2.

## TABLE 5-21
## MODIFIED EPLEY MANEUVER, STEP 2

| PATIENT POSITION | PATIENT INSTRUCTIONS |
|---|---|
| With the patient in sitting, instruct him to move his head to 45 degrees in the direction of the ear to be tested. While the patient is in sitting, stand behind him with one hand on his shoulder on the side to be tested. After the patient turns his head to the test side, correct his position as needed and then return your hand to the dorsal shoulder. Make sure you are not gripping the shoulder but just touching it. | Once in the long-sitting position, tap the patient's shoulder on the side you wish to test as a tactile cue. Instruct the patient, "Turn your head halfway to this side."<br><br>Once in the correct position, instruct the patient, "Keep your head turned and lie back as quickly as you can, keeping your eyes open. Tell me if you feel dizzy or nauseous." |

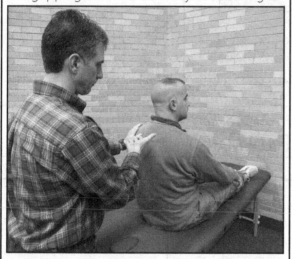

**Figure 5-11.** Modified Epley 3.

While maintaining rotation, move the patient into supine, with his head in 20 to 30 degrees of extension off the end of the treatment surface.

As the patient moves into supine, the clinician releases touch to the shoulder with one hand and catches the patient's head with the other hand. Use the hand that is supporting the head to correct and guide the head position as needed. The hand not supporting the head is now free to open the patient's eyelids if he is holding them closed owing to symptoms of vertigo.

*(continued)*

## TABLE 5-21 (CONTINUED)
## MODIFIED EPLEY MANEUVER, STEP 2

| PATIENT POSITION | PATIENT INSTRUCTIONS |
|---|---|
| 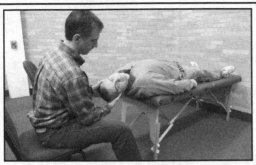 **Figure 5-12.** Modified Epley 4. Hold this position for 45 seconds, or until the nystagmus stops. If nystagmus lasts more than 1 minute, return the patient to sitting. | |

## TABLE 5-22
## MODIFIED EPLEY MANEUVER, STEP 3

| PATIENT POSITION | PATIENT INSTRUCTIONS |
|---|---|
| While keeping the head in extension, rotate the head to 45 degrees past neutral away from the side being tested. (This is a 90-degree movement from sequence 2 to sequence 3.) Allowing the patient to turn his own head, the clinician may guide this movement using the support hand as needed. *Hold* this position until the nystagmus stops and then add 30 seconds. If you do not see nystagmus, hold for 30 seconds. 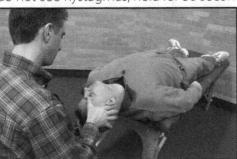 **Figure 5-13.** Modified Epley 5. | "Keep your head back, and turn it halfway to the other side. Tell me if you feel dizzy or nauseous." |

## TABLE 5-23
## MODIFIED EPLEY MANEUVER, STEP 4

| PATIENT POSITION | PATIENT INSTRUCTIONS |
|---|---|
| Rotate the head and body away from the test ear so that the head is pointed nose-down toward the ground at 135 degrees from supine. During the verbal instructions, the clinician taps the patient's shoulder as a tactile cue to indicate the side toward which the patient should roll. As the patient rolls onto that side, allow his head to roll off of the supporting hand. Adjust the patient's head position as needed so that he is looking at the ground at about a 45-degree angle. If the patient has head control, you do not have to hold his head in this position. | "Keep your head turned and roll onto your side so that you are looking slightly toward the ground." |

Keep in mind that you can rotate the trunk to accommodate a lack of cervical range of motion. Unless the patient lacks head control or has special cervical issues, you do *not* need to hold his head during this motion. While allowing the patient's head to roll off your supporting hand as he turns onto his side, place a hand on the patient's uppermost shoulder and move to stand on the patient's side and facing him so as to guard him.

*Hold* this position until the nystagmus stops, then add 30 seconds. If you do not see nystagmus, hold for 30 seconds.

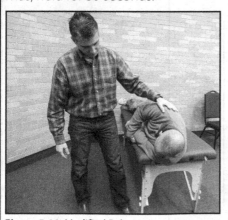

**Figure 5-14.** Modified Epley 6.

## TABLE 5-24
# MODIFIED EPLEY MANEUVER, STEP 5

| PATIENT POSITION | PATIENT INSTRUCTIONS |
|---|---|
| With the head maintaining its rotated position, return the patient to sitting. | "Keep your head turned and push up into sitting. You may get dizzy for a moment." |
| *The clinician should keep one hand on the patient's shoulder for 30 seconds after he returns to sitting.* | Once the patient is in sitting, he may straighten his head. |
| Initially, the patient may not be dizzy, but as the otoconia move into the utricle and back onto the otolithic membrane where they belong, the patient may suddenly experience a brief episode of vertigo. | |

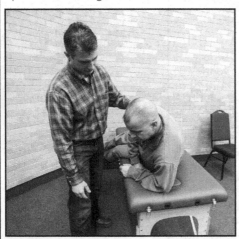

**Figure 5-15.** Modified Epley 7.

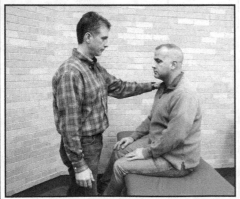

**Figure 5-16.** Modified Epley 8.

## TABLE 5-25
## MODIFIED EPLEY MANEUVER, STEP 6

**PATIENT POSITION**

Repeat maneuver as needed within patient tolerance.

If the patient is tolerating the intervention, wait 5 minutes and then repeat the Dix-Hallpike test. If the patient still tests positive, repeat your maneuver until there is resolution or the patient becomes too nauseous to continue. There is supporting evidence for superior remission rates by repeating repositioning maneuvers during the same treatment.[48] If the test is negative after the intervention, schedule the patient to come back another day to be retested.

## TABLE 5-26
## MODIFIED EPLEY MANEUVER SEQUENCE, NO CLINICIAN

Patient seated with head turned to test side

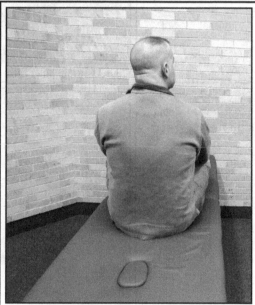

**Figure 5-17.** Modified Epley 1.

*(continued)*

TABLE 5-26 (CONTINUED)
# MODIFIED EPLEY MANEUVER SEQUENCE, NO CLINICIAN

| | |
|---|---|
| Patient lying down with head extended | 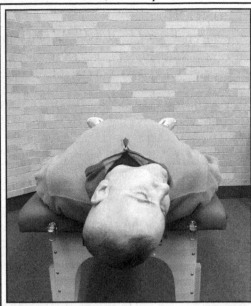<br>**Figure 5-18.** Modified Epley 2. |
| Head rotated to contra-lateral side 45 degrees from neutral | 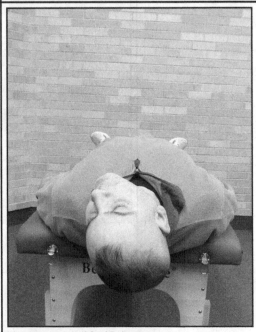<br>**Figure 5-19.** Modified Epley 3. |

*(continued)*

### TABLE 5-26 (CONTINUED)
## MODIFIED EPLEY MANEUVER SEQUENCE, NO CLINICIAN

| | |
|---|---|
| Patient rolls to contra-lateral side keeping the head rotated | 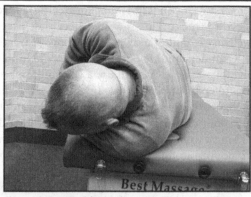 **Figure 5-20.** Modified Epley 4. |
| Maintaining head posi-tion, patient pushes into sitting | 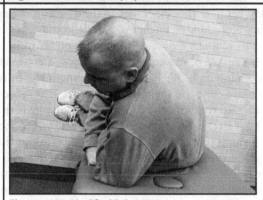 **Figure 5-21.** Modified Epley 5. |
| Once seated, the patient may straighten his head | 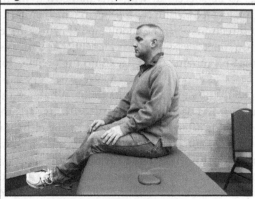 **Figure 5-22.** Modified Epley 6. |

Semont Liberatory Maneuver

The Semont liberatory maneuver may be used to treat canalithiasis (loose crystals) or cupulolithiasis (stuck crystals). When used to treat cupulolithiasis, it is called a *liberatory maneuver*, since it is liberating (or freeing) otoconia (crystals) from the cupula (where they are stuck). This is a maneuver that uses the inertia of endolymphatic flow as well as the pull of gravity as a means of treating cupulolithiasis.[49] You will gain a better understanding of the mechanics behind the maneuver by understanding endolymphatic flow. We will use a common household example and then apply the concept to endolymphatic flow. Imagine that we have a glass pitcher and plan to make lemonade. We fill it with lemon juice and water but want to mix sugar into the drink. If we pour our sugar into the pitcher, it will collect on the bottom, so we have to stir it. Using a wooden spoon, we begin to stir clockwise. As we stir, we are getting the liquid moving around inside of the pitcher in a clockwise direction. We do this as a means of moving the sugar granules. If we didn't have a spoon, another way we could get the lemonade moving around inside of the pitcher would be to pick up the entire pitcher and start moving it in a clockwise circular fashion. Again, the lemonade would begin to flow clockwise in the direction we are moving the pitcher. We are using the motion of the pitcher to get the liquid that is contained within the pitcher to move. Now that we have this image in our minds, let's consider this in terms of the inner ear. We have a canal that is almost a complete circle, and the canal is full of liquid endolymph. We have crystals lying loose in the liquid-filled canal that we want to move (like the sugar crystals in the lemonade). Obviously our spoon won't fit, so how can we move the crystals? The answer is that we move the *entire patient* very quickly in the direction we want the crystals to move and thereby move the liquid endolymph that is inside, so that it is flowing in the direction of the utricle, just as we moved the entire pitcher to move the lemonade clockwise inside the pitcher. The movement of the liquid will carry the crystals along with the liquid flow (called *endolymphatic flow*) back to the utricle where they belong.

For us to be successful with this maneuver, we have to think about *where* the crystals are located within the ear (ie, in which canal), so we can move the patient in the right direction to get the endolymph flowing in the direction of the utricle. If the crystals are stuck, we can use this maneuver as a means of forcefully pulling them off the cupula and moving them back into the utricle. Some researchers do not believe that all cases of cupulolithiasis involve stuck crystals but instead that the crystals are trapped in the short arm of the canal. Whatever the true situation (stuck or not), this maneuver has been found to be an effective treatment and can be performed by the patient alone after a demonstration by the clinician or with the assistance of the clinician. When the clinician is involved, it is a very hands-on maneuver. Patient positioning for this maneuver depends on the canal you wish to treat. You need to think about where the crystals are assumed to be and in which direction you need the endolymph to flow, which will be in the direction of the patient's body "flip" from the initial side-lying position to the contralateral side. In the following example, we will assume treatment of a posterior canal.

Steps to perform the Semont liberatory maneuver[23] are listed in Tables 5-27 through 5-30. Table 5-30 shows the sequence with the clinician guiding the maneuver.

## TABLE 5-27
# SEMONT LIBERATORY MANEUVER, STEP 1

| PATIENT POSITION | PATIENT INSTRUCTIONS |
|---|---|
| While sitting on the side of the table/bed, the patient's head is rotated 45 degrees away from the ear to be treated.<br><br>Next, with head rotated, the patient moves into side-lying onto the side of suspected involvement. (He should now be side-lying on the involved side with his nose rotated up to the ceiling 45 degrees.)<br><br>For the treatment of posterior canal BPPV, while in side-lying, rotate the head as if looking toward the ceiling at a 45 degree angle. If you are assisting/guiding the maneuver, your hands will be on each side of the patient's head at ear level while the patient crosses his arms and holds your forearms to assist during the moving parts of the maneuver. | Position the patient in side-lying, and instruct, "Hold onto my forearms. On three, we will flip to lie on your other side. We need to do this quickly, so you need to help me. Your head will stay in this position. I need you to help me while you change sides. Are you ready? One... two... three!" |

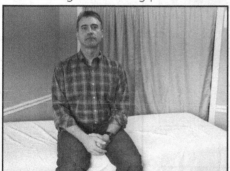

**Figure 5-23.** Semont 1.

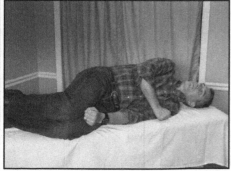

**Figure 5-24.** Semont 2.

## TABLE 5-28
# SEMONT LIBERATORY MANEUVER, STEP 2

| PATIENT POSITION | PATIENT INSTRUCTIONS |
|---|---|
| While maintaining head position, move the patient rapidly and forcefully into side-lying on the opposite side *without stopping* in the upright sitting position. When he comes to rest, he should be side-lying and looking toward the ground with his head still rotated at 45 degrees. | Once moved into the new position, "We need to stay in this position for at least 30 seconds." |

*Hold* this position. Hold times vary from 30 seconds to 2 minutes.

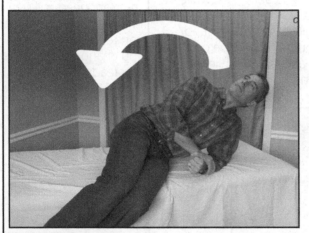

**Figure 5-25.** Semont 3.

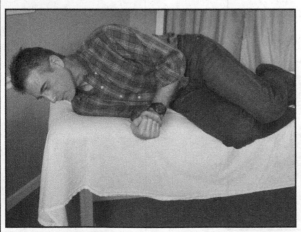

**Figure 5-26.** Semont 4.

## TABLE 5-29
## SEMONT LIBERATORY MANEUVER, STEP 3

| PATIENT POSITION | PATIENT INSTRUCTIONS |
|---|---|
| Patient maintains head rotation while returning to a sitting position. Once seated, he may straighten his head. The clinician should keep a hand on the patient's shoulder for about 30 seconds once he is sitting to guard him in case he becomes vertiginous. | "Keep your head turned and push back to sitting. Once you are seated, you may straighten your head." |

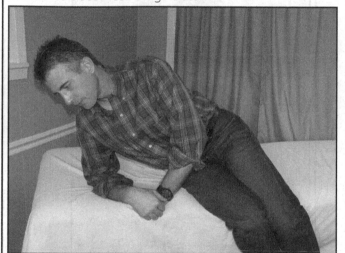

**Figure 5-27.** Semont 5.

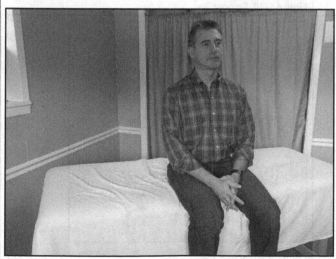

**Figure 5-28.** Semont 6.

## TABLE 5-30
# SEMONT LIBERATORY MANEUVER SEQUENCE WITH CLINICIAN

| | |
|---|---|
| The patient's head is rotated 45 degrees away from test ear and then is positioned into side-lying on the side of the test ear. | 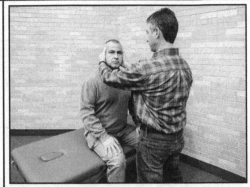 **Figure 5-29.** Semont 1a. |
| | 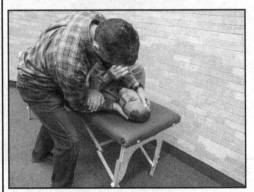 **Figure 5-30.** Semont 2a. |
| While maintaining head position, the patient is rapidly and forcefully flipped into side-lying on the opposite side. | 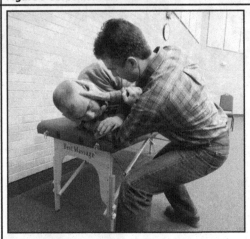 **Figure 5-31.** Semont 3a. |

*(continued)*

## TABLE 5-30 (CONTINUED)
## SEMONT LIBERATORY MANEUVER SEQUENCE WITH CLINICIAN

| | |
|---|---|
| Keeping the head rotated, the patient is returned to sitting. Once seated, the patient is allowed to return the head to a neutral position. | 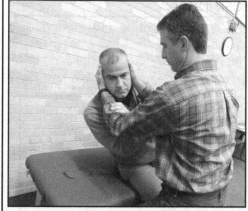<br>**Figure 5-32.** Semont 4a. |
| | 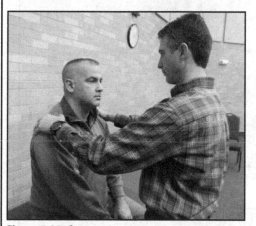<br>**Figure 5-33.** Semont 5a. |

 Gans Repositioning Maneuver

The Gans repositioning maneuver (GRM) is another technique for treating posterior canalithiasis. In a study of 207 patients diagnosed with BPPV of the posterior canal (121 with right ear involvement, 76 with left ear involvement, and 10 with bilateral ear involvement). All patients were treated using the GRM. Subjects returned at 1-week intervals for follow-ups until the posterior canal was cleared. Results showed resolution rates of 80.2% after one treatment and 95.6% after 2 treatments.[50]

Tables 5-31 through 5-35 give directions for performing the GRM (personal communication with Dr. Richard Gans, 2013).

# TABLE 5-31
# GANS REPOSITIONING MANEUVER, STEP 1

## PATIENT POSITION

The patient sits on the side of the treatment table/bed facing forward (head/neck neutral). Rotate the head 45 degrees away from the involved ear, and move the patient into side-lying onto the involved side.

*Crystal movement:* Otoconia move to center of posterior canal.

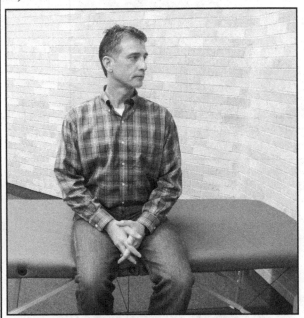

**Figure 5-34.** Gans 1.

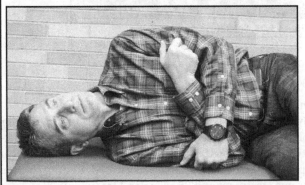

**Figure 5-35.** Gans 2.

## TABLE 5-32
## GANS REPOSITIONING MANEUVER, STEP 2

**PATIENT POSITION**

Instruct the patient to roll onto his other side (if needed, the clinician can roll the patient), maintaining head position so that the patient is now looking toward the ground at 45 degrees of head rotation.

*Crystal movement:* Otoconia move to common crus.

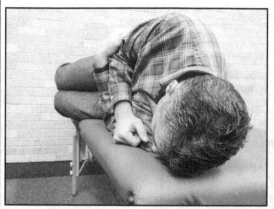

**Figure 5-36.** Gans 3.

## TABLE 5-33
## GANS REPOSITIONING MANEUVER, STEP 3

**PATIENT POSITION**

Staying in the position described in step 2, instruct the patient to perform a head shake (as if saying "no") 3 or 4 times rapidly. When his head stops shaking, the patient should once again be in the nose-down 45-degree position.

*Crystal movement:* Debris from the otoconia traverses the common crus.

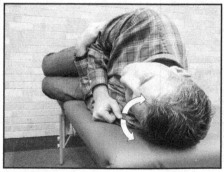

**Figure 5-37.** Gans 4.

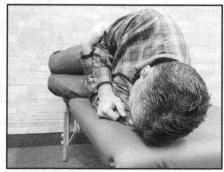

**Figure 5-38.** Gans 5.

## TABLE 5-34
# GANS REPOSITIONING MANEUVER, STEP 4

### PATIENT POSITION

While maintaining the 45 degrees of rotation, return the patient to sitting. Then return to head-neutral position (ie, zero cervical rotation), and flex the head/neck for about 15 seconds. Finally, the patient resumes a neutral neck posture.

*Crystal movement:* Debris from the otoconia enters the utricle.

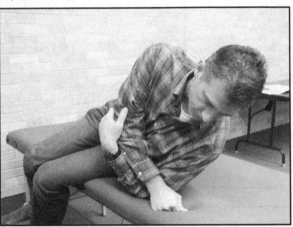

**Figure 5-39.** Gans 6.

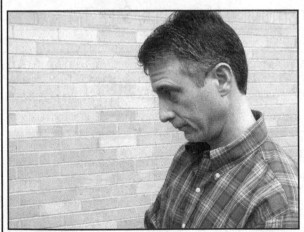

**Figure 5-40.** Gans 7.

| TABLE 5-35 |
|---|
| **GANS REPOSITIONING MANEUVER, STEP 5** |
| **PATIENT POSITION** |
| Finally, instruct the patient to resume a neutral neck posture. |

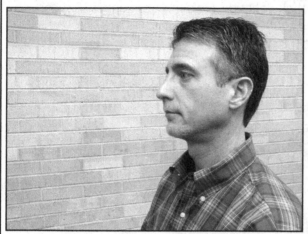

**Figure 5-41.** Gans 8.

 Brandt-Daroff Exercise

The Brandt-Daroff exercise is a home repositioning exercise intended to promote loosening and movement of the otoconia toward the utricle[19,51]; it is also useful for treating motion sensitivity as a habituation exercise. As a repositioning maneuver, it does not target any one specific canal and is less effective as a BPPV intervention than other maneuvers.[19] However, it has utility in some instances. Self-administered canalith repositioning (eg, specific maneuvers used by patients on their own at home, like the Semont or modified Epley maneuvers) have been found to be much more effective than having patients perform the Brandt-Daroff (64% vs 23%).[52]

When is this exercise/maneuver useful? Instances where choosing the Brandt-Daroff instead of another maneuver or as an adjunct intervention may prove beneficial include the following:

- If for some reason patients cannot tolerate another maneuver, they may perform this exercise.
- If the patient cannot remember how to do a repositioning maneuver or has difficulty reading and following directions, this is a good alternative as it is simple to perform.

## TABLE 5-36
# BRANDT-DAROFF EXERCISE, STEP 1

### PATIENT INSTRUCTIONS

The patient sits on the edge of a bed and rotates their head *left* 45 degrees, and quickly lies down on their *right* side. *Hold* this position for 30 seconds after vertigo stops (or 30 seconds if no vertigo is present).

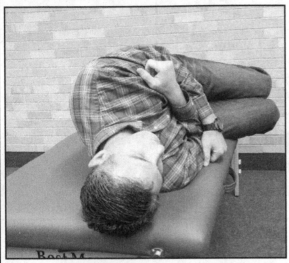

**Figure 5-42.** Brandt-Daroff 1.

- When patients are frail or you are afraid that they may be at risk of injury during another maneuver, you may instruct them to perform this exercise on their own without being touched by clinician or having the clinician direct the movements.
- If you have tried repositioning maneuvers that have not yielded good results, this exercise can be useful as an adjunctive home exercise.
- Since the movements are dynamic and progress through a wide range of head positions, this exercise is useful for motion habituation.

The Brandt-Daroff is not a hands-on exercise with regard to the clinician. Patients perform it by using verbal cues or written instructions. It is always good to first demonstrate this exercise and to provide a handout that includes pictures or drawings showing how to perform it.

Directions for the Brandt-Daroff exercise are given in Tables 5-36 through 5-40.

## TABLE 5-37
# BRANDT-DAROFF EXERCISE, STEP 2

**PATIENT INSTRUCTIONS**

The patient returns to sitting (30 seconds).

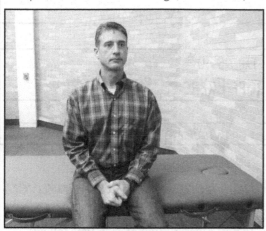

**Figure 5-43.** Brandt-Daroff 2.

## TABLE 5-38
# BRANDT-DAROFF EXERCISE, STEP 3

**PATIENT INSTRUCTIONS**

The patient rotates his head to the right 45 degrees and quickly lies down on his *left* side, *holding* this position for 30 seconds after the vertigo stops (or 30 seconds if no vertigo is present).

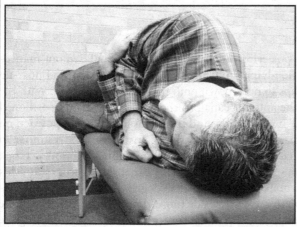

**Figure 5-44.** Brandt-Daroff 3.

| TABLE 5-39 |
|---|
| **BRANDT-DAROFF EXERCISE, STEP 4** |
| **PATIENT INSTRUCTIONS** |
| Return to sitting.<br>(Sequences 1 through 4 represent one cycle of the exercise.) |

| TABLE 5-40 |
|---|
| **BRANDT-DAROFF EXERCISE, STEP 5** |
| **PATIENT INSTRUCTIONS** |
| Do 5 cycles in a row 3 times daily until symptoms resolve. |

## *Anterior Semicircular Canals Repositioning Maneuvers*

Some repositioning maneuvers for targeting the anterior semicircular canals require cervical extension and some do not. A description of each type follows.

### Anterior Canal Repositioning Maneuvers Not Requiring Cervical Extension

Korres et al[53] reviewed a variety of maneuvers to treat BPPV of the anterior canals. Their conclusion was that further studies were needed before clinical significance could be established for one maneuver over another. In other words, there aren't enough studies comparing these maneuvers to say if any are superior over others, and currently no "best practice" is established for treating the anterior canal variety of BPPV. The following repositioning maneuvers treat the anterior semicircular canal: modified Epley, reverse Epley, Radko, prolonged positioning, and modified Dix-Hallpike.

 **Reverse Semont Maneuver**

Remember, in treating the posterior canals with the traditional Semont maneuver, the patient is positioned side-lying on the side of the involved ear and nose-up 45 degrees; the patient then flips to nose-down onto the contralateral side. With the reverse Semont, the target is the anterior canal, so the patient is initially positioned a 45 degrees nose-down on the involved side, and then flips to a nose-up position on the contralateral side while maintaining head position. Instructions are similar to those for the Semont except that you reverse the direction of quick motion to target the anterior canal. Let's use an example of left anterior canalithiasis to explain this maneuver. The patient would rotate his or her head 45 degrees toward the symptomatic ear and then move into side-lying on that side (nose-down 45 degrees toward the floor). Next, the patient would quickly flip to the contralateral side, maintaining the head position so that when stopped, the patient is lying with the unaffected ear closer

| | |
|---|---|
| **TABLE 5-41** | |

# REVERSE SEMONT MANEUVER

| PATIENT INSTRUCTIONS | |
|---|---|
| Begin that patient positioned with the head rotated 45 degrees to the ground on the involved ear. | 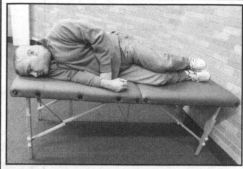**Figure 5-45.** Reverse Semont 1. |
| The patient flips (or is flipped) onto the uninvolved side without changing his head position. | 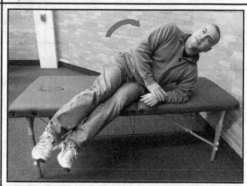**Figure 5-46.** Reverse Semont 2. |
| The patient remains in the 45-degree nose-up position between 30 second and 2 minutes. | 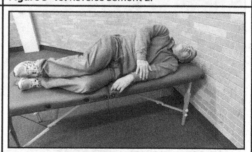**Figure 5-47.** Reverse Semont 3. |

*(continued)*

to the ground and is looking nose-up 45 degrees to the ceiling. After the required hold time, the patient returns to sitting. Hold times are the same as described for the Semont (30 seconds to 2 minutes). Table 5-41 gives directions for the reverse Semont maneuver.

## TABLE 5-41 (CONTINUED)
# REVERSE SEMONT MANEUVER

### PATIENT INSTRUCTIONS

The patient maintains his head position and returns to sitting. Once sitting, he may straighten his head.

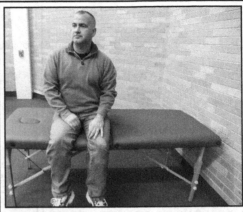

**Figure 5-48.** Reverse Semont 4.

## TABLE 5-42
# RAHKO MANEUVER, STEP 1

### PATIENT INSTRUCTIONS

Position the patient side-lying for 30 seconds with the uninvolved (healthy) ear closer to the ground.

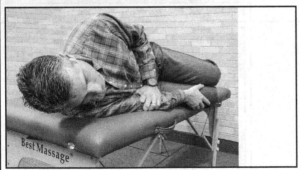

**Figure 5-49.** Rahko 1.

### Rahko Maneuver

Rahko maneuver[54] for treating the anterior canal (canalithiasis) uses gravity to move the crystals. In his study, Rahko treated 57 cases of anterior canal BPPV using his described technique and reported that 53 of 57 had complete remission of symptoms. The steps of the Rahko maneuver are shown in Tables 5-42 through 5-46.[53]

## TABLE 5-43
# RAHKO MANEUVER, STEP 2

### PATIENT INSTRUCTIONS

Next, rotate the patient's head nose-down toward the ground at 45 degrees. *Hold* this position for 30 seconds.

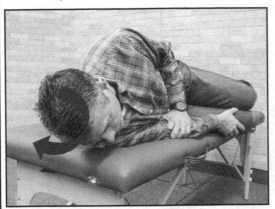

**Figure 5-50.** Rahko 2.

## TABLE 5-44
# RAHKO MANEUVER, STEP 3

### PATIENT INSTRUCTIONS

Continuing to move away from the involved ear, maintain the head position in the 45 degrees of rotation and roll the patient 180 degrees until he is lying supine with his head turned 45 degrees toward the involved ear. *Hold* this position for 30 seconds.

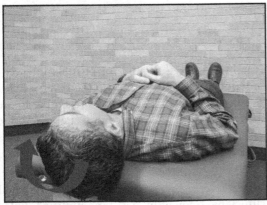

**Figure 5-51.** Rahko 3.

| TABLE 5-45 |
| :---: |
| **RAHKO MANEUVER, STEP 4** |
| **PATIENT INSTRUCTIONS** |
| Keeping the patient supine, position the patient's head in neutral rotation (eg, supine with nose to ceiling). *Hold* this position for 30 seconds. |

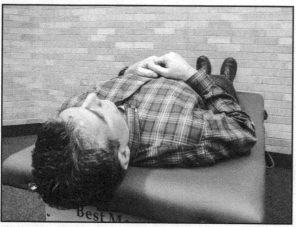

**Figure 5-52.** Rahko 4.

| TABLE 5-46 |
| :---: |
| **RAHKO MANEUVER, STEP 5** |
| **PATIENT INSTRUCTIONS** |
| Return the patient to sitting with his head in neutral. *Hold* the sitting position, supporting the patient, for 3 minutes. |

## Anterior Canal Repositioning Maneuvers With Cervical Extension

If cervical extension is not an issue, there are a number of possible intervention choices. One intervention for anterior canal BPPV is to use the reverse Epley maneuver. There are also a couple of repositioning maneuvers that are similar to the Dix-Hallpike. Kim et al[55] describe such a maneuver, while Yacovino et al[56] describe similar maneuver (called the *deep head-hanging treatment*). The treatments are similar but do have some differences.[57] Let's review these maneuvers.

### Reverse Epley Maneuver

Some authors have proposed using a reverse Epley to treat the anterior canal (canalithiasis).[53] As mentioned, clinicians frequently use the modified Epley

## TABLE 5-47
# KIM'S DEEP HEAD HANG, STEP 1

### PATIENT INSTRUCTIONS/POSITION

The patient starts in a long-sitting position on the treatment table.

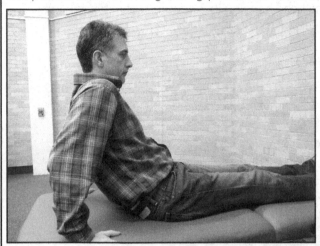

**Figure 5-53.** Kim 1.

maneuver to treat canalithiasis of the anterior canals. Perform the *reverse Epley* using the same steps as the modified Epley maneuver; however, the ear contralateral to the identified anterior canal affected by BPPV is treated. Let's use an example of left anterior canal BPPV (canalithiasis) to demonstrate this maneuver. Dix-Hallpike findings may include a positive left Dix-Hallpike with downbeating and *left-torsional* nystagmus (less than 1 minute) *or* a positive *right* Dix-Hallpike with downbeating and *left-torsional* nystagmus (less than 1 minute). Remember, the torsional direction of the quick phases of the nystagmus should indicate the involved ear. Now that you had established a left anterior canal BPPV (canalithiasis), you would perform the modified Epley *as if* you were treating the right posterior canal (eg, the patient turns his or her head to the right 45 degrees and moves into a supine head-hang to begin the repositioning maneuver).

 *Kim's Head-Hanging Maneuver*

Kim et al[55] reported a 96.7% success rate in their uncontrolled study of 30 subjects. These results were questioned by Hain, who found such a high success rate for the anterior canal unlikely and pointed out that this study was uncontrolled.[57]

Directions for Kim's deep head hang are given in Tables 5-47 through 5-50.

## TABLE 5-48
# KIM'S DEEP HEAD HANG, STEP 2

### PATIENT INSTRUCTIONS/POSITION

Turn the patient's head to 45 degrees toward the symptomatic ear and place him into supine with the head hanging in 30 degrees of extension (while maintaining the 45 degrees of rotation).

*Hold* this position for 2 minutes.

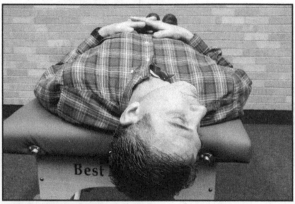

**Figure 5-54.** Kim 2.

## TABLE 5-49
# KIM'S DEEP HEAD HANG, STEP 3

### PATIENT INSTRUCTIONS/POSITION

While maintaining the supine with the 45-degree head-rotation position, elevate the patient's head out of extension to neutral (zero degrees of flexion/extension).

*Hold* this position for 1 minute.

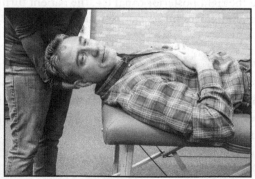

**Figure 5-55.** Kim 3.

| TABLE 5-50 |
| --- |
| ## KIM'S DEEP HEAD HANG, STEP 4 |
| **PATIENT INSTRUCTIONS/POSITION** |
| Return the patient to sitting while maintaining the rotation; once in sitting, the patient returns to neutral rotation with his chin tilted down 30 degrees. Hold time for the tilt is not specified. 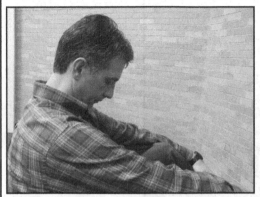 **Figure 5-56.** Kim 4. |

### The Deep Head-Hanging Maneuver

Yacovino et al[56] reported 85% remission of symptoms in a study of 13 patients. In this study, the maneuver had to be repeated overall 1.97 times for symptoms resolution. As with Kim's study, this was an uncontrolled study and it had a small sample size. Another study was performed by Al Saif and Alsenany using the deep head-hanging maneuver with 28 subjects. These investigators found a success rate of 82.1% after one treatment. Another 14.2% of patients had success after a second treatment, and 3.5% required a third treatment for symptom resolution. 100% of subjects had symptom resolution in 3 treatments or less.[58]

The treatment steps as described by Yacovino et al[56] are listed in Tables 5-51 through 5-54.

## Lateral Canal Repositioning Maneuvers

As with the anterior canal maneuvers, there are variations of the lateral canal maneuvers. We will categorize these maneuvers as rolling and nonrolling maneuvers.

### Rolling Maneuvers

There are a number of canalith repositioning maneuvers for BPPV of the lateral canal. They are used for canalithiasis (loose crystals), which your test will show when the patient demonstrates geotropic nystagmus (eyes beating toward the ground) while in the roll-test positions. These maneuvers are pretty much alike with minor

## TABLE 5-51
# YACOVINO DEEP HEAD HANG, STEP 1

**PATIENT INSTRUCTIONS/POSITION**

The patient starts in a long-sitting position on the treatment table.

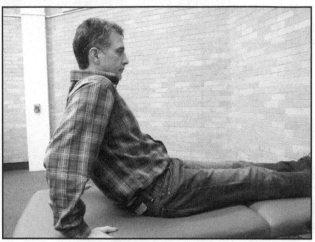

**Figure 5-57.** Yacovino 1.

## TABLE 5-52
# YACOVINO DEEP HEAD HANG, STEP 2

**PATIENT INSTRUCTIONS/POSITION**

The patient is moved into a supine position with his head extended off the treatment table 30 degrees. This position is *held* for at least 30 seconds.

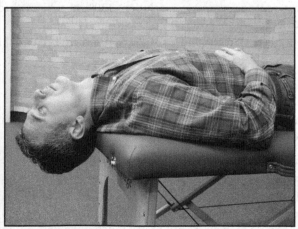

**Figure 5-58.** Yacovino 2.

## TABLE 5-53
# YACOVINO DEEP HEAD HANG, STEP 3

### PATIENT INSTRUCTIONS/POSITION

The patient is moved into a supine position with his head extended off the treatment table 30 degrees. This position is *held* for at least 30 seconds.

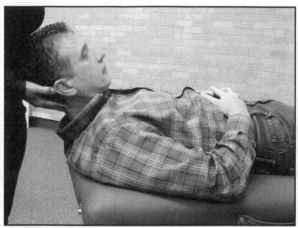

**Figure 5-59.** Yacovino 3.

## TABLE 5-54
# YACOVINO DEEP HEAD HANG, STEP 4

### PATIENT INSTRUCTIONS/POSITION

Return the patient to sitting while keeping the 45 degrees of flexion. Once the patient is sitting, return the head to neutral.

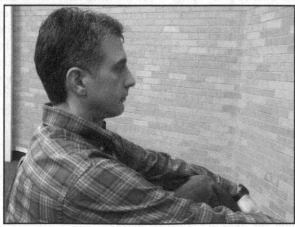

**Figure 5-60.** Yacovino 4.

## TABLE 5-55
# BARBECUE ROLL, STEP 1

### PATIENT INSTRUCTIONS

Position the patient supine with the head rotated (90 degrees) toward the involved ear. *Hold* until nystagmus/dizziness stops plus 30 seconds.

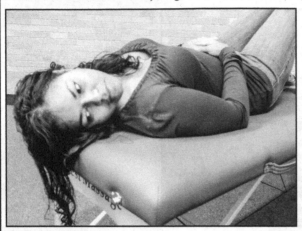

**Figure 5-61.** BBQ 1.

variations; all of them begin with the patient supine with the head turned toward the affected ear (which is now closer to the ground) and then progressively turning away from the affected ear. The barbecue roll and log-roll maneuvers move the patient progressively away from the affected ear into a nose-down toward the ground position (270 degrees of total maneuver head rotation around the yaw axis). The patient is then returned to a sitting position. The difference between these 2 maneuvers is that the log-roll positions the patient's entire body prone to get the head nose-down and then has the patient push up into a kneeling position. The barbecue roll, on the other hand, relies on cervical rotation and trunk positioning (avoiding prone) by rotating the entire trunk to just past side-lying to position the head nose-down. Keeping in mind that the head position is what is important (and not what the rest of the body is doing), you may find it easier to avoid getting patients in prone, as it is sometimes difficult to assist them out of the prone position into sitting. The Lempert maneuver rolls the patient's body completely in 360 degrees (and the head 270 degrees) and then returns the patient to a sitting position. Let's review these maneuvers.

###  Barbecue Roll

This maneuver relies on gravity to move the crystals after the patient's head is placed into the desired position. Some clinicians use quick head turns while moving the patient from position to position, but this is not a required part of the maneuver.

Tables 5-55 through 5-59 show the steps of the barbecue roll.[13]

## TABLE 5-56
## BARBECUE ROLL, STEP 2

### PATIENT INSTRUCTIONS

Rotate the patient's head to neutral (no rotation, with nose to ceiling). *Hold* until nystagmus/dizziness stops plus 30 seconds.

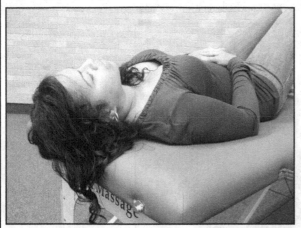

**Figure 5-62.** BBQ 2.

## TABLE 5-57
## BARBECUE ROLL, STEP 3

### PATIENT INSTRUCTIONS

Rotate the patient's head 90 degrees from neutral away from the involved ear. *Hold* until nystagmus/dizziness stops plus 30 seconds.

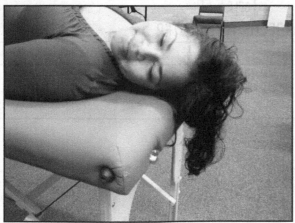

**Figure 5-63.** BBQ 3.

## TABLE 5-58
## BARBECUE ROLL, STEP 4

**PATIENT INSTRUCTIONS**

Maintaining the head rotation, instruct the patient to roll onto her side away from the involved ear until she has her nose directly toward the ground.

*Hold* until nystagmus/dizziness stops plus 30 seconds.

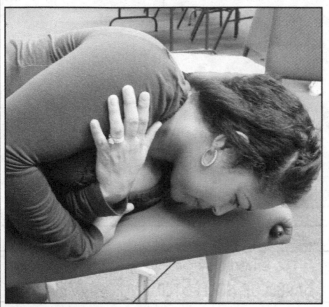

**Figure 5-64.** BBQ 4.

## TABLE 5-59
## BARBECUE ROLL, STEP 5

**PATIENT INSTRUCTIONS**

Keeping the patient's head in rotation, instruct her to push into sitting. Once in sitting, she may straighten her head. The examiner should then guard the patient for 30 seconds.

 **Log Roll**

Similar to the barbecue roll is the log roll, shown in Tables 5-60 through 5-64.

### TABLE 5-60
# LOG ROLL, STEP 1

**PATIENT INSTRUCTIONS**

Position the patient supine with the head rotated 90 degrees toward the involved ear. *Hold* until nystagmus/dizziness stops plus 30 seconds.

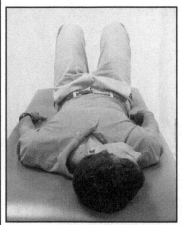

**Figure 5-65.** Log Roll 1.

### TABLE 5-61
# LOG ROLL, STEP 2

**PATIENT INSTRUCTIONS**

Rotate the patient's head to neutral with nose to ceiling.
*Hold* until nystagmus/dizziness stops plus 30 seconds.

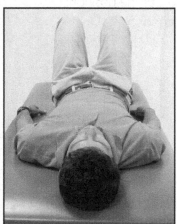

**Figure 5-66.** Log Roll 2.

## TABLE 5-62
# LOG ROLL, STEP 3

### PATIENT INSTRUCTIONS

**Keeping the patient's head in neutral**, instruct him to roll onto his side 90 degrees away from the involved ear (which is now closer to the ceiling).

*Hold* until nystagmus/dizziness stops plus 30 seconds.

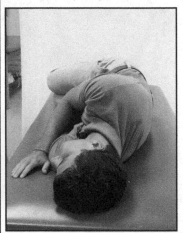

**Figure 5-67.** Log Roll 3.

## TABLE 5-63
# LOG ROLL, STEP 4

### PATIENT INSTRUCTIONS

Keeping his head in neutral, the patient rolls into a prone position.

*Hold* until nystagmus/dizziness stops plus 30 seconds.

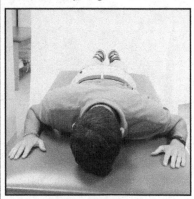

**Figure 5-68.** Log Roll 4.

| TABLE 5-64 |
| :---: |
| **LOG ROLL, STEP 5** |
| **PATIENT INSTRUCTIONS** |
| Instruct the patient to push into kneeling and then straighten his trunk and head. |

| TABLE 5-65 |
| :---: |
| **LEMPERT MANEUVER, STEP 1** |
| **PATIENT INSTRUCTIONS** |
| Position the patient supine. <br> *Hold* for 30 to 60 seconds until all nystagmus subsides. <br><br> 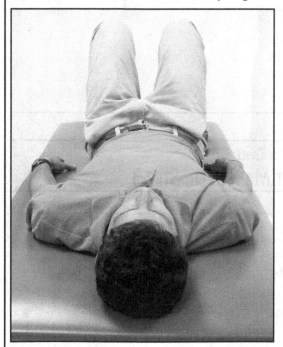 <br><br> **Figure 5-69.** Lempert 1. |

 *Lempert Maneuver*

For the Lempert maneuver, the patient performs each 90-degree position change rapidly and within a half second. Directions for the Lempert maneuver[58] are given in Tables 5-65 through 5-70. *Hold* each position for 30 to 60 seconds until all nystagmus subsides.[59]

## TABLE 5-66
# LEMPERT MANEUVER, STEP 2

**PATIENT INSTRUCTIONS**

The patient rotates his head to the unaffected ear 90 degrees. (The unaffected ear is now down toward the ground.)

*Hold* for 30 to 60 seconds until all nystagmus subsides.

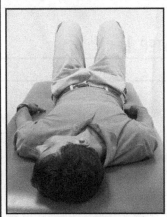

**Figure 5-70.** Lempert 2.

## TABLE 5-67
# LEMPERT MANEUVER, STEP 3

**PATIENT INSTRUCTIONS**

Turn *the patient's body* from supine to prone away from the affected ear while the head maintains its relative position (with respect to the ground) as described in step 2. In other words, don't allow the patient's head to move as you turn the body into prone.

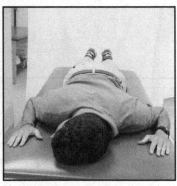

**Figure 5-71.** Lempert 3.

## TABLE 5-68
## LEMPERT MANEUVER, STEP 4

### PATIENT INSTRUCTIONS

Once prone, rapidly turn the patient's head to a nose-to-ground position. *Hold* for 30 to 60 seconds until all nystagmus subside.

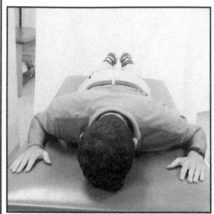

**Figure 5-72.** Lempert 4.

## TABLE 5-69
## LEMPERT MANEUVER, STEP 5

### PATIENT INSTRUCTIONS

While in prone, the head is rotated 90 degrees away from the affected ear. (The affected ear is now down toward the ground.)

*Hold* for 30 to 60 seconds until all nystagmus subsides.

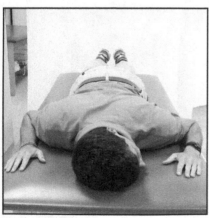

**Figure 5-73.** Lempert 5.

## TABLE 5-70
# LEMPERT MANEUVER, STEP 6

### PATIENT INSTRUCTIONS

Return the patient to sitting.

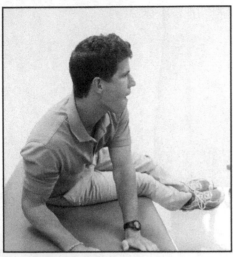

**Figure 5-74.** Lempert 6.

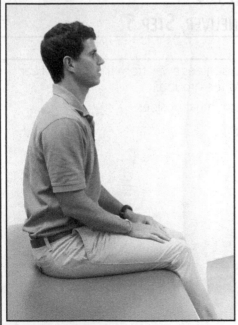

**Figure 5-75.** Lempert 7.

| TABLE 5-71 |
| --- |
| **GUFONI MANEUVER, STEP 1** |
| **PATIENT INSTRUCTIONS** |
| Position the patient in sitting on the edge of the treatment table/bed, arms by his sides. |

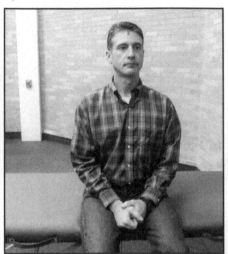

**Figure 5-76.** Gufoni 1.

## Nonrolling Maneuvers (Lateral Canals)

 ***Gufoni Maneuver—Geotropic Variant***

This maneuver uses gravity as the force to move the crystals and is an intervention to treat BPPV of the lateral canals that present with geotropic nystagmus.

The treatment sequence of the Gufoni maneuver is listed in Tables 5-71 through 5-73.[60]

***Gufoni Maneuver—Apogeotropic Variant***

Follow the same procedure as in the geotropic type but perform it on the affected.[60]

***Vannucchi Prolonged Positioning Maneuver***

The Vannucchi prolonged positioning maneuver really is not a "maneuver" in the sense that a clinician is assisting in the performance of a sequence of position changes. Instead, it is a form of prolonged positioning. Vannucchi et al suggest that having a patient sleep on the side with the affected ear up will resolve lateral canal BPPV. In their study, they report a 75% success rate.[61] Hain suggests that this maneuver would not be expected to work for the apogeotropic variant of lateral canal BPPV and further suggests that in theory, side-lying for 10 minutes is plenty, rather than holding that position all night.[62]

# Table 5-72
# Gufoni Maneuver, Step 2

## PATIENT INSTRUCTIONS

Instruct the patient to move quickly into side-lying on the unaffected (healthy) side. One side-lying, his head is immediately rotated 45 degrees toward the floor (nose down).

*Hold* for 2 minutes.

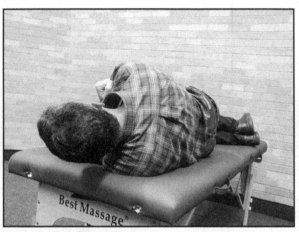

**Figure 5-77.** Gufoni 2.

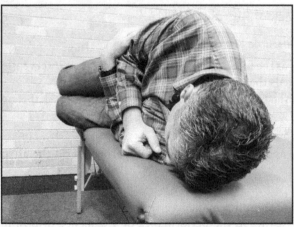

**Figure 5-78.** Gufoni 3.

| TABLE 5-73 |
| :---: |
| **GUFONI MANEUVER, STEP 3** |
| **PATIENT INSTRUCTIONS** |
| Keeping his head turned, the patient returns to sitting. Once sitting, he may straighten his head. |
| 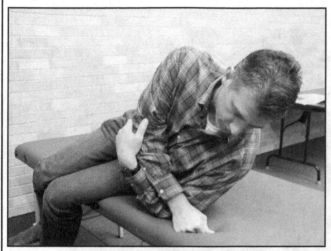 |
| **Figure 5-79.** Gufoni 4. |

 *Vannucchi-Asprella Maneuver*

The Vannucchi-Asprella maneuver is described as being effective for both geotropic and apogeotropic variants of lateral canal BPPV. In a study of lateral canal BPPV maneuvers comprising 40 subjects with geotropic forms of PPV, the Vannucchi-Asprella maneuver successfully cleared 30 subjects of BPPV in the first session, with maneuvers repeated until the nystagmus disappeared. The remaining 10 patients were cleared using the Vannucchi-Asprella maneuver followed by the Lempert maneuver. The author reports, in the same study, resolving 6 cases of apogeotropic lateral canal BPPV with this maneuver,[63] also saying that this maneuver is always repeated a minimum of 5 times. The research article for this study does not specify hold times for the position changes. Given information from other maneuvers, you may wish to try this with the 30-second hold times (for sequences 1 and 2) if the maneuver is not successful without holding each step.

Steps of the Vannucchi-Asprella maneuver are shown in Tables 5-74 through 5-77.

## TABLE 5-74
# VANNUCCHI-ASPRELLA MANEUVER, STEP 1

### PATIENT INSTRUCTIONS

The patient begins in long-sitting (or with knees bent for comfort) with the head in neutral (looking straight ahead) and is moved into supine.

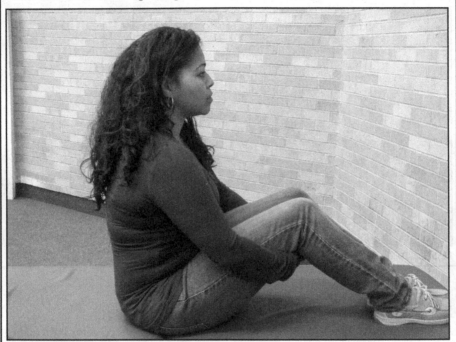

**Figure 5-80.** Vannucchi 1.

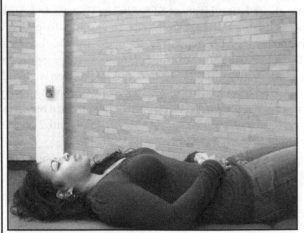

**Figure 5-81.** Vannucchi 2.

## TABLE 5-75
# VANNUCCHI-ASPRELLA MANEUVER, STEP 2

### PATIENT INSTRUCTIONS

Briskly turn the patient's head 90 degrees toward the healthy side.

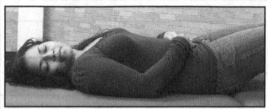

**Figure 5-82.** Vannucchi 3.

## TABLE 5-76
# VANNUCCHI-ASPRELLA MANEUVER, STEP 3

### PATIENT INSTRUCTIONS

Return the patient to sitting, keeping the head turned. Once sitting, the patient slowly bring it back to neutral.

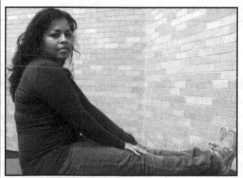

**Figure 5-83.** Vannucchi 4.

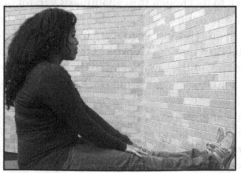

**Figure 5-84.** Vannucchi 5.

| TABLE 5-77 |
| :---: |
| **VANNUCCHI-ASPRELLA MANEUVER, STEP 4** |
| **PATIENT INSTRUCTIONS** |
| Repeat this sequence 5 times. |

| TABLE 5-78 |
| :---: |
| **HEAD-SHAKE CONVERSION, STEP 1** |
| **PATIENT INSTRUCTIONS** |
| Position the patient in supine with head flexed 30 degrees. |

| TABLE 5-79 |
| :---: |
| **HEAD-SHAKE CONVERSION, STEP 2** |
| **PATIENT INSTRUCTIONS** |
| Rotate the patient's head in the yaw plane (head shake "no") to 30 degrees past neutral on each side (back and forth) at a frequency of 2 Hz (720 degrees per second). The research article does not specify the duration of the head shake but it was most likely brief (eg, less than 20 seconds). |

##  Apogeotropic Conversion to Geotropic

There are differing theories on the causes of apogeotropic nystagmus. One thought is that crystals are actually stuck (adhered to) the cupula. These stuck crystals weigh it down and deflect the cupula when the patient's head is in a position where gravity can bend the cupula owing to the added weight. The other school of thought is that the crystals are loose but very close to the cupula in the short arm of the canal and perhaps trapped there. When the patient moves into a test position, the effect of the moving crystals and endolymph in the short arm of the canal acts in the same manner on the cupula as a crystal that is stuck to it. Though the canalithiasis variant (ie, loose crystals) is easier to resolve, clinicians want to convert the nystagmus to the geotropic variant, which will be evident upon retesting when the patient has geotropic nystagmus. Once liberated, the crystals can move freely within the canal, so that the now loose crystals can be repositioned out of the canal and into the utricle where they belong. In common terms, you need to free (liberate) the stuck crystals before you can reposition them back to the utricle.

Casani et al describe 2 treatment interventions to convert apogeotropic nystagmus to geotropic nystagmus.[60] If these conversion maneuvers didn't work, then Casani suspected true cupulolithiasis (stuck crystals). Let's review 2 different methods of making this conversion, the head-shake conversion and head-rotation conversion methods (Tables 5-78 through 5-82).

| TABLE 5-80 |
|---|
| **HEAD-ROTATION CONVERSION, STEP 1** |
| **PATIENT INSTRUCTIONS** |
| Position the patient in supine with the head turned toward the affected ear (which is down). |

| TABLE 5-81 |
|---|
| **HEAD-ROTATION CONVERSION, STEP 2** |
| **PATIENT INSTRUCTIONS** |
| Rapidly rotate the head 180 degrees toward the healthy side. |

| TABLE 5-82 |
|---|
| **HEAD-ROTATION CONVERSION, STEP 3** |
| **PATIENT INSTRUCTIONS** |
| Slowly rotate the head back to the starting position. |

# BENIGN PAROXYSMAL POSITIONAL VERTIGO STUDIES

Vestibular therapy encompasses more than just exercises for the vestibular system. Examples of research that supports vestibular therapy, including balance interventions, follow. These studies clearly do not represent the total sum of research on these subjects but highlight some findings that may have an impact on clinical decision making.

## Canalith Repositioning Efficacy

We refer to maneuvers that move crystals within the vestibular canals as canalith repositioning maneuvers. You may see these abbreviated as *CRM* or *CRP* in literature, but in writing a clinical note in a chart, it is better to write out the title to avoid confusing other clinicians who may read your note.

### Benign Paroxysmal Positional Vertigo of the Posterior Canal

In a study of 965 patients treated with canalith repositioning, symptoms subsided immediately in 85% of patients by the first repositioning; 2% required more than 3 repositioning treatments. Elderly subjects had significantly higher recurrence rates.[64]

A 2004 Cochrane review found that the Epley maneuver (a canalith repositioning maneuver) was well tolerated and effective for treating posterior canal BPPV when compared with controls.[65]

The patients treated for BPPV with the Epley maneuver were compared with a control group who received no repositioning maneuver or treatment. Subjective improvement at 1 month was 89% for the Epley-treated group vs 10% for the no treatment group. At 6 months, subjective improvement was 92% for the Epley-treated group vs 50% for the no-treatment group. The authors concluded that the Epley maneuver provides effective and long-term control of symptoms in patients with BPPV.[45]

A review by Helminski and colleagues[42] of studies published between 1966 and September 2009 found the following:

- Randomized controlled trials provided strong evidence that the canalith repositioning procedure resolves posterior canal benign paroxysmal positional nystagmus.

- Quasi-random controlled trials suggested canalith repositioning procedure or the liberatory maneuver performed by a clinician or with proper instructions as a home treatment resolves posterior canal benign paroxysmal positional nystagmus.

In a review of BPPV interventions, Herdman[66] reports 2 studies that effectively treated BPPV of the posterior canal using the Semont (liberatory) maneuver. Each study compared this maneuver with sham treatment groups. Mandalá et al reported 86.8% resolution using the Semont,[67] while Chen et al reported an 84% resolution.[68]

Brandt-Daroff exercises have been reported as being effective in 98% of subjects after 14 days of exercises.[51] Other studies have found this approach to be less effective than more canal-specific maneuvers (such as the Semont). Criticisms of this exercise are that it is not canal-specific and that canalith repositioning has quicker resolution rates. The Brandt-Daroff does have uses as an alternative to other maneuvers when forceful motions are not an option, and it is an easy home exercise to perform when the patient has difficulty following multiple-step maneuvers.

## Benign Paroxysmal Positional Vertigo of the Lateral Canal

Traditionally, clinicians use the roll test to diagnose lateral canal BPPV. You identify the affected side (ear) in cases of canalithiasis as the more symptomatic side during testing. For cupulolithiasis, the affected side is the side of lesser symptoms.[66] The Bow-and-Lean test is used to determine which ear is involved in cases of lateral canal BPPV.[39] Use of this test increases treatment efficacy from 67.4% to 83.1% for the canalithiasis form of lateral canal BPPV and from 61.1% to 74.7% for the cupulolithiasis form.[13]

Testa et al[69] studied the efficacy of 2 variations of the Gufoni maneuver for lateral canal BPPV, dividing subjects between these intervention options ($n = 87$). They found resolution rates of 93% after the first session of the modified Gufoni and 88% after treatment using the standard Gufoni maneuver.

## Benign Paroxysmal Positional Vertigo of the Anterior Canal

There are significantly fewer studies of anterior canal BPPV compared with those of other canals. As discussed earlier in the section on repositioning maneuvers for the anterior semicircular canals:

- Rahko's maneuver[54] for anterior canal canalithiasis uses gravity to move the crystals. In his study, Rahko treated 57 cases of anterior canal BPPV using his described technique and reported that 53 of 57 patients had complete remission of symptoms.
- Kim et al, using a head-hanging maneuver, reported a 96.7% success rate in their uncontrolled study of 30 subjects.[55] These results were questioned by Hain, who found such a high success rate for the anterior canal unlikely and pointed out that this study was uncontrolled.[57]

# Recurrence of Benign Paroxysmal Positional Vertigo

In a study by Do et al, 138 patients diagnosed with BPPV in the emergency room and ear, nose and throat outpatient clinics were classified by how quickly they were treated with canalith repositioning maneuvers, either in less than 24 hours (early group) from symptom onset or in more than 24 hours (delayed repositioning group). A total of 33.3% had recurrence. The early group's recurrence rate was 19.7%, while the *delayed* group had a recurrence rate of 45.8%. This was a significant difference, suggesting that early treatment after initiation of symptoms may affect recurrence.[9]

# Vibration

Some believe that by applying vibration to the mastoid, the crystals are helped to move; however, there are studies refuting this claim. In one such study of 94 subjects, the researcher found that vibration did not significantly affect short- or long-term outcomes.[46] Fife et al reviewed 5 such studies, 4 of which showed no further benefit when mastoid vibration was added.[23]

A recent Cochrane review of 11 trials states that there is "insufficient evidence to support the routine application of mastoid oscillation during the Epley maneuver, or additional steps in an 'augmented Epley' manoeuvre.'" The review also states that no adverse outcomes were reported for these treatments.[70]

# Postmaneuver Restrictions

In a review of studies that examined the utility of restrictions following canalith repositioning, the American Academy of Neurology found that 5 studies supported no post-treatment restrictions, and one study supported restrictions. Their conclusion: There is insufficient evidence to determine efficacy of restrictions.[23]

While some still recommend post-maneuver instructions such as sitting upright, avoiding supine positions, sleeping at 45 degrees, or wearing soft-collars, most research articles agree they are not needed.

A study reported by Fife et al[23] found no difference between success rates of 88% to 96% for those given and not given posttreatment instructions.[71]

A Cochrane review of trials involving 855 participants found that "There is evidence supporting postural restrictions post-Epley maneuver; however, the 'statistically significant' effect only highlights a small improvement in efficacy. An Epley maneuver alone is effective in just under 80% of patients with typical BPPV."[70]

Based on this information, when might you use postmaneuver restriction instructions? Perhaps, if you have a patient who is not responding well to repositioning interventions. In such a case you may wish to add some postmaneuver restrictions to see if they make a difference in that patient's outcomes. Should you use postmaneuver restrictions routinely for most patients? Not according to the research.

## Spontaneous Resolution

Within 7 days of posterior canal BPPV onset, 30% of patients will experience spontaneous remission.[3,42]

# REFERENCES

1.  von Brevern M, Radtke A, Lezius F, et al. Epidemiology of benign paroxysmal positional vertigo: a population based study. *J Neurol Neurosurg Psychiatry*. 2007;78:710-715.
2.  Helminski J, Zee D, Janssen I, Hain T. Effectiveness of particle repositioning maneuvers in the treatment of benign paroxysmal positional vertigo: a systematic review. *Physical Therapy*. 2010;90:663-678.
3.  Imai T, Ito M, Takeda N, et al. Natural course of the remission of vertigo in patients with benign paroxysmal positional vertigo. *Neurology*. 2005;64:920-921.
4.  Rabie A, Foster C, Chang A, Windle M. Canalith-repositioning maneuvers—contraindications. Available at http://emedicine.medscape.com/article/82945-overview#a05. Updated 2012. Accessed October 4, 2014.
5.  Fife D, Fitzgerald JE. Do patients with benign paroxysmal positional vertigo receive prompt treatment? Analysis of waiting times and human and financial costs associated with current practice. *Int J Audiol*. 2005;44:50-57.
6.  Dorigueto R, Mazzetti K, Gabilan Y, Hanaca F. Benign paroxysmal positional vertigo recurrence and persistence. *Otorhinolaryngology*. 2009;75(4):565-572.
7.  Del Rio M, Arriaga M. Benign positional vertigo: prognostic factors. *Otolaryngol Head Neck Surg*. 2004;130(4):426-429.
8.  Nunez R, Cass S, Furman J. Short- and long-term outcomes of canalith repositioning for benign paroxymsal positional vertigo. *Otolaryngol Head Neck Surg*. 2000;122(5):647-652.
9.  Do Y, Kim J, Yang H-S, et al. The effect of early canalith repositioning on benign paroxysmal positional vertigo on recurrence. *Clin Exp Otorhinolayngol*. 2011;4(3):113-117.
10. Herdman S, Tusa R. Physical therapy management of benign paroxysmal postional vertigo. In: Herdman SJ, ed. *Vestibular rehabilitation* (3rd ed).. Philadelphia: FA Davis; 2007:233-260.
11. Halker R, Barrs D, Wellik K, Wingerchuck D, Demaerschalk B. Establishing a diagnosis of benign paroxysmal positional vertigo through the Dix-Hallpike and side-lying maneuvers. *The Neurologist*. 2008;14:201-204.
12. Baloh R, Jacobson K, Honrubia V. Horizontal semicirucular canal variant of benign positional veritgo. *Neurology*. 1993;43:2542-2549.
13. Lee S, Kim J. Benign paroxysmal positional veritgo. *J Clin Neurol*. 2010;6:51-63.
14. Blatt P, Georgakakis G, Herdman S, Clendaniel R, Tusa R. The effect of canalith repositioning maneuver on resolving postural instability in patients with benign paroxysmal postional vertigo. *Am J Otol*. 2000;21:356-363.
15. Giacomini P, Alessandrini M, Magrini A. Long-term postural abnormailities in benign paroxysmal positional veritgo. *ORL J Otorhinolayngol Relat Spec*. 2002;64:237-241.

16. Hain T. Cupulolithiasis. Available at http://dizziness-and-balance.com/disorders/bppv/cupulo-lithiasis.htm. Updated 2013. Accessed October 1, 2014.
17. Radtke A, Berlin C, Lempert T. Response to Honrubia. Re: Self-treatment of benign paroxysmal positional veritgo: Semont vs Epley procedure. Available at http://www.neurology.org/content/63/1/150.figures-only/reply#neurology_el_1944. Updated 2004. Accessed October 4, 2014.
18. Kasse C, Santana G, Branco-Barreiro F, et al. Postural control in older patients with benign paroxysmal positional vertigo. *Otolaryngol Head Neck Surg.* 2012;146(5):809-815.
19. Bhattacharyya N, Baugh RF, Orvidas L, et al. Clinical practice guideline: benign paroxysmal positional vertigo. *Otolaryngol Head Neck Surg.* 2008;139(5 Suppl 4):S47-S81.
20. Bertholon P, Tringali S, Faye M, Antoine J, Martin C. Prospective study of positional nystagmus in 100 consecutive patients. *Ann Otol Rhinol Laryngol.* 2006;115:587-594.
21. Von Brevern M, Seelig T, Neuhauser H, Lempert T. Benign paroxysmal positional vertigo predominantly affects the right labyrinth. *J Neurol Neurosurg Psychiatry.* 2004;75:1487-1488.
22. Baloh R, Honrubia V, Jacobson K. Benign positional vertigo: clinical and oculographic features in 240 cases. *Neurology.* 1987;37:371-378.
23. Fife T, Iverson D, Lempert T, et al. Practice parameter: therapies for benign paroxysmal positional vertigo (an evidence-based review). Report of the quality standards subcommittee of the American Academy of Neurology. *Neurology.* 2008;70(22):2067-2074.
24. Riga M, Bibas A, Enellis J., Korres S. Inner ear disease and benign paroxysmal positional vertigo: a critical review of incidence, clinical characteristics, and management. *Int J Otolaryngol.* 2011:1-7.
25. Gross E, Ress B, Viirre, Nelson J, Harris J. Intractable benign paroxysmal positional vertigo in patients with Meniere's disease. *Laryngoscope.* 2000;110(4):655-659.
26. Mandala M, Awrey J, Nuti D. Vestibular neuritis: recurrence and incidence of secondary benign paroxysmal positional vertigo. *Acta Otolaryngol.* 2010;130(5):565-567.
27. Ishiyama A, Jacobson K, Baloh R. Migraine and benign positional vertigo. *Ann Otol Rhinol Laryngol.* 2000;109(4):377-380.
28. Ogun OA, Buki B, Cohn ES, Janky KL, Lundberg YW. Menopause and benign paroxysmal positional vertigo. *Menopause: J North Am Menonpause Soc.* 2014;21(8):1-4.
29. Korres S, Balatsouras DG, Kaberos A, Economou C, Kandiloros D, Ferekidis E. Occurence of semiciruar canal involvement in benign paroxysmal positional vertigo. *Otol Neurotol.* 2002;23:926-932.
30. Leopardi G, Chiarella G., Serafini G, et al. Paroxysmal positional vertigo: short- and long-term clinical and methodological analysis of 794 patients. *Acta Otorhinolaryngol Ital.* 2003;23:155-160.
31. Balatsouras DG. Benign paroxysmal positional vertigo with multiple canal involvement. *Am J Otolaryngol.* 2012;33(2):250-258.
32. Cakir B, Cakir Z, Civelek S, Sayin I, Turgut S. What is the true incidence of horizontal semicircular canal benign paroxysmal positional vetigo? *Otolarynagol Head Neck Surg.* 2006;126(2):451-454.
33. Shim DB, Kim JH, Park KC, Song MH, Park HJ. Correlation between the head-lying side during sleep and the affected side of benign paroxysmal positional veritgo involving the posterior or horizontal semicircular canal. *Laryngoscope.* 2012;122(4):873-876.
34. Crevits L. Treatment of anterior canal benign paroxysmal positional vertigo by a prolonged forced position procedure. *J Neurol Neurosurg Psychiatry.* 2004;75(5):779-781.
35. Cohen H. Side-lying as an alternative to the Dix-Hallpike test of the posterior canal. *Otol Neurol.* 2004;25:130-134.
36. Nuti D, Agus G, Barbieri M, Passali D. The management of horizontal-canal paroxysmal positional vertigo. *Acta Otolaryngol (Stockh).* 1998;118:445-460.
37. Fife T. Recognition and management of horizontal canal benign paroxysmal positional vertigo syndrome. *Am J Otolaryngol.* 1998;19:345-351.
38. Casani A, Vannucci G, Fattori B, Berrettini S. Treatment of horizontal canal positional vertigo: our experience in 66 cases. *Laryngoscope.* 2002;112:172-178.
39. Choung Y, Shin Y, Kahng H, Park K, Choi S. "Bow and lean test" to determine the affected ear of horizontal canal benign paroxysmal positional vertigo. *Laryngoscope.* 2006;116:1776-1781.
40. Soto-Varela A, Satons-Perez S, Rossi-Izquierdo M., Sanchez-Sellero I. Are the three canals equally susceptible to benign paroxysmal postional vertigo? *Auidol Neurotol.* 2013;18(5):327-334.
41. Steddin S, Brandt T. Unilateral mimicking bilateral benign paroxysmal positioning vertigo. *Arch Otolaryngol Head Neck Surg.* 1994;120:1339-1341.

42. Helminski J, Zee D, Janssen I, Hain T. Effectiveness of particle repostioning maneuvers in the treatment of benign paroxysmal postional vertigo: a systematic review. *Phys Ther.* 2010;90(5):663-678.
43. Rashad UM. Patients with benign paroxysmal positional vertigo and cervical spine problems: is Epley's manoeuvre contraindicated, and is a proposed new manoeuvre effective and safer? *J Laryngol Otol.* 2010;124:1167-1171.
44. Epley J. The canalith repositioning procedure for treatment of benign paroxysmal positional vertigo. *Otolaryngol Head Neck Surg.* 1992;107(3):399-404.
45. Richard W, Bruinties T, Oostenbrink P, van Leeuwen R. Efficacy of the Epley maneuver for posterior canal BPPV: a long-term, controlled study of 81 patients. *Earn Nose Throat J.* 2005;84(1):22-25.
46. Hain T, Helminski J, Reis I, Uddin M. Vibration does not improve results of the canaltih repositioning procedure. *Arch Otolaaryngol Head Neck Surg.* 2000;126(5):617-622.
47. Marcias J, Ellensohn A, Massingale S, Gerkin R. Vibration does not improve results of the canalith repositioning procedure. *Arch Otolaryngol Head Neck.* 2000;126(5):617-622.
48. Herdman S, Tusa R, Zee D, Proctor L, Mattox D. Single treatment approaches to benign paroxysmal positional vertigo. *Arch Otolaryngol Head Neck.* 1993;119:450.
49. Faldon ME, Bronstein AM. Head accelerations during particle repositioning manoeuvres. *Audiol Neurootol.* 2008;13:345-356.
50. Roberts R, Gans R, Montaudo R. Efficacy of a new treatment maneuver for posterior canal benign paroxysmal positional vertigo. *J Am Acad Audiol.* 2006:598-604.
51. Brandt T, Daroff R. Physical therapy for benign paroxysmal positional vertigo. *Arch Otolaryngol.* 1980;106:484-485.
52. Sargent EW, Bankaitis AE, Hollenbeak CS, et al. Mastoid oscillation in canalith repositioning for paroxysmal positional vertigo. *Otol Neurotol.* 2001;22(2):2205-2209.
53. Korres S, Riga M, Sandris V, Danielides V, Sismanis A. Canalithiasis of the anterior semicircular canal (ASC): treatment options based on the possible underlying pathogenetic mechanisms. *Int J Audiol.* 2010;49:606-612.
54. Rahko T. The test and treatment methods of benign paroxysmal positional vertigo and an addition to the management of vertigo due to the superior vestibular canal (BPPV-SC). *Clin Otolaryngol Alllied Sci.* 2002;27(5):392-397.
55. Kim Y, Shin J, Chung J. The effect of canalith repositioning for anterior semicircular canal canalithiasis. *ORL J Otorhinolaryngol Relat Spec.* 2005;67:56-60.
56. Yacovino D, Hain T, Stone H. New therapeutic manoeuvre for anterior canal benign paroxysmal positional vertigo. *J Neurol.* 2009;256:1851-1855.
57. Hain TC. Anterior BPPV. Available at http://dizziness-and-balance.com/disorders/bppv/acbppv/anteriorbppv.htm. Updated 2014. Accessed October 1, 2014.
58. Al Saif A, Alsenany S. Physical therapy management of anterior canal benign paroxysmal positional vertigo by the deep head hanging maneuver. *J Health Sc.* 2012;2(4):29-32.
59. Lempert T, Tiel-Wilck K. A positional maneuver for treatment of horizontal-canal benign positional vertigo. *Laryngoscope.* 1996;106:476-478.
60. Casani A, Nacci A, Dallan I, et al. Horizontal semicircular canal benign paroxysmal positional vertigo: effectiveness of two different methods of treatment. *Audiol Neurotol.* 2011;16:175-784.
61. Vannucchi P, Giannoni B, Pagnini P. Treatment of horizontal semicircular canal benign paroxysmal vertigo. *J Vestib Res.* 1997;7:1-6.
62. Hain TC. Lateral canal BPPV. Available at http://dizziness-and-balance.com/disorders/bppv/lcanalbppv.htm. Updated 2013. Accessed October 1, 2014.
63. Libonati GA, Gagliardi D, Cifarelli D, Larotonda G. "Step by step" treatment of lateral semicircular canalolithiasis under videonystagmoscopic examination. *ACTA Otorhinolaryingol Ital.* 2003;23(1):10-15.
64. Prokopakis E, Vlastos IM, Tsagournisakis M, Christodoulou P, Kawauchi H, Velegrakis G. Canalith repositioning procedures among 965 patients with benign paroxysmal positional vertigo. *Audiol Neurootol.* 2013;18(2):83-88.
65. Hilton M, Pinder D. The Epley (canalith repositioning) manoeuvre for benign paroxysmal positional vertigo (review). *Cochrane Database Syst Rev.* 2004;2:CD003162.
66. Herdman S. Vestibular rehabilitation. *Curr Opin Neurol.* 2013;26(1):96-101.
67. Mandalá M, Santoro GP, Asprella Libonati C, et al. Double-blind randomized trial on short-term efficacy of the Semont maneuver for the treatment of posterior canal benign paroxysmal positional vertigo. *J Neurol.* 2012;259:882-885.
68. Chen Y, Zhuang J, Zhang L, et al. Short-term efficacy of Semont maneuver for benign paroxysmal positional vertigo: a double-blind randomized trial. *Otol Neurotol.* 2012;33:1127-1130.

69. Testa D, Castaldo G, De Santis C, Trusio A, Motta G. Treatment of horizontal canal benign paroxysmal positional vertigo: a new rehabilitation technique. *Scientific World J.* 2012;2012:160475. doi: 10.1100/2012/160475. Epub 2012 Apr 19.

70. Hunt W, Zimmerman E, Hilton M. Modifications of the Epley (canalith repositioning) manoeuvre for posterior canal benign paroxysmal positional vertigo (BPPV). *Cochrane Database Syst Rev.* 2012(4): CD008675.

71. Massoud E, Ireland D. Post-treatment instructions in the nonsurgical management of benign paroxysmal positional vertigo. *J Otolaryngol.* 1996;25:121-125.

# 6

# Vision (Oculomotor) System

**CHAPTER GOALS**

1. Name the cardinal directions of eye motion.
2. Review the terminology used in describing eye position and motion.
3. Identify eye motions that direct eyes to objects.
4. Identify eye motions that hold images steady.
5. List tests of ocular alignment.
6. Discuss disorders affecting eye motion.
7. List oculomotor interventions.

We use our eyes to see the world. If we plan to get up from a chair, walk to the kitchen and get a drink, we can use the visual information to help us plan our motor actions. We can see what is in our path, and plan to step around or over things as needed, and adjust our movements based on unexpected things we see, such as surface changes we have to negotiate.

Testing of vision, for our purposes, will focus on how the eyes move and less so on visual acuity (or how sharply the patient sees). When the eyes do not align or move properly, the patient may have a variety of complaints, such as blurred vision, headache, dizziness, oscillopsia (shaking vision), or diplopia (double vision). These visual

Plishka CM.
*A Clinician's Guide to Balance and Dizziness:*
*Evaluation and Treatment* (pp 191-236).
© 2015 Taylor & Francis Group.

disturbances often may affect the patient's function, balance, and ability or willingness to perform activities of daily living, ambulate, and socialize.

By assessing eye motion and alignment, the examiner can gain insight into conditions that may be impacting function, causing complaints, or contributing to the overall consequences of a balance condition. Examination of the oculomotor system typically includes motions that bring the eye to a target, and then hold it on the target. This includes *fixation* (gaze holding), ocular range of motion (ROM), ocular alignment, and examination of how the eyes move conjunctively (together).[1]

For more complex cases, you may wish to consult ophthalmology, neuro-ophthalmology, or a behavioral optometrist. Ophthalmology is a branch of medicine that specializes in the eyes. Neuro-ophthalmology is a subspecialty of both neurology and ophthalmology dealing with visual problems caused by nervous system issues. Behavioral optometrists create treatment programs to correct visuomotor and perceptual-cognitive deficits. They look at things like eye alignment, tracking, eye teaming, eye motions, eye focus, and visual processing.

Before reviewing the examination of eye movements, we need to review some new terminology that describes eye movements.[1] Table 6-1 lists the terminology we may need to use in discussing eye motions.

A common description of *visual acuity* is "how sharply we see." Examinations may be performed at bedside or in an office using an eye chart (eg, Snellen chart). While visual acuity certainly may play a role in a person's balance, we are going to focus on the motions of the eye (oculomotor system). For us to see clearly, we have to be able to move our eyes to place the image of objects we are interested in on the *retinas*. The center portion of the retina is the *fovea*, and it is here that we see the sharpest. You may read in a journal or hear in a lecture the term *foveal vision*. It refers to the patient's ability to keep the image of the visual target on the fovea. That is, the patient has the ability to move the eyes to the target, and hold the image on the fovea to see it clearly.

To have the opportunity to see objects clearly, we have to direct our eyes to an object of interest (the thing we want to see) and then be able to hold the image of that object on our foveae. We have different eye motions to accomplish these tasks[2] (Table 6-2).

# VISUAL FIELDS

The visual field is the area of space that is visible to a steadily fixed eye.[3] The *central visual field* has 30 degrees of vision and central fixation. The *peripheral visual field* is everything outside of the 30 degrees of the central visual field. Table 6-3 describes the normal visual field from the point of fixation.

| TABLE 6-1 |
|---|
| **TERMINOLOGY OF EYE MOVEMENTS** |

| TERM | MOVEMENT |
|---|---|
| Ductions | Movement of a single eye alone |
| • Abduction | Movement of the cornea away from midline (temporally) |
| • Eso- | Turning inward |
| • Adduction | Movement of the cornea towards midline (nasally) |
| • Exo- | Turning outward |
| • Elevation, or sursumduction | Movement of the cornea upward |
| • Depression, or deosumduction | Movement of the cornea downward |
| • Intorsion, or incyclotorsion | Rotation of the upper cornea toward midline |
| • Extorsion, or excyclotorsion | Rotation of the upper cornea away from midline |
| Versions | Conjugate movements of both eyes |
| • Dextroversion | Movement of both eyes to the right (abduction of the right eye, adduction of the left eye) |
| • Levoversion | Movement of both eyes to the left (abduction of the left eye, adduction of the right eye) |
| • Upgaze, or supraversion | Movement of both eyes upward |
| • Downgaze, or infraversion | Movement of both eyes downward |
| Vergence | Both eyes move, but in equal and opposite directions |
| • Convergence | Both eyes adduct |
| • Divergence | Both eyes abduct |

# EYE POSITION AND DIRECTION OF MOTION

The term *gaze* indicates that the eyes are looking in a certain direction. Gaze directions are as follows[4]:

<table>
<tr><td colspan="2">TABLE 6-2<br>EYE MOTIONS USED TO SEE OBJECTS</td></tr>
</table>

| | |
|---|---|
| Saccades<br>Smooth pursuit<br>Vergence | Direct the eyes |
| Fixation<br>Vestibulo-ocular reflex<br>Optokinetics | Hold the images steady |

<table>
<tr><td colspan="2">TABLE 6-3<br>VISUAL FIELD</td></tr>
</table>

| AREA | DEGREES OF VISION |
|---|---|
| Nasal | 60 degrees medially |
| Superior | 60 degrees upward |
| Inferior | 70 to 75 degrees downward |
| Temporal | 100 degrees laterally |

**Figure 6-1.** Primary gaze.

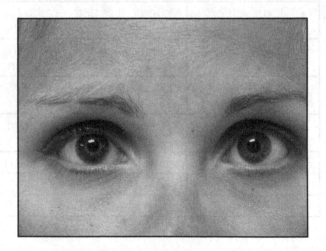

- Primary gaze: The eyes are looking straight ahead (Figure 6-1)
- Secondary gaze: Up, down, left or right (Figure 6-2)
- Tertiary gaze (for each eye): Up + in, up + out, down + in, down + out (Figure 6-3)

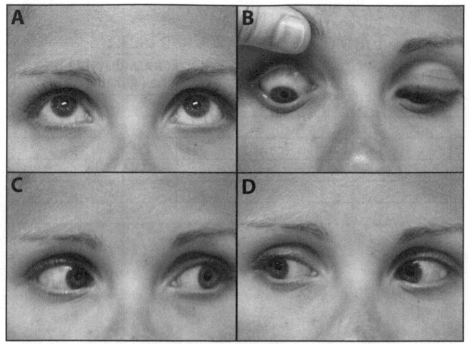

**Figure 6-2.** Secondary gaze: (A) up, (B) down, (C) left, and (D) right.

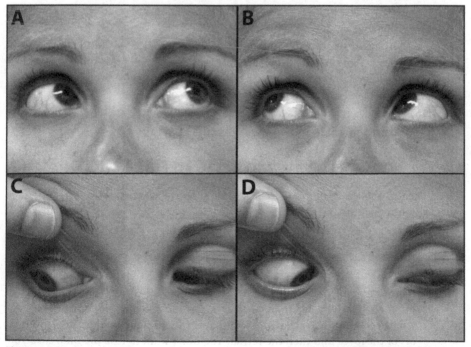

**Figure 6-3.** Tertiary gaze: (A) up and left, (B) up and right, (C) down and right, and (D) down and left.

| | TABLE 6-4 | |
|---|---|---|
| | EYE MOTION INNERVATION AND MUSCLES | |
| MOTION | PRIMARY MUSCLE | CRANIAL NERVE INNERVATION |
| Adduction | Medial rectus | III Oculomotor |
| Abduction | Lateral rectus | VI Abducens |
| Elevation | Superior rectus | III Oculomotor |
| Depression | Inferior rectus | III Oculomotor |
| Intorsion | Superior oblique | IV Trochlear |
| Extorsion | Inferior oblique | III Oculomotor |

## Cardinal Gaze

Clinicians refer to the following 6 gaze positions as the *cardinal gaze positions*:

1. Right + upgaze
2. Right gaze
3. Right + downgaze
4. Left + upgaze
5. Left gaze
6. Left + downgaze

The activity of different eye muscles or combinations of eye muscles produces these motions.[1,5] Table 6-4 lists the eye motions along with the innervation and muscles that produce the motions.

As a general rule[6]:

- Horizontal eye movements are generated in the pons
- Vertical eye movements are generated in the midbrain

## Eye Motions That Direct the Eyes to Objects

As listed in Table 6-2, motions we use to direct our eyes to an object include saccades, smooth pursuit, and vergence.

### Saccades

Saccades are jumping motions of our eyes, and we use them for different reasons:

- To correct our eye position.
  - An example of this would be if you were trying to track an object that is moving slightly faster than your eyes can move using smooth pursuit. As you try to visually track the object that is moving, the image starts to move off of the fovea and then the retina. You don't want to lose the image, so you use a saccade to jump ahead and catch up with the object.

- To substitute for smooth pursuit.
  - If you do not have smooth pursuit and you want to track a moving object, you may string a bunch of saccades together to move the eyes repetitively in one direction. This is not uncommon in people over 60 years of age but would be a concerning finding in middle-aged patient populations.
- To look quickly back and forth between 2 objects.

Saccade latency, speed, and amplitude[7]:
  - Latency of saccades, 200 to 250 ms
  - Peak velocity range, 30 degrees per second to 800 degrees per second
  - Peak duration range, 20 to 140 ms
  - Amplitude range, 0.5 to 40 degrees

There are actually different types of saccades with different instructions for testing each type. We will only be discussing how to assess voluntary (volitional) saccades. To test these, the clinician presents the patient with 2 visual targets, such as the examiner's finger and nose, or by holding up a finger on each hand. The patient is then instructed to look alternately at the 2 targets on command.[2]

For visual targets within the patient's visual field (about 45 degrees on each side of his or her center), a normal test would result in either 1 or 2 saccades to get from one target to the other.

In testing saccades, we look to see if the patient can perform accurate saccades and are careful to observe how many saccades are required to move between 2 targets. Positive findings of saccades testing include the following:

- *Hypometric saccades*, which undershoot the target, requiring an increased number of saccades to reach the target. Causes include visual deficits and cerebellar or brainstem lesions.[8]
- *Hypermetric saccades*, which overshoot the visual target. The saccades move too far and miss the target, and the patient has to add a corrective saccade in the opposite direction to reach the target. Causes include visual deficits and cerebellar or brainstem lesions.[8]
- *Velocity of saccades*. Remember, saccades are the quickest eye motions. If a patient cannot generate quick enough saccades, it appears as if the patient were performing smooth pursuit. Slow saccades are caused by peripheral oculomotor nerve or muscle weakness, internuclear ophthalmoplegia, lesions of the paramedian pontine reticular formation, and degenerative neurological diseases (eg, supranuclear palsy).[5,8]
- *Initiation of saccades*. Delayed initiation of saccades occurs with some metabolic and degenerative disorders, such as Parkinson's disease.[8]

Repeat tests when you observe positive findings. As with the example of the first saccade, which may overshoot, we may see some hyper- or hypometric saccades as the patient tries to locate the target. However, after a few repetitions, the saccades should be accurate and on target.[8] Tables 6-5 through 6-7 provide instructions for testing saccades.

---

### TABLE 6-5
## VOLITIONAL SACCADES TEST, STEP 1

**Instruction:** "I want you to look at the tip of this finger. When I say the word *swap*, look at the other finger." The examiner then uses a chosen word, like *swap*, to command the patient to perform volitional saccades. Avoid using *left* and *right* as commands, as this may confuse some patients.

**Clinician:** The patient is typically in a sitting position (although this will not alter the test) with the examiner facing her. The examiner presents the patient with 2 stationary visual targets. For example, you may use a finger and your nose as targets, or 2 of your fingers (one each from hand— eg, your index fingers) held about 90 degrees apart with each finger at 45 degrees on opposite sides of the patient's center of vision. Direct the patient to look at one of the targets and then *on command* to move her eyes to the other target. Instruct the patient to switch or jump from target to target several times without moving her head.

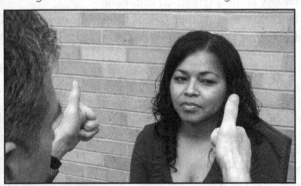

**Figure 6-4.** Saccades test.

---

### TABLE 6-6
## VOLITIONAL SACCADES TEST, STEP 2

**Clinician:** In testing saccades, the clinician should assess saccadic velocity, latency, accuracy, trajectory, and conjugacy (to determine whether the eyes move together).

---

 *Saccades Testing Instructions*

Common terms used to describe the accuracy of the saccades include *hypometric* and *hypermetric*.

Hypometric saccades: If we break the word *hypometric* down, we see *hypo* (less than) and *metric* (referring to distance). A hypometric eye movement would be a saccadic movement that spans less than a normal distance. If your eye movements

| TABLE 6-7 |
| --- |
| ## INTERPRETATION OF THE VOLITIONAL SACCADES TEST |

*Interpretation*

*Negative test:* The eye movements are conjugate (symmetrical) and quick; they move from target to target in either 1 or 2 saccades. Allow for overshooting on the first commanded saccade, but realize that repetitive overshooting is abnormal.

*Positive test:* Positive signs include consistent hypermetric or hypometric saccades, disconjugate saccades, excessively slow saccades, or increased latency during the generation of saccades (ie, if there is a long pause between the command to perform the saccades and the actual initiation of eye movement).

fall short of the normal distance while performing a saccade, you will need more saccades to get from point A to point B. While examining saccades, if the patient consistently uses more than 2 saccades to look between targets within the visual field, describe these saccades as being hypometric.

Hypermetric saccades: If we break the word *hypermetric* down, we see *hyper* (more than) and *metric* (distance). A hypermetric saccade moves too far and overshoots the target. When this happens, the patient needs to make a corrective saccade in the opposite direction to go back to the target. It is not uncommon to see a hypermetric saccade during the first saccade that is tested (ie, the first command you give the patient to look at the other target); however, if the patient consistently presents hypermetric (overshooting) saccades, the test would be considered positive for a saccadic deficit. Table 6-8 lists common saccadic impairments and their causes.

## Smooth Pursuit

Smooth pursuit is the slow tracking motion of the eye while the head is still and one watches something move across the visual field. When objects move across our visual fields fairly slowly, we can watch them by using smooth pursuit motions. An example of smooth pursuit is when you are sitting in a chair and watching someone walk across the room. The motion your eyes make to do this is a slow, smooth motion of tracking that follows a target as it is moving. Intuitively we try to keep the visual target on the fovea (retina) so we can see it clearly. Basic information about smooth pursuit includes the following:

- Latency: 100 to 130 ms.[2,7]
- Velocity: For most of us, smooth pursuit can compensate for head movements up to a velocity of 100 degrees per second.[10] Higher velocities are available for large-amplitude, full-field, or self-moved target motions[7] and for top athletes who have trained themselves to watch fast-moving objects and may generate pursuit as fast as 130 degrees per second.[10]

| TABLE 6-8 | |
|---|---|
| **CAUSES OF SACCADIC IMPAIRMENTS[9]** | |
| **IMPAIRMENTS** | **CAUSES** |
| Slow saccades, often with hypometria | • Medications (eg, anticonvulsants, benzodiazepines)<br>• Neurodegenerative disorders |
| Slow horizontal saccades | Brainstem lesions |
| Slow vertical saccades | • Midbrain lesions<br>• Ischemic diseases<br>• Inflammatory diseases<br>• Neurodegenerative diseases (especially supranuclear palsy) |
| Hypermetric saccades | Cerebellar lesions |
| Delayed-onset saccades | Supratentorial cortical dysfunction |

Most people cannot generate pursuit unless there is some type of target. This target may be visual, auditory, tactile, proprioceptive, or cognitive.[2] Try it! Without watching a moving object (and in a quiet room), try using smooth pursuit to look from one side of the room to the other. If you have a camera in your phone, record your eyes as you do this. You will find that you can't generate smooth pursuit eye motions without a target. If you observe carefully (or play back your video), you will realize you are using a series of saccades.[2] Use your smart phone to videotape your eye movements as you try this and then repeat it by watching someone walk across the room.

Smooth pursuit is a normal motion, but it may change with age. It is not unusual to see patients in their late 50s or 60s who do not have smooth pursuit. Not every person of that age loses smooth pursuit, however. When smooth pursuit is not available, the person cannot perform the eye motion to track slowly and must use a different motor program to see things that are moving across the visual field. Usually this means using saccades; when we observe this, we call it *saccadic smooth pursuit*. For a middle-aged or early adult patient, a finding of saccadic smooth pursuit would be concerning, but for patients over 60 years of age or so it is an age-related change that is not in itself concerning.

Do the eyes move conjugately (together) and are the motions smooth? You check smooth pursuit with both vertical and horizontal pursuit motions. Causes of pursuit abnormalities include medications (tranquilizers and anticonvulsants), lesions of the cerebellum, and diffuse disease of one cerebral hemisphere.[8] Tables 6-9 through 6-11 provide instructions for testing smooth pursuit.

| TABLE 6-9 |
| :---: |
| **SMOOTH PURSUIT TESTING, STEP 1** |
| **Instruction:** "Follow my pen tip using only your eyes. Keep your head still." <br> **Clinician:** A visual target (eg, fingertip or fat end of a pen) is presented 12 to 15 inches from the patient and in the center of the visual field. Slowly and smoothly move the target horizontally within the patient's visual field to about 45 to 50 degrees alternately to either side of center. Observe eye motions as the patient tracks the target. |

| TABLE 6-10 |
| :---: |
| **SMOOTH PURSUIT TESTING, STEP 2** |
| **Clinician:** Repeat step 1, only this time use vertical motions as you move the target. Make sure you raise the target above the primary position, forcing the patient into upward gaze. Be on guard for compensatory head or neck motions to assist tracking. If the patient does substitute neck motions for eye motions, use one hand to hold the head still while you retest smooth pursuit. |

| TABLE 6-11 |
| :---: |
| **INTERPRETATION OF SMOOTH PURSUIT TESTING** |
| *Interpretation* <br> *Negative test:* The patient uses smooth motions of the eye (not jumping saccades), and the eyes move conjugately. <br> *Positive test:* Saccadic smooth pursuit, disconjugate eye motions, or a lack of ocular ROM. |

 ***Smooth Pursuit Testing Instructions***

There are numerous central anatomical structures involved in smooth pursuit. Impaired smooth pursuit occurs with structural lesions, intoxications from medications (eg, anticonvulsants, benzodiazepines) or alcohol, and degenerative disorders of the cerebellum or extrapyramidal system.[9]

## Vergence

Vergence is the eye motion we use to change the focal point of our vision either closer or farther away from its current point of fixation (using both eyes, it is called *binocular fusion*). We can do this once, as when looking at a stationary object that is either further or closer than the *last* object we were looking at, or we may do it continuously, as when tracking at an object that is moving toward or away from us (depth tracking). Vergence information includes the following[7]:

- Latency of vergence, about 160 milliseconds
- Maximum velocity, about 20 degrees per second.

We classify vergence motions as either *convergence* or *divergence*. Convergence is when our eyes move in opposite directions of each other but each is moving toward midline. To use a common term, it is when we go "cross-eyed." We use convergence in focusing on a closer object or in tracking something that is moving toward us. Divergence is when the eyes rotate visual lines of sight away from each other (and away from midline). We use this motion in focusing on an object that is farther away or in visually tracking an object that is moving away from us.

We also classify motions as either *conjunctive* (the eyes move in the same direction) or *disjunctive* (the eyes move in opposite directions).

### Convergence Insufficiency

*Convergence insufficiency* is the inability to maintain binocular function (keeping the 2 eyes working together) while viewing at a near distance.[11] Convergence insufficiency is identified when a patient cannot do one of the following: converge to 6 cm, or comfortably and without fatigue converge to 10 cm (from the tip of the nose).[12] Symptoms of convergence insufficiency include some or all of the following: diplopia (double vision), headaches while reading, difficulty concentrating on near work (eg, computers, reading), or blurring words when reading. Patients with convergence insufficiency often try to compensate by squinting or closing one eye while reading.

*Convergence sufficiency* is the ability to maintain binocular fusion (which is the ability to see one image while using both eyes). We assess it by *slowly* moving a visual target from 3 feet away toward the patient's nose. By using a discrete target, such as one end of a pen or pencil, you give the patient a small target on which to fix his or her gaze. The patient is instructed to report seeing double (diplopia) at any point of the test. In testing vergence, the examiner watches the eyes as they converge. When an eye can no longer converge sufficiently to track a target, it loses fixation and deviates outward. The point where this occurs is called *maximum convergence*.[8] Typically, after losing binocular fusion, it takes the patient a moment to report seeing double (diplopia), and you usually see the eyes lose fixation before you hear the patient report diplopia. For this reason, you must do this test with a very slow moving target. If you rely only on the patient's report and are moving your target quickly, you will have moved past the point where the patient lost fixation by the time he or she reports having done so and you will have an inaccurate measurement. While some people have the ability to converge as close as the tip of the nose, maximum convergence is usually 8 to 10 cm distant (tip of patient's nose to visual target); however, it increases with age.[8]

Vergence is often the first visual system affected by fatigue, alcohol, or drugs, and a defective vergence system is commonly the cause of the following symptoms: diplopia, strabismus, eye strain, periocular headache, and blurred vision after short periods of reading.[2] Tables 6-12 through 6-14 present instructions for testing vergence.

Convergence is disturbed in the following conditions: rostral midbrain lesions and tumors of the pineal region and thalamus.[9]

# TABLE 6-12
## VERGENCE TESTING, STEP 1

**Instruction:** "Look at the tip of my (finger, pen). Do you see 1 or 2? As I move the pen toward your nose, keep your eyes on it. Tell me right away if you begin seeing double or if the image is too blurry to see."

**Clinician:** The clinician faces the patient. Present the patient with the tip of your index finger (as if pointing at the patient) or with the fat end of a pen as a visual target. Hold the target about 3 feet away from and directly in front of the patient's nose. *Very slowly* move the target toward the patient's nose tip. Stop when the target reaches the tip of the patient's nose or when the patient reports that the target looks double or is blurry. Measure the distance from the stopped target to the end of the patient's nose.

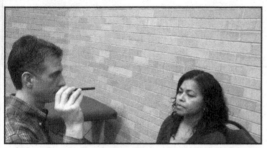

**Figure 6-5.** Vergence test 1.

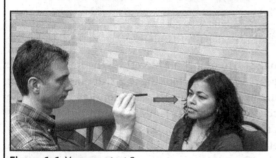

**Figure 6-6.** Vergence test 2.

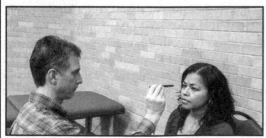

**Figure 6-7.** Vergence test 3.

| TABLE 6-13 |
|---|
| **VERGENCE TESTING, STEP 2** |
| **Clinician:** Repeat step 1 three times. As you are moving the target toward the patient's nose, watch the eyes. At the moment binocular vision is lost you will see one eye leave the target. You may see this before you hear the patient report it. Assess the distance from the point of maximum convergence to the tip of the patient's nose. |

| TABLE 6-14 |
|---|
| **INTERPRETATION OF VERGENCE TESTING** |
| *Interpretation* |
| *Negative test:* The patient is able to converge from about 50 cm to 10 cm or better. |
| *Positive test:* The patient loses fixation prior to 10 cm. |

## Eye Motions That Hold Images Steady

Using the eye motions we have just reviewed (saccades, smooth pursuit, and vergence), we can find our target. Now that we have found it, we need to have the ability to keep our eyes on it. To hold images steady, we need fixation, the vestibulo-ocular reflex (VOR), and optokinetics (OPK).

 Fixation (Gaze Holding) and Range of Motion

The fixation system holds the image of an object of interest on the fovea. The eye is never truly still, even when it appears to be, as in looking at a still object. In order to create fixation, we use 3 miniature eye movements that are not detectable by the naked eye: microsaccades (tiny saccades), microdrift (small smooth pursuit movements), and microtremor (which is the underlying motor activity driving microsaccades and microdrift).[2] When something disrupts fixation, the patient may complain of oscillopsia, which is the perception of a moving environment. Deficits in the fixation system itself or intrusions of other motions such as nystagmus disrupt fixation.

Fixation is tested not just in the primary positions of the eyes (looking straight ahead) but also at or near endpoints around the ocular ROM. During the assessment of fixation at these various eye positions (we will discuss 11 such points), you may also assess the alignment of the eyes by asking the patient to report if he or she has diplopia. During fixation at each test point, the examiner watches the patient's eyes to see if they are relatively held still on the target or unable to remain on the target. When visual fixation with a near target is being tested, the patient fixates for about 5 to 15 seconds on a target (such as a fingertip or the end of a pen) that is

---

### TABLE 6-15
# OCULAR RANGE-OF -MOTION TESTING, STEP 1

**Instruction:** "Follow my pen tip using only your eyes. Keep your head still."

**Clinician:** A visual target (e.g. fingertip or fat end of a pen) is presented 12 to 15 inches from the patient and in the center of the visual field. Move the visual target to each of the points represented in Figure 6-8 (cardinal positions, up- and downgazes, 45 degree positions, and the primary position). Hold the patient's gaze at each point for a minimum of 5 seconds.

---

### TABLE 6-16
# OCULAR RANGE-OF-MOTION TESTING, STEP 2

**Clinician:** Observe if the patient can reach the visual target by moving only the eyes and not substituting head motion. Then, while holding gaze fixed at each target stop, observe if the patient develops any nystagmus.

---

12 to 15 inches away from the patient's eyes. Avoid giving the patient a visual target that is too large. For example, avoid holding the pen vertically and asking the patient to look at the pen, or similarly holding a finger vertically as a target. When using a pen/pencil or finger, make sure to hold it such that only one end (usually the fat end of the pen or a fingertip) is visible to the patient in order to have the patient direct gaze at a discrete point. Alternatively, if you prefer to hold the pen vertically, instruct the patient to "look at the *end* of my pen/pencil/finger." Illuminating your fingertip by using a penlight is another great way to present a visual target and may hold the attention of younger patients or those with attention deficits. If you are also using an ophthalmoscope during the exam, have the patient fixate on a visual target with the contralateral eye while you are observing other eye. You will see some normal movements of the optic nerve while the patient fixates with the contralateral eye, including microsaccades, continuous drift, and microtremor.[8,13]

During tests of fixation assess the following:

- Can the patient maintain visual fixation on a target?
- When fixating on a target, does the patient develop nystagmus or suppress existing nystagmus?
- Does the patient complain of diplopia?

The lack of ocular ROM may point to palsy, muscle weakness, or central pathologies. It is important to determine whether the patient has normal gross ocular ROM as well as to note whether there is any difficulty maintaining certain ranges. Observations of nystagmus may be indicative of pathology. The steps in testing ocular ROM are explained in Tables 6-15 and 6-16.

**Figure 6-8.** Eye ROM Diagram.

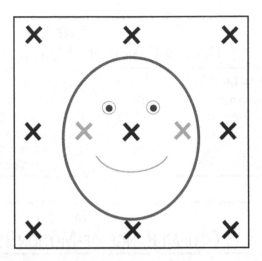

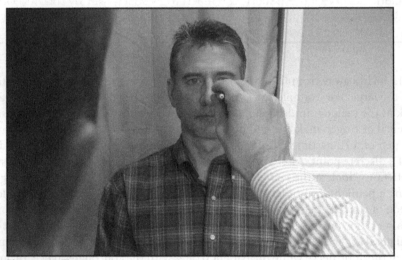

**Figure 6-9.** Fixation.

 *Ocular Range of Motion Testing Instructions*

Use the depiction in Figure 6-8 as a guide to place your visual targets for ROM and fixation testing. The oval represents the patient's face. There are 9 darker X's at points representing the cardinal positions, up- and downgaze, as well as the primary position. There are 2 lighter Xs at 45 degrees to either side of the primary position. You will direct the patient's gaze toward each of these positions.

Here are some examples of testing ocular ROM. First let's discuss testing the middle row of the chart we just reviewed. Start in the primary position of centered gaze and observe the patient's ability to fixate. Another important observation, if it occurs, is the development of nystagmus while the patient is fixating on the visual target (Figure 6-9).

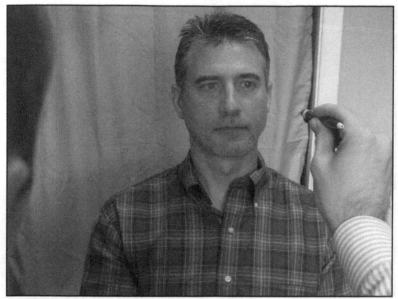

**Figure 6-10.** Gaze L 45 degrees.

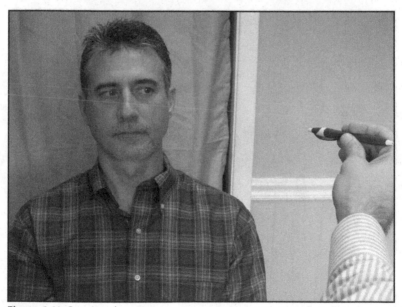

**Figure 6-11.** Gaze L end-range.

Next, move your pen until the patient's eyes are 45 degrees laterally from primary gaze. In our example, we first have the patient gaze left. After holding this position, the target is moved to the patient's end-range laterally on the same side (Figures 6-10 and 6-11).

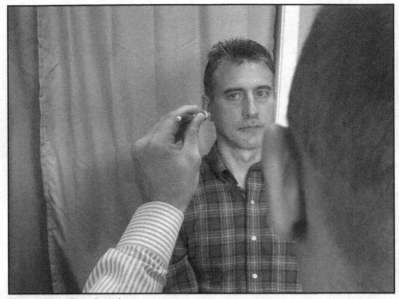

**Figure 6-12.** Gaze R 45 degrees.

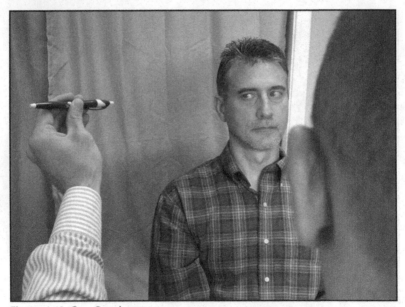

**Figure 6-13.** Gaze R end-range.

Next, observe the patient's gaze on his or her right at 45 degrees and at end-range (Figures 6-12 and 6-13).

After you have observed the right side, the middle line of the chart is completed. There is no reason to bring the visual target back to any of these points unless you

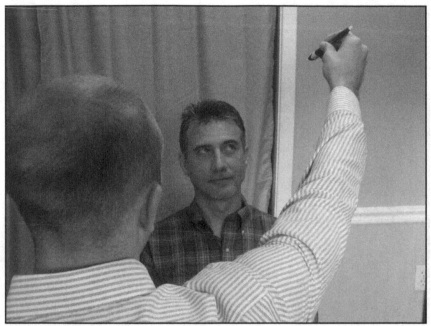

**Figure 6-14.** Gaze left up.

wish to retest it. At end-ranges (or near end-ranges) of motion, you may see nystagmus. If there are more than 3 beats, this should be reported as an abnormal finding. For some, more than 3 beats may still be a normal finding. However, as a screening technique, it is a good practice to report more than 3 beats as an abnormal finding and request further examination by neurology. Some clinicians do not direct the patient's gaze to complete extreme end ranges but near those points. No nystagmus should be seen at the 45-degree test spots.

Now move the visual target up as far as the patient can visually track it. You will place the visual target in 3 places, as depicted on the top line of the chart: up + left end-range, straight up (center), and up + right end-range. Remember to hold each position. Again, we are using extreme upward gaze, so you may see nystagmus at any of these test points (more than 3 beats being abnormal). Also keep in mind that a lack of upward gaze is a central sign. Patients who lack upward gaze will compensate by extending the head, neck, trunk, or a combination. Do not allow the patient to move the head or trunk during testing (Figures 6-14 through 6-16).

Note that many optometrists do not check the centered up- or downgaze positions but that medical physicians do. In our examination we include these positions.

Now that you have examined the first 2 lines of the chart, we will test the bottom line, which includes end-ranges down + left, straight down (center), and down + right (Figures 6-17 through 6-19).

While the patient is in downgaze, it is sometimes difficult to see the eyes. When this occurs, you will need to lift the eyelids. There are pathologies that will cause

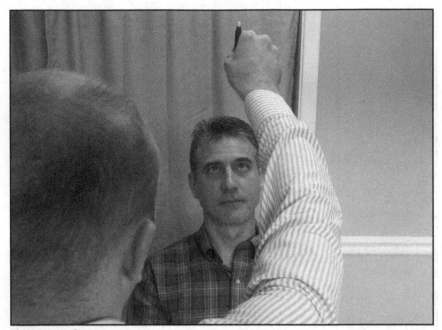

**Figure 6-15.** Gaze up.

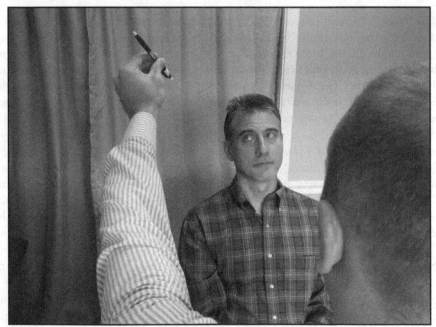

**Figure 6-16.** Gaze right up.

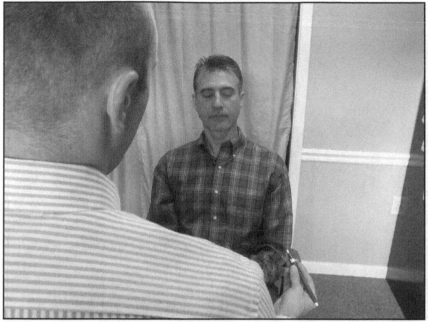

**Figure 6-17.** Gaze left down.

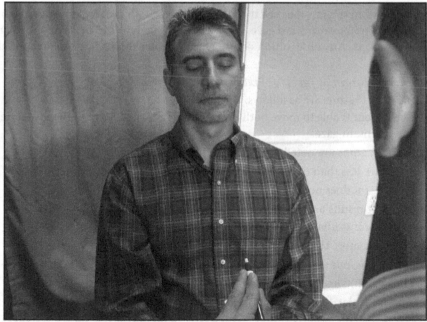

**Figure 6-18.** Gaze down.

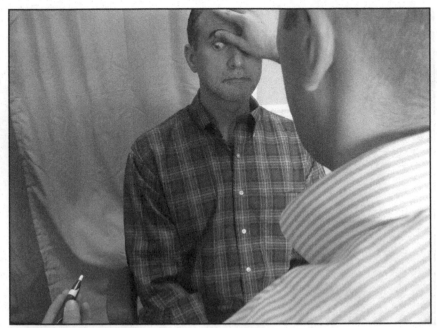

**Figure 6-19.** Gaze right down.

one eye to have nystagmus but not the other, so check both eyes for downward gaze. Since this is extreme downward gaze, you may see nystagmus of 3 beats or less in any of these positions. Any observation of nystagmus greater than 3 beats may represent pathology.

### Interpretation of Tests for Fixation and Range of Motion

Negative test results are as follows:

- The patient is able to move both eyes to each indicated point of the visual field and maintain gaze.
- No nystagmus are noted in less than end-range motions.
- There are less than or equal to 3 beats at extreme endpoints.
- The patient does not complain of diplopia.

Positive test results are as follows:

- The patient is unable to move into certain ocular ranges.
- There are more than 3 beats at end-range positions.
- Any nystagmus at 45 degrees indicates possible pathology.
- The patient complains of diplopia.

Testing of ocular ROM examines cranial nerves and eye muscles. Upward gaze may decrease somewhat (but not completely) with advanced age.[14] Disruption of the ability to maintain fixation in general may be due to central or peripheral dysfunction. Examples of central lesions that may disrupt fixation include seizures or occipital lobe infarct,[2] infranuclear lesions and supranuclear lesions,[15] and certain brainstem and cerebellar syndromes.[9]

## Nystagmus

The following are some important points regarding nystagmus you may observe:

- Toxins, drugs, alcohol intoxication, peripheral dysfunction, or central dysfunctions/lesions may cause spontaneous nystagmus.
- Direction-changing nystagmus (eg, quick phases beating left with leftward gaze and right with rightward gaze) is an indication of central pathology.
- Nystagmus brought on by fixing the gaze is an indication of central pathology.
- Rebound nystagmus (which occurs after bringing the eyes back to center following lateral gaze, and with quick phases in the opposite direction of the held gaze) generally indicates cerebellar dysfunction or damage.[9]
- Existing nystagmus that is suppressed by fixing the gaze is an indication of peripheral pathology.
- Nystagmus that begins or increases with gaze in one horizontal direction but decreases or stops with gaze in the opposite direction is most often an indication of peripheral pathology. While peripheral issues are more likely the cause of unilateral gaze nystagmus, there are central issues that may cause this, such as brainstem or cerebellar lesions.[16]
- Vertical nystagmus is typically an indication of central pathology[9]:
  - *Down-beating nystagmus* may be caused by bilateral lesions of the flocculus or paraflocculus (eg, due to anticonvulsant drugs) or lesions at the bottom of the fourth ventricle.[17] It is most often drug-induced or congenital (as by the Arnold-Chiari malformation) but may also be caused by cerebellar degeneration, a paramedian lesion in the medulla oblongata,[18] multiple sclerosis, hemorrhage, infarction, or tumors. Downbeat nystagmus syndrome is a condition where patients with signs of fixation-induced downbeating nystagmus also have other signs of falling backward and past-pointing upward.[17,19]
  - *Upbeating nystagmus* (fixation-induced) is the result of damage to the pontomesencephalic brainstem. The main etiologies of these brain-stem lesions are ischemia, tumors, Wernicke's encephalopathy, cerebellar degeneration, and intoxication. Other accompanying signs may include falling backward and past-pointing downward.[19,20]

## The Vestibulo-ocular Reflex

The next eye motion we need to hold images steady is the use of the VOR. As described previously, the VOR moves the eyes in the opposite direction but at the same speed as that of head movements. More information is available in Chapters 1 and 4.

## Optokinetics

Optokinetic eye movements stabilize the eyes when they are tracking a large moving scene.[2] *Optokinetics* in general is abbreviated OPK, while *optokinetic nystagmus* are abbreviated OKN. When our eyes detect constant motion in our environment due to constant motion of our world, ourselves, or both, OKN becomes active, allowing us to see clearly. The nystagmus activate reflexively, and we refer to this as the *optokinetic reflex*. If we did not use these nystagmus, the visual environment would be blurry while the world moved around us. An example of a situation where you use OKN would be if you were standing along railroad tracks and a train were quickly moving by. As the train cars sped by, the OPK system would detect a moving environment across the visual field and turn on the OPK reflex (nystagmus), which would now allow you to see individual cars as they moved by.

While the resulting nystagmus looks the same, the VOR and OKN differ. The stimulus for the VOR is head motion; in the case of the OKN, however, the eyes detect constant motion initiated by self-motion.[7] The latency for the OKN is 100 ms.[7]

You can see another good example of the OPK reflex by watching someone who is looking out of a car or train window as the world goes by. As the scenery moving across the visual field is tracked, the oculomotor system, using the OPK reflex, turns on OKN. The eyes begin a reflexive beating motion that moves quickly in the direction of the car's or train's direction of motion and somewhat more slowly to follow the scene as it moves by (slow phase of nystagmus). Once the eyes track as far as they can and are at their end ROMs, they very quickly move back to the other side using a saccade (quick phase of the nystagmus) in order to start the visual tracking all over again.

A bedside test of OPK involves moving a striped piece of paper in front of the patient's eyes horizontally and vertically. Smart phone and tablet apps are available to provide moving lines for OPK testing. Tables 6-17 through 6-19 provide instructions for OPK testing.

 ***Optokinetics Testing Instructions***

To see an object in 3 dimensions, we have to have both eyes point at it and focus on it. While doing this, we actually see 2 images, one from each eye. The brain takes the images from each eye and fuses them into one conscious image, which we see. This process is called *binocular fusion*. When the eyes temporarily or acutely misalign, the patient may complain of dizziness, double vision, headaches, and nausea. However, when the condition is chronic, the brain may suppress the foveal vision or entire vision of the misaligned eye. As a result, the patient does not necessarily see double (diplopia) but may lose the sense of depth perception. The patient may not even be aware that the images from one of the eyes are not being used. The causes of ocular misalignment may be muscular or central. A complaint of diplopia obviously necessitates an eye examination; however, the patient who constantly trips or seems clumsy does not always stand out as possibly experiencing ocular misalignment. Any patient who complains of balance problems and/or dizziness warrants an examination of ocular alignment. When a patient has a misalignment, you may wish to consult with someone more specialized to perform a more in-depth assessment, such a neurologist, ophthalmologist, neuro-ophthalmologist, or behavioral optometrist.

| TABLE 6-17 |
| :---: |
| **OPTOKINETIC TESTING, STEP 1** |

**Instruction:** "Look at this first line. I am going to move this piece of paper past your eyes. Keep your head still and count the lines as they go by."

**Clinician:** Hold an edge of the paper in front of one of the patient's eyes and instruct her to look at the first line. If you are using a phone or tablet, hold it in front of her eyes.

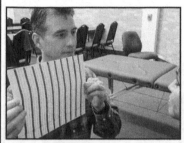

**Figure 6-20.** OPK 1.

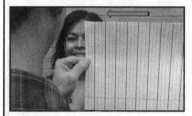

**Figure 6-21.** OPK 2.

## *Ocular Alignment*

 Cover Tests

The Cover test is composed of 2 tests commonly used as screens for ocular alignment: the Cover-Uncover test (also known as the *Unilateral Cover test*) and the Alternating Cover test (also known as the *Cross-Cover test*). Always perform the Unilateral Cover test first. Directions for these tests are as follows.[21]

### *Cover-Uncover Test (Unilateral Cover Test) Instructions*

The first test—the *Unilateral Cover test*, also known as the *Cover-Uncover test* (Table 6-20)—tests the patient for heterotropia (also known as *manifest strabismus*), which is an abnormal eye deviation. This test answers the question, "Are the eyes consistently pointing at the same object?"

Figure 6-26A shows a diagram to help explain this test further. Here we are looking down on top of our patient and the dark pointed lines show the direction in which each eye is pointing. Ideally both eyes would be pointing at the same object:

## TABLE 6-18
## OPTOKINETIC TESTING, STEP 2

**Clinician:** *Slowly* move the paper across the patient's visual field. You need to be able to see the patient's eyes, so do not block your own view as you do this. Repeat in each direction (L → R, R → L, Up → Down, Down → Up).

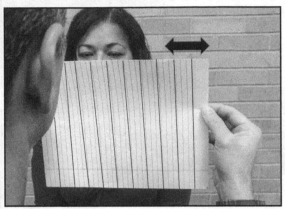

**Figure 6-22.** OPK 3.

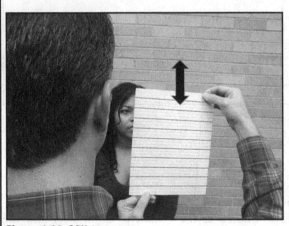

**Figure 6-23.** OPK 4.

## TABLE 6-19
## INTERPRETATION OF THE OPTOKINETIC TEST

*Interpretation*

*Negative test:* Rhythmic nystagmus are noted as the patient visually tracks the lines moving past her eyes.

*Positive test:* Nystagmus are present, or not consistently rhythmic.

# TABLE 6-20
# INSTRUCTIONS FOR THE UNILATERAL COVER TEST

**Instruction:** "Look at the tip of my nose. I'm going to cover and uncover one of your eyes. Make sure you keep focused on the tip of my nose."

**Clinician:** The clinician faces the patient and instructs her to focus both eyes on a target (the clinician's nose). The visual target should be about 40 cm (15.7 inches) from the patient. If the patient normally wears eyeglasses, she should wear them during the test. As the patient looks at the target, cover one of her eyes with an occluder (such as the solid end of a Maddox rod or your hand). Observe the *uncovered eye* for about 5 seconds during this test, noting any eye motions needed to find the visual target. Corrective eye motions indicate a positive test. Test each eye independently. Repeat the test a couple times for each eye.

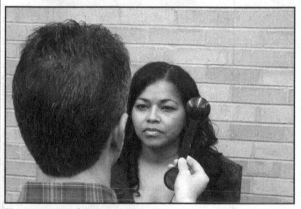

**Figure 6-24.** Left uncover.

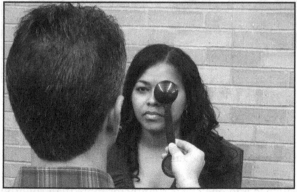

**Figure 6-25.** Left cover.

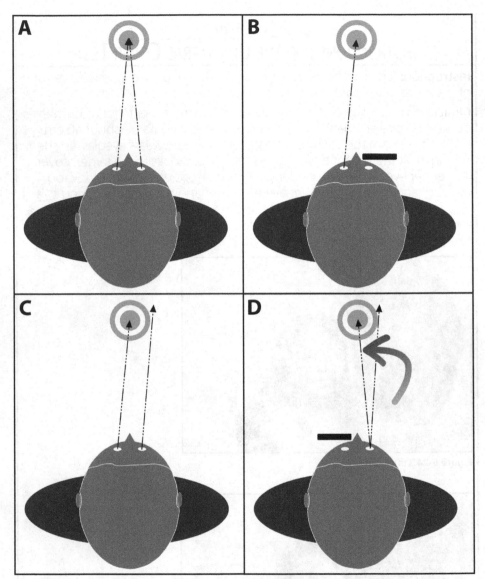

**Figure 6-26.** (A) Binocular fusion. (B) Cover test 1. (C) Strabismus. (D) Cover test 2.

During the test we cover one eye while observing the uncovered eye. If the observed uncovered eye is already pointing at the target, it will not move during the test (Figure 6-26B).

Sometimes the eyes are misaligned and one eye is slightly (or more than slightly) off target (Figure 6-26C).

If we cover the contralateral eye (which is pointed at the target), the patient will be able to look at the target only with the eye that is pointed in the wrong direction. As we cover the "good eye," the patient will realize that he or she is not looking in the right place and move the eye to the correct position to see the target (Figure 6-26D).

Looking at the uncovered eye, we will observe the correction as it moves its position. This indicates a positive test for manifest strabismus (heterotropia).

### Unilateral Cover Test Interpretation

If the uncovered eye moves to acquire the visual target after the contralateral eye is covered, the test is positive for heterotropia. Note the direction of uncovered eye's deviation.

- If it moves inward, an exotropia is present.
- If it moves outward, an esotropia is present.
- If it moves downward, a hypertropia is present.
- If it moves upward, a hypotropia is present.

An observation of vertical eye movements indicates a more serious finding; in that case the clinician should refer the patient for tests to rule out central pathologies.

### Alternating Cover Test (Cross-Cover Test) Instructions

The Alternating Cover test is a test of heterophoria (also known as *latent strabismus*). This condition allows for binocular fusion, but when fusion is broken, as when one eye is covered, the eyes lose alignment (ie, the covered eye moves away from the target and instead moves to a resting position). Table 6-21 provides instructions for the Alternating Cover test.

Test Interpretation: Movement of the eye just after it is uncovered is a positive test for heterophoria. Observations of vertical eye movements may indicate a more serious finding; in such a case the clinician should refer the patient for tests to rule out central pathologies. Note the direction of the covered eye's movement just after it is uncovered.

- If it moves inward, an *exophoria* is present. When the eye was covered, it drifted outward; when uncovered, a correction was needed to reacquire the target.
- If it moves outward, an *esophoria* is present. When the eye was covered, it drifted inward; when uncovered, a correction was needed to reacquire the target.
- If it moves downward, a *hyperphoria* is present. When the eye was covered, it drifted upward; when uncovered, it had to make a correcting downward motion to reacquire the target.
- If it moves upward, a *hypophoria* is present. When the eye was covered, it drifted downward. When uncovered, it had to make a correcting upward motion to reacquire the target.

## Maddox Rod Test

The Maddox Rod test uses dissimilar images to test ocular alignment. This test measures heterophoria or tropia but does not differentiate between the presence of phorias or tropias. For this reason, the cover tests should be performed prior to the Maddox Rod test. The Maddox rod has a lens comprising of rows of glass or plastic rods that produce the image of a line. Depending on how the lens is held (the direction of the rods) the red line will be either horizontal or vertical. From the uncovered eye, the patient will see a dot. Table 6-22 provides instructions for the Maddox Rod test.

## TABLE 6-21
# INSTRUCTIONS FOR THE ALTERNATING COVER TEST

**Instruction:** "Look at the tip of my nose. I'm going to cover and uncover each of your eyes several times. Make sure you keep focused on the tip of my nose."

**Clinician:** The clinician faces the patient and instructs her to focus both eyes on a target (the clinician's nose). If she normally wear eyeglasses, she should wear them during the test. The clinician is interested in the *covered* eye during this test and wants to observe what happens to the position of the eye when it is covered. During the test, cover each eye alternately in order to break binocular fusion. Hold the cover at least 5 seconds or longer, then quickly move the occluder to cover the contralateral eye. Do not move so slowly as to allow the patient to once again focus on the target with both eyes. Always keep one eye covered during this test. Watch the *covered eye*. Just after it was uncovered, did it move to reacquire the target? Movement of the eye just after it is uncovered indicates a positive test for heterophoria.

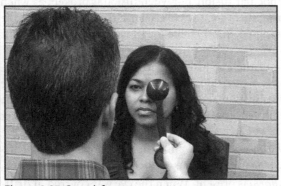

**Figure 6-27.** Cover left.

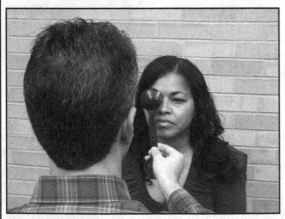

**Figure 6-28.** Cover right.

| TABLE 6-22 |
| :---: |
| **INSTRUCTIONS FOR THE MADDOX ROD TEST** |

1. Reduce the room light.
2. Decide whether to measure the horizontal or vertical deviation and then place the Maddox rod in front of the patient's right eye. The patient will view with both eyes open.
3. The light is focused on the midline of the patient's face.
4. Explanation given to the patient: "You will see a red line and a white dot. Describe the dot and line. Is the dot touching or on top of the line? If not, describe the position of the line compared with the dot."

### Interpretation of the Maddox Rod Test[22]

To determine horizontal deviations, the cylinders of the lens are held horizontally and the red line will be seen as vertical. For this example, the lens is held in front of the patient's right eye. If the patient sees:

- The dot and line superimposed, there is no deviation.
- The red line to the left and white dot on the right, an *exodeviation* is present.
- The red line is to the right and the dot is to the left, an *esodeviation* is present.

The amount of deviation can be assessed by placing a prism bar in front of the eye, with the strength of the prism indicating the amount of deviation.

To determine vertical deviations, the cylinders of the lens are held vertically in front of the patient's eye, and the red line will be seen as horizontal. For this example, the lens is held in front of the patient's right eye. If the patient sees:

- The dot and line superimposed, there is no deviation.
- The red line above the dot, a right *hypodeviation* is present.
- The red line below the dot, a right *hyperdeviation* is present.

# DISORDERS AFFECTING EYE MOTION

During the examination, we looked at different motions of the eyes. Positive findings for eye motion are as follows:

- Fixation (gaze holding): Is the patient able to hold the eyes still while looking at a visual target? If not, you see the patient's eyes moving all around the target as he or she tries to fixate on it.

- Gaze nystagmus:
  Is any observed? Typically we look for nystagmus
  - At rest (spontaneous)
  - At 45 degrees of lateral gaze
  - At (or near) end-ROMs around the edges of ocular range

Without sophisticated clinical tests provided by an audiologist or even a computed tomography or magnetic resonance imaging examination, we do not know from a bedside exam if the causes of observed nystagmus are central or peripheral. There are clues as to which may be causing the nystagmus, but electronystagmography/audiography testing gives more definitive findings.

## Possible Peripheral Signs

- Positional nystagmus following classic benign paroxysmal positional vertigo latency, duration, and direction of eye motions.
- If a patient has gaze nystagmus in one horizontal direction of motion (eg, gaze left) but not during the contralateral motion (eg, gaze right), we typically begin to suspect a peripheral problem, such as a unilateral vestibular loss (using Alexander's law). This is especially true if nystagmus diminishes with visual fixation (looking at a target such as a light). If nystagmus either does not suppress or actually increases while the patient is fixating on a light target, a central pathology becomes more likely. Keep in mind that this is not always 100% accurate but does greatly increase the likelihood of a central pathology.

## Possible Central Signs

- Suspect central pathology when a patient has rebound nystagmus.
  - This type of nystagmus is gaze-evoked (that is, activated with gaze). Nystagmus either disappears or reverses direction when lateral gaze is held. When the eyes return to the primary position, a brief burst of nystagmus occurs in the opposite direction. The causes of rebound nystagmus include cerebellar atrophy, tumors, and focal cerebellar structural lesions.[16]

- Gaze nystagmus
  - Vertical nystagmus (central issues more likely)
  - Direction-changing nystagmus (ie, left gaze nystagmus with left gaze and right gaze nystagmus with right gaze). This type generally reflects dysfunction of gaze-holding structures in the brainstem and cerebellum.[23]
  - Dissociated nystagmus (one eye has nystagmus but not the other eye). Common causes: multiple sclerosis and myasthenia gravis.[16]
- Positional nystagmus with only one component (pure vertical or rotational nystagmus)
- Pure torsional nystagmus
- Positional nystagmus that do not follow classic benign paroxysmal positional vertigo latency, duration, and direction of eye motions
- Nystagmus elicited by visual fixation
- Abnormal smooth pursuit: Do the eyes move smoothly and conjugately (together in unison)? Or are their movements jerky or saccadic (when the patient uses saccades instead of smooth pursuit)? Are the movements impaired

in one direction but not the other (eg, left to right, but not right to left)? Are movements intact vertically and horizontally?

- ○ Remember, smooth pursuit changes with age and may not be present until age 10. Moreover, it may degrade or disappear in the sixth decade of life. We should still note "saccadic smooth pursuit" if it is observed in these age groups, but may wish to note the "age appropriateness."
- ○ Smooth pursuit is influenced by alertness, age, medications, intoxicants, and degenerative disorders of the cerebellum or extrapyramidal systems.
- Impaired saccades: Are saccades accurate? Do they undershoot targets (hypometric), or overshoot targets (hypermetric)? Test these during horizontal and vertical motions. Are saccades impaired in one direction but not the other?
- Convergence insufficiency: Does the patient see 1 or 2 targets? Can the patient accommodate visually when objects are moving toward or away from his or her nose? At what point, if at all, do things go "double"? Can the patient's eyes converge to at least 10 cm?
- Skew: You may find skews (vertical misalignments) of the eyes during the alternate-cover test. Skew deviations are the result of a right-left imbalance in otolith and graviceptive inputs from the vestibular system to the oculomotor system; except for rare exceptions, skews are central in origin.[24] A brainstem or cerebellar injury from stroke, multiple sclerosis, or trauma may cause a skew deviation. Skew deviations are usually accompanied by binocular torsion (both eyes rotate in one direction), torticollis, and tilt (in combination called the *ocular tilt reaction*).[24]

If the eyes do not move properly, dizziness is often one of the patient's complaints. Other complaints may include blurred vision, headaches, or difficulty reading. Neurologic lesions will cause different oculomotor signs and deficits depending on the location of the lesion. These are classified as follows[25] (Table 6-23):

Always inform the referring physician of abnormal eye motions.

## Oculomotor Complications of Multiple Sclerosis

There are different oculomotor issues with the MS patient population depending on the location of the lesions. Some commonly seen oculomotor abnormalities include nystagmus, internuclear ophthalmoplegia, saccadic dysmetria or oscillations, impairment of smooth pursuit, VOR cancellation deficits, and impaired OPK reflex.[26]

## Oculomotor Complications of Parkinson's Disease

Commonly seen ocular issues in the Parkinson's patient population include fixation deficits, hypometric saccades, impaired smooth pursuit, and impaired convergence.[26]

| TABLE 6-23 OCULOMOTOR SIGNS OF NEUROLOGIC LESIONS ||
|---|---|
| **DISORDER** | **EXAMPLES** |
| Infranuclear disorders | • Oculomotor nerve palsy<br>• Trochlear nerve palsy<br>• Abducens nerve palsy<br>• Miswiring (eg, Duane's syndrome) |
| Supranuclear disorders | • Internuclear ophthalmoplegia<br>• Skew deviation<br>• Dissociated vertical deviation<br>• Dorsal midbrain syndrome<br>• Horizontal and vertical gaze palsies |
| Disorders of eye movement modulation | • Nystagmus<br>• Neuromyotonia of abducens or oculomotor fibers |

# Nystagmus

## Pathologic Nystagmus

There are *many* different types of nystagmus. As we learned in Chapter 1, jerk nystagmus are an involuntary, reflexive movement of the eye that usually has a fast and a slow phase in opposite directions. The fast phase is a quick resetting motion that allows the patient to quickly reposition the eye so that it may track again. The saccadic system mediates the fast phase of the nystagmus. The slow phase is a visual tracking motion run by the smooth pursuit system; this allows the fovea to maintain the image of what we wish to see.[3]

Nystagmus are either physiological or pathological. As we have learned, we use nystagmus every day to help us see clearly. When the brain "turns on" nystagmus to allow us to see clearly, we classify them as physiological. When nystagmus occur when not needed or in a way that does not help us position our eyes to assist in clear vision, the nystagmus are pathological.

## Congenital Nystagmus

This type of nystagmus is present from birth or early infancy, symmetrically affects both eyes (binocular), and is typically horizontal in all gaze positions. The patient does not complain of oscillopsia, and this nystagmus is not physiological. That is to say, it does not help us to function or see.

### Gaze-Evoked Nystagmus

This occurs while maintaining an eccentric gaze position (movement *away from* the primary position of the eye) and usually occurs on lateral or upward gaze. The most common etiologies include sedatives, tranquilizers, anticonvulsants, and alcohol. This type of nystagmus also often occurs owing to vestibular imbalance and follow Alexander's Law (increased nystagmus when looking in the direction of the quick phase).[26]

### Downbeat (Vertical) Nystagmus

This may be caused drugs, brainstem and cerebellar lesions, bilateral internuclear ophthalmoplegia, and lesions affecting the posterior commissure.[27]

### Rebound Nystagmus

Rebound nystagmus is a reversal of the direction of nystagmus, usually after a person has been holding eccentric gaze. This may occur in healthy subjects but is most frequently observed in patients with cerebellar disease.[26]

## OCULOMOTOR INTERVENTIONS

When do we use oculomotor exercises? If we see oculomotor deficits during the evaluation, many times we may use the deficit as the exercise. We may need to consult other specialists if the deficit is moderate or severe. Theoretically, oculomotor exercises can help to improve oculomotor function or to stimulate an adaptive process where the brain will find alternative movements or information from other systems as substitutions for the impaired eye motion. For example, if the patient has a positive saccades test, as when he or she has hypometric or hypermetric saccades, we could have the patient perform saccades as an exercise. Barozzi et al compared the effects of oculomotor exercises on static balance and perceived disability (using the dizziness handicap) for patients with persistent disequilibrium and found that the added oculomotor exercises reduced the "perceived overall impairment and postural sway" in patients who had documented unilateral vestibular loss.[28]

You may also choose oculomotor exercises as part of your plan of care to address certain pathologies. For example, the use of OPK stimulation has been found to improve vestibular function as well as having beneficial effects for stroke patients. Let's look at some examples of oculomotor exercises.

## *Examples of Oculomotor Exercises*

### Saccades

A study of 46 subjects with vestibular disorders (both of peripheral and central origin) who performed 12 consecutive training sessions based on repeated visually guided saccades showed improvements for all subjects in postural control and saccadic performance.[29]

**Figure 6-29.** Tragal Compression test.

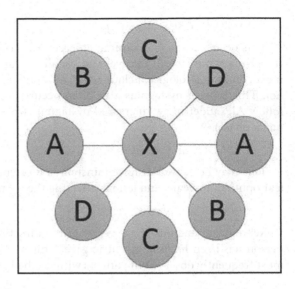

For saccade exercises, visual targets are often preprinted lines or hash marks on a piece of paper. You may also simply use 2 objects in the room as visual targets. Targets on a circle (corresponding pairs 180 degrees apart) are helpful to encourage and train saccades in different directions. Instructions for saccades exercises are as follows:

- Present the patient, who is sitting with a stationary head, with various visual targets that are within the field of view. Instructions are to look quickly back and for the between the targets using saccades but without head movement. Both vertical and horizontal saccades are performed. A typical progression of these exercises moves the patient from performing them in sitting, to standing, then standing on a compliant surface such as foam.

- Another variation includes a head turn. With this exercise, the patient looks at a visual target that can be seen without turning the head. This target should not be directly in front of the patient. The patient acquires the target using a saccade, and then turns the head toward it. This continues as the patient acquires new targets that are placed in a variety of directions and angles within the field of view.

### *Examples of Saccades Charts*

Refer to the saccades chart below. Instruct the patient to sit in front of the chart and look at one target, then to the X in the middle, to the corresponding target on the other side of the circle, and then back to the X, and finally the starting point again. Using the letter "A" as an example, the patient would look A (left)-X-A (right) (counts as 1 repetition), then back to X, then A (left) again (counts as another repetition). Repeat for the prescribed number of repetitions (commonly 20 to 40 repetitions, or timed), then move to the next letter. An example of an entire round of exercises would be (Figure 6-29):

A-X-A-X-A (X10), B-X-B-X-B (X10), C-X-C-X-C (X10), D-X-D-X-D (X10), etc.

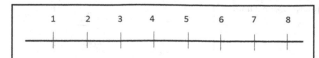

**Figure 6-30.** Valsalva.

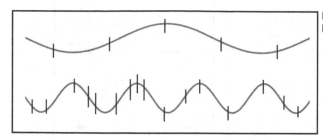

**Figure 6-31.** Saccades exercise horizontal lines.

You may also use different types of lines marked at either even or varied intervals. Refer to the following charts. The lines do not all have to be straight. By varying the lines to use waves or zigzags, you increase the variety of angles the patient must use during the exercise. Here are a few examples (Figures 6-30 and 6-31):

Just draw or print a line and put hash marks along it. The hash marks may have even or varying spaces between them. If you are trying to train saccades of a certain size to use as a substitute for the loss of other motions (like a VOR), you would want evenly spaced hash marks. If you are trying to challenge the brain to improve the saccades themselves, you may wish to use a mix of evenly spaced and varyingly spaced hash marks. Using the lines with hash marks, have the patient scan each line L→R, and R→L. Then turn the chart and have the patient scan the lines vertically, top→bottom and then bottom→top. Figure 6-32 shows a vertical line chart.

A great exercise to teach scanning of the environment, which is an intervention often used in treating visuospatial neglect in stroke patients, involves hiding easily identified objects (like tennis balls) in a room and then having the patient visually scan the room using saccades until he or she finds the objects. Make sure you incorporate vertical eye motions, not just left and right scanning. Prompt the patient to scan the environment using saccades and a still head. Make sure that all targets are within the patient's visual field.

## Smooth Pursuit

Keep in mind that a deficit in smooth pursuit may be an age-related change in your patient. These are simple tracking exercises done while the head is still and the visual target is moving *slowly* within or across the field of view without the patient's head moving. With children or patients who have difficulty maintaining attention, the use of a penlight or toy that lights up as a visual target is often helpful.

A survey of leadership members of the Vestibular Special Interest Group of the American Physical Therapy Association asking to how they use smooth pursuit as an exercise yielded the following answers: following acquired brain injury (first monocular, then binocular tracking); as habituation exercise for patients who complain of vertigo in visually stimulating environments; when there is a noted smooth pursuit

**Figure 6-32.** Saccades exercise vertical lines.

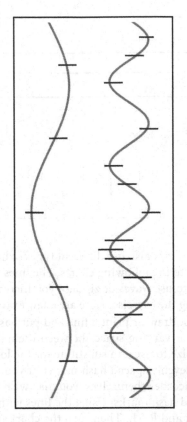

deficit upon examination; and for central disorders or post-concussion. The respondents described various ways to stimulate smooth pursuit tracking, from following a slow-moving target on a plain background to the use of more visually complex backgrounds, monocular to binocular, and games such as catch-toss or smartphone/tablet games requiring visual tracking.[30] More than one respondent mentioned using behavioral optometry techniques or actually referring to a behavioral optometrist for added guidance or evaluation.

## Orthoptic Exercises

Orthoptic exercises address binocular vision abnormalities. Such exercises can be helpful in addressing *convergence insufficiency,* for example, which is the inability to maintain binocular function (keeping the 2 eyes working together) at a near distance.[11] Examples of orthoptic exercises include pencil push-ups and jump convergence exercises like the Brock string or dot card (explanations of these exercises are given further on). It is important to use these exercises only when there is certainty of binocular vision potential, so that the patient improves and the exercises do not exacerbate the problem. In applying these exercises to the wrong patient there is a risk of causing accommodative or convergence spasm by overdoing the exercise or insuperable (unable to overcome/control) diplopia, as when these exercises are given

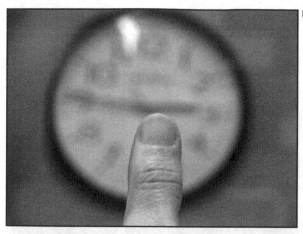

**Figure 6-33.** Vergence Jump 1.

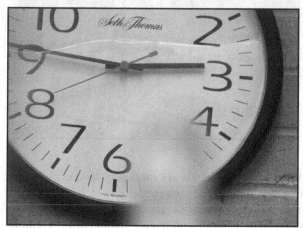

**Figure 6-34.** Vergence Jump 2.

to a patient who is suppressing vision from one eye. If you are unsure whether your patient is suitable for these types of exercises, consult a neurologist or ophthalmology specialist prior to beginning these types of interventions.

### Two-Target Jump Convergence

One method is to have the patient focus on something close (like a thumb) held close to the breakpoint of convergence (ie, the closest distance at which the patient can see one target) while the other target is something across the room (at least 10 feet) in front of the patient that is visually behind the thumb (without moving the head). The patient alternately changes focus from the near to the far target and back, holding each target for at least 3 seconds. This is repeated several times (Figures 6-33 and 6-34).

### Brock String

The Brock string is a string a few feet long that has a few colored beads on it. One end of the string is tied to something, such as a doorknob, while the other end is held

**Figure 6-35.** Brock string near-vergence.

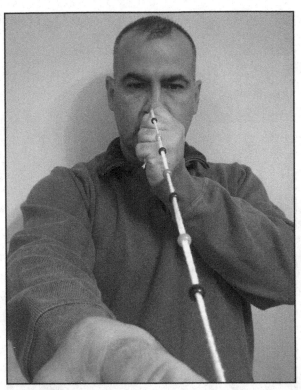

close to the tip of the patient's nose. Colored beads are randomly spaced along the string and the patient is instructed to change focus sequentially to each bead for the prescribed amount of time or repetitions. For near-vergence work, you may wish to use a small piece of yarn held by the patients, one end in each hand, with one end to the nose and the other at arm's length. As in the other example, colored beads are randomly spaced along the string and the patient performs focal changes to each bead. The beads may be moved to different places along the string to vary the focal points, thus performing the exercise with different target distances. Repeat 3 to 5 cycles. Repetition number may vary depending on your plan of care or how many other orthoptic exercises the patient is performing (Figures 6-35 and 6-36).

In performing this exercise, whenever the patient is looking at one target, all targets that are either closer or farther away should be seen in double. The patient should also see 2 strings that cross at the point of fixation. If the patient sees only one string, visual suppression is present, and the practitioner should decide whether these exercises should be continued.[12] Suppression is when the brain suppresses conscious awareness of the image from one eye so as to prevent diplopia.

### Dot Card

The dot card is similar to the Brock string, but instead of using a string that has beads spaced along it, a rectangular piece of paper is used that has a line drawn down

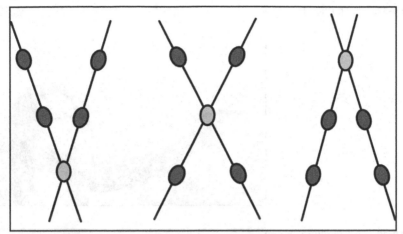

**Figure 6-36.** Brock string diagram. Lighter colored beads indicate the point of visual fixation.

the length, and dots or X's marked evenly along the line. The paper is held just below the patient's nose with the line moving away and in slight depression. Instruct the patient to focus on the farthest dot, and ask if the target is seen as a single or double image (it should be a single image). Next, the patient changes the fixation point to the next-closest dot along the line. This continues, holding each target at least 3 seconds, until the patient reaches a target that cannot be seen as a single image. Repeat this exercise for 3 to 5 cycles. Repetition number may vary depending on your plan of care, or if the patient has other orthoptic exercises to perform.

As with the Brock string, in using the dot card the patient should see 2 of each dot except the one that is the current visual target. If this is not the case, then the patient may be suppressing foveal vision in one eye, and the clinician must decide whether these exercises should be continued.[12]

### Pencil Push-ups

So far, we have discussed the use of visual targets that are static (not moving). Another way to perform vergence exercises is to track a *moving* visual target. The patient holds a pencil so that the fat (eraser) end is closer to the face. This end of the pencil is used as the visual target. Starting with the pencil held at arm's length, it is very slowly moved towards the nose. While it moves, the patient is instructed to maintain fixation on the fat end of the pencil as a visual target. When the target becomes either blurred or doubled, the patient changes the direction of the pencil's movement so that it is now slowly moving away (again while maintaining visual fixation). When needed, the patient may look away and then back at the target to regain fusion (ie, stop seeing 2 images). These moving vergence exercises are sometimes called *pencil push-ups*, and the patient usually repeats them for 3 to 5 cycles of repetition. Repetition number may vary depending on your plan of care or how many other orthoptic exercises the patient is performing (Figures 6-37 through 6-39).

**Figure 6-37.** Pencil pushup 1.

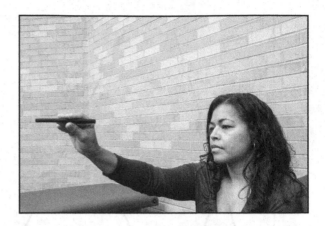

**Figure 6-38.** Pencil pushup 2.

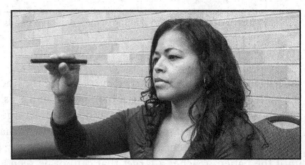

**Figure 6-39.** Pencil pushup 3.

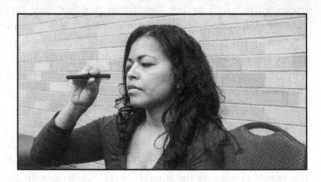

There are mixed study results on the efficacy of the pencil push-up exercise. In smaller studies these exercises were found to be effective in addressing convergence insufficiency.[31,32] In at least one study of 46 adults, while a group of subjects who used pencil push-ups as an intervention had significantly reduced symptoms, only the group using a different orthoptic exercise intervention achieved statistically significant changes in near point of convergence and positive fusional vergence (ie, they could see a near target without seeing double).[33]

## Optokinetic Stimulation

Many clinicians use OPK stimulation to effectively treat motion sickness as well as to improve vestibular function. The OPK system is stimulated when our environment is moving around us, when we are turning/spinning in our environment, or both. Traditional opinion dictates that the optimal way to stimulate this system is with a full-field effect, although recently there is evidence that puts this belief into question. During clinical testing, specialist clinicians create a full-field type of stimulation by using a rotary chair. The patient sits in a rotary chair that spins at a certain rate and direction, which the clinician controls. For OPK testing, this chair is in a booth that has vertical alternating white and black stripes on the wall. As the chair spins, the stripes stimulate the OPK system.

Obviously most clinics do not have rotary chairs available to them, but a relatively inexpensive alternative method of achieving a full-filed stimulus is by having the patient sit or stand in a dark room while a disco ball projects moving points of light against the walls. If this is your method of choice, make sure you have a disco ball that can change the direction of spin so that you can target specific directions of eye motions. Treatment for motion sickness has been described by Berthoz, who used an OPK stimulation protocol.[34] Patients may experience momentary sensations where they feel as if they are moving; at other times they may sense that the room is moving. These sensations are both normal and expected. If your patient becomes overly nauseous, turn off the machine, bring up the lights, and allow for time to recover. Continue once symptoms have subsided. The goal is to have the patient gradually increase tolerance to OPK stimulation up to 15 to 20 minutes, although some recent studies suggest that even brief stimulation is helpful and effective.

You may wish to target a specific direction of OKN (eg, left to right, right to left, up to down, or down to up) based on your evaluation findings. If you are interested only in stimulating the OPK system as a whole, make sure you include different directions of stimuli to force the use of OKN in different directions.

In the disco ball example, the patient may begin in sitting or standing (guarded) in a darkened room, and is instructed to watch the rotating lights. Give the patient control of stopping the stimulus. The clinician should remain nearby to turn up the lights or provide assistance. Viewing the stimulus is to the patient's tolerance, and breaks are given as needed to recover. The goal is to increase the patient's tolerance to viewing the moving environment. The clinician should document the length of time during which the patient is tolerant to this intervention and also note the patient's subjective complaints regarding the stimulation. This will make it possible to demonstrate improvement over time.

### Striped Lines for Optokinetic Stimulus

Examples of using striped lines include having the patient view moving lines on a smart phone/table app. Or you can simply draw lines on a piece of paper that can be moved in front of the patient's field of view. Instruct the patient to view this stimulus either using a set number of repetitions or by measuring the duration of tolerance to the stimulus. Either method is useful to demonstrate increasing tolerance to the

**Figure 6-40.** OPK vertical.

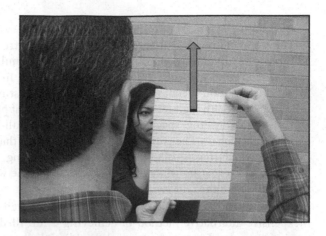

**Figure 6-41.** OPK horizontal.

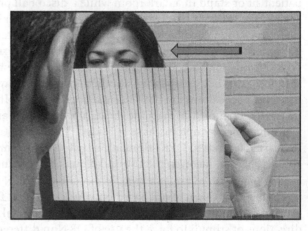

stimulus. If a piece of paper is being used, the clinician moves the paper across the patient's field of view and the patient is instructed to count the lines as they go by (Figures 6-40 and 6-41).

These "less than full-field" interventions (eg, striped lines on paper or phone apps) are convenient for smaller clinics and for use by home health clinicians, in hospital settings, or as a home exercise. In fact, a recent study of 60 subjects compared OPK exercises using 3 different intervention groups:

1. A supervised full-field approach
2. A supervised group using a CD that displayed an OPK disc or drum rotating at 40 or 60 degrees per second
3. An unsupervised group who used the CD at home.

Treatment effect was assessed after 8 weeks. All groups showed significant improvements for vestibular symptoms, visual vertigo, and autonomic symptoms. Posturography and functional gait assessment improved significantly for both supervised groups but not significantly for the unsupervised group. Condition-related anxiety was reduced in the supervised CD group, while condition-related depression was improved for the supervised full-field group. This study demonstrated the effectiveness of less than full-field OPK stimulation while also showing the added benefits of supervised interventions.[35]

In one study, brief periods of unidirectional OPK stimulation lasting for 30 seconds 10 times daily for 10 days produced VOR gain changes after a vestibular loss.[36]

OPK stimulation is beneficial in a number of conditions, including for the treatment of hemineglect (visual neglect) following a stroke,[37] for the suppression of motion sickness among airline pilots and flight attendants,[38] and to improve VOR function for the treatment of vestibular loss.

## Nonvestibular Dizziness and Disequilibrium

Patients who had disequilibrium and dizziness not stemming from a vestibular etiology improved their conditions using vestibular therapy. A 6-week study of these subjects found that balance exercises incorporating gaze stabilization led to significantly greater improvement in fall risk compared with the balance exercise only without gaze stabilization.[39]

# REFERENCES

1. Borchert MS. Principles and techniques of the examination of ocular motility and alignment. In: *Walsh & Hoyt's Clinical Neuro-ophthalmology*. 6th ed. Philadelphia: Lippincott WIllilams & Wilkins; 2005:887-905.
2. Wong A. *Eye Movement Disorders*. Oxford, UK: Oxford University Press; 2008.
3. University of Arizona Department of Neurology. Unit 10. Available at http://www.neurology.arizona.edu/training/UNIT10.pdf. Updated 2005. Accessed March 16, 2013.
4. Parks M. Eye movements and positions. Available at http://80.36.73.149/almacen/medicina/oftalmologia/enciclopedias/duane/pages/v1/v1c002.html. Updated 2006. Accessed October 15, 2014.
5. Leigh RJ, Zee D. *The Neurology of Eye Movements*. 4th ed. New York: Oxford University Press; 2006.
6. Kardon R. Introduction to anatomy and neural pathways. *Am Orthopt J*. 2005;55:2-9.
7. Dell'Osso LF, Daroff RB. Eye movement characteristics and recording techniques. In: Glaser JS, ed. *Neuro-ophthalmology*. 3rd ed. 2006:327-343.
8. Walker H, Hall W, Hurst J, eds. *Clinical Methods: The History, Physical, and Laboratory Examinations*. 3rd ed. Boston: Butterworths; 1990.
9. Brandt T, Dieterich M, Strupp M. *Vertigo and Dizziness*. London: Springer; 2005.
10. Rine RM, Wiener-Vacher S. Evaluation and treatment of vestibular dysfunction in children. *NeuroRehabilitation*. 2013;32(3):507-518.
11. American Association for Pediatric Ophthalmology and Strabismus. Convergence insufficiency. Available at http://www.aapos.org/terms/conditions/38. Updated 2012. Accessed October 4, 2014.
12. Maqsud MA. Orthoptic exercises: a forgotten art? Available at http://www.optometry.co.uk/uploads/articles/cet-2013/april-5-2013-cet-1.pdf. Updated 2013. Accessed October 4, 2014.
13. Miller N. *Walsh and Hoyt's Clinical Neuro-ophthalmology*. Vol 2. 4th ed. Baltimore: Williams & Wilkins; 1985.
14. Chamberlain W. Restriction in upward gaze with advancing age. *Am J Ophthalmol*. 1971;71:341-346.
15. Borchert MS. Principles and techniques of the examination of ocular motility and alignment. In: *Walsh & Hoyt's Clinical Neuro-ophthalmology*. 6th ed. Philadelphia: Lippincott Williams & Wilkins; 2005:887-905.

16. Baloh R, Honrubia HV. *Clinical neurophysiology of the vestibular system.* 2nd ed. Philadelphia: FA Davis; 1979.
17. Baloh RW, Spooner JW. Downbeat nystagmus. A type of central vestibular nystagmus. *Neurology.* 1981;31:304-310.
18. Cox TA, Corbett JJ, Thompson S, et al. Upbeat nystagmus changing to downbeat nystagmus with convergence. *Neurology.* 1981;31:891-892.
19. Dieterich M, Grünbauer M, Brandt T. Direction-specific impairments of motion perception and spatial orientation in downbeat and upbeat nystagus in humans. *Neurosci Lett.* 1998;245:29-32.
20. Janssen JC, Larner AJ, Morris H, et al. Upbeat nystagmus: clinical coanatomical correlation. *J Neurol Neurosurg Psychiatry.* 1998;65:380-381.
21. Schmidt P, Maguire M, Dobson V, et al. Comparison of preschool vision screening tests as administered by licensed eye care professionals in the vision in preschoolers study. *Ophthalmology.* 2004;111(4):637-650.
22. Fakhruddin A. Maddox rod. Available at http://www.slideshare.net/aliasgerfakhruddin9/maddox-rod. Updated 2013. Accessed October 4, 2014.
23. Baier B, Dieterich M. Incidence and anatomy of gaze-evoked nystagmus in patients with cerebellar lesions. *Neurology.* 2011;76:361-365.
24. Brodsky M, Donahue S, Vahiades M, et al. Skew deviation revisited. *Surv Ophthalmol.* 2006;51:105-128.
25. Kardon R. Introduction to anatomy and neural pathways. *Am Orthopt J.* 2005;55:2-9.
26. Leigh RJ, Zee DS. *The Neurology of Eye Movements.* 4th ed. New York: Oxford University Press; 2006.
27. Bhidayasiri R, Plant G, Leigh R. A hypothetical scheme for the brainstem control of vertical gaze. *Neurology.* 2000;54:1985-1993.
28. Barozzi S, Di Berardino F, Arisi E, Cesarani A. A comparison between oculomotor rehabilitation and vestibular electrical stimulation in unilateral peripheral vestibular deficit. *Int Tinnitus J.* 2006;12(1):45-49.
29. Monzani D, Setti G, Marchioni D, Genovese E, Gherpelli C, Presutti L. Repeated visually-guided saccades improves postural control in patients with vestibular disodrders. *Acta Otorhinolaryngol Ital.* 2005;25:224-252.
30. Dransfield M, Fuller K, Galgon AK, Heusel-Gillig L, Holmberg J. Email communication by Charles Plishka: survey question regarding smooth pursuit exercise. 2014.
31. Kim KM, Chun BY. Effectiveness of home-based pencil push-ups (HBPP) for patients with symptomatic convergence insufficiency. *Korean J Ophthalmol.* 2011;25(3):185-188.
32. Gallaway M, Scheiman M, Malhotra K. The effectiveness of pencil pushups treatment for convergence insufficiency: a pilot study. *Optom Vis Sci.* 2002;79(4):265-267.
33. Scheiman M, Mitchell GL, Cotter S, et al. A randomized clinical trial of vision therapy/orthoptics versus pencil pushups for the treatment of convergence insufficiency in young adults. *Optometry Vision Sci.* 2005;82(7):E583-E995.
34. Berthoz A. *The brain's sense of movement.* Cambridge, UK: Harvard University Press; 2000.
35. Pavlou M, Bronstein AM, Davies RA. Randomized trial of supervised versus unsupervised optokinetic exercise in persons with peripheral vestibular disorders. *Neurorehabil Neural Repair.* 2013;27(3):208-218.
36. Pfaltz CR. Vestibular compensation. Physiological and clinical aspects. *Acta Otolaryngol.* 1983;95:402-406.
37. Kerkhoff G, Keller I, Ritter V, Marquardt C. Repetitive optokinetic stimulation induces lasting recovery from visual neglect. *Restorative Neurol Neurosci.* 2006;24(4-6):357-369.
38. Vitte E, Berthoz A. Repeated optokinetic stimulation in conditions of active standing facilitates recovery from vestibular deficits. *Exp Brain Res.* 1994;102:141-148.
39. Hall CD, Heusel-Gillig L, Tusa RJ, Herdman SJ. Efficacy of gaze stability exercises in older adults with dizziness. *J Neurol Phys Ther.* 2010;34:64-69.

# 7

# Musculoskeletal and Somatosensory Systems

---

## CHAPTER GOALS

1. Name different methods to test muscle strength.
2. Explain a scale used to grade muscle strength.
3. Name 2 instruments used to measure angular motion of joint movement.
4. List different types of somatosensory sensations.
5. Name different methods of testing proprioception.
6. Describe monofilament testing.
7. List methods to improve somatosensation.

---

## MUSCULOSKELETAL SYSTEM

Strength and range of motion (ROM) deficits that are common among those who are balance-impaired often involve weakness in the hip muscles, kyphotic postures, and limitations to ankle ROM. For the patient with Parkinson's disease, symptoms often include rigidity, freezing, stooped/flexed posture, reduced trunk rotation, and balance impairment. To get accurate data, the clinician must examine the musculoskeletal system carefully.

Plishka CM.
*A Clinician's Guide to Balance and Dizziness:*
*Evaluation and Treatment* (pp 237-248).
© 2015 Taylor & Francis Group.

## Strength Testing

Methods available to test muscle strength include the following[1]:

- Isometric dynamometry
  - Examples: Handheld dynamometry, fixed dynamometry, sphygmo-manometry
  - Sensitive for all muscle grades
  - Good reliability
- Isokinetic dynamometry
  - Examples: Biodex, Cybex, and others
  - Not recommended for strength below 3/5
  - Good reliability
- Manual muscle testing
  - Most commonly used method
  - Reliability ranges from poor to good
  - Reliability affected by
    - Examiner strength, technique, bias, commands, judgment, feedback
    - Patient strength, arousal, motivation, comprehension
  - To be reproducible, operational definitions for grading criteria need to be refined and validated

There are different types of manual muscle tests,[2] including the following:

- Break test—Resistance is applied at the end of the tested range
- Make test—Resistance is applied throughout the range

For each of these, resistance should be applied and released gradually.

The most commonly used scale[2] to grade muscle strength is a 5-point scale modified by Daniels and Worthingham in 1946 and Kendall in 1949. The following grades are from the Medical Research Council[3] (Table 7-1). Grades 0, 1, and 2 are tested in gravity-minimized positions. All other grades are tested in antigravity positions.

Weak muscles of the elderly patient with balance problems commonly include hip extensors and hip abductors. Be sure to test these against gravity and watch for substitution patterns, such as hip flexion instead of abduction. This substitution is easily observed when the patient is supine and instructed to only abduct the hip.

During transfers from sitting to standing, patients with hip abductor weakness sometimes substitute the use of knee extension (quadriceps muscles) to assist in getting out of a chair. When you are interacting with a patient who has hip extensor weakness, you may observe him or her pushing against the chair with the back of the legs to assist. Such a patient uses the weight of his or her body to anchor the distal lower limbs and the muscle action of the quads to pull the rest of the body out of the chair. This is likely a substitution pattern to compensate for weak hip extensors.

| | TABLE 7-1 |
|---|---|

## GRADES OF THE MANUAL MUSCLE TEST

| GRADE | FUNCTION OF THE MUSCLE |
|---|---|
| 0 | No palpable or observable muscle contraction |
| 1 | No visible movement; palpable or observable tendon prominence/flicker contraction |
| 2- | Moves through partial ROM, gravity eliminated |
| 2 | Able to move through full ROM, gravity eliminated |
| 2+ | Moves through partial ROM against gravity or moves through complete ROM with gravity eliminated and holds against pressure |
| 3- | Gradual release from test position |
| 3 | Holds test position against gravity |
| 3+ | Holds test position against slight resistance |
| 4- | Holds test position against slight to moderate pressure |
| 4 | Holds test position against moderate resistance |
| 4+ | Holds test position against moderate to strong pressure |
| 5 | Holds test position against maximal resistance |

## *Range of Motion*

Be sure to assess the patient's posture from the front, back, and side. For objective measures, use a goniometer to measure any joint limitations for ROM. Two instruments are commonly used to measure joint angular ranges of motion[4]:

- The bubble inclinometer
  - Has a fluid-filled 360-degree rotating dial and scale with degrees marked along the dial edge. The dial has a visible bubble inside that indicates the angular position of the targeted body part and the ROM as it moves.
  - Measures flexion, extension, abduction, adduction, and rotation.
  - Joints measured: neck, shoulder, elbow, wrist, hip, knee, ankle, and spine.
- The goniometer
  - Consists of either a half circle (180 degrees) or full circle (360 degrees), called the body, with degrees marked along the circle. A stationary arm is attached to the body. A moving arm is attached to the center of the goniometer body (fulcrum). This moving arm aligns with the moving limb or segment.
  - Measures flexion, extension, abduction, adduction, and rotation.
  - Joints measured: shoulder, elbow, wrist, hip, knee, and ankle.

Once muscle weakness or ROM issues have been identified, appropriate interventions may be added to the plan of care. Sometimes stretching and/or strengthening will be used as interventions. At other times assistive devices will be needed to compensate for functional loss.

In assessing the balance-impaired patient, the clinician should pay close attention to ankle ROM and control. Limited dorsiflexion that compromises toe clearance during the gait cycle may lead to tripping and falling. Orthotics designed to limit ankle motion have been found to have positive effects on balance in certain populations. Ankle-foot orthoses limit ankle motion in one or more planes.

With regard to balance, there is evidence indicating that ankle-foot orthoses do not compromise balance for the normal-balanced population and have positive effects on various balance-related outcome measures.[5] In a review of 37 studies (most with neurologically impaired subjects), it was concluded that rigid designs seem to be beneficial in static balance tasks while more flexible designs seem to be superior under dynamic balance conditions.[5]

A study of orthotics in subjects with a history of inversion ankle sprains found[6] the following:

- This group had poorer balance than uninjured subjects.
- Molded orthotics improved balance scores.
- Unmolded orthotics did not improve balance scores.

A study of the effects of insoles in subjects ($n = 45$) older than 65 years of age found that use of a heel cup with an arch support worn for at least 4 hours a day for 8 weeks enhanced standing balance.[7]

## Posture

Ideal posture provides a body position that balances the body's mass around the center of gravity,[8] so that minimal energy expenditure from postural muscles is needed.[9] As discussed earlier, if the body segments are not sufficiently supported by the base of support, the patient may have compromised balance. As with the example of stacking boxes, if each box is stacked directly on top of the one below, the stack is more stable. In terms of the human, do the boxes line up? When patients lean or bend, they shift their center of gravity. If muscle weakness or tightness causes postural changes, the center of gravity may be moved away from the base of support. Examine your patient's posture from the front, back, and side. Do postural changes place the patient at risk? If so, will stretching contracted muscles and strengthening weaker, overstretched muscles help?

A study of healthy computer-based workers ($n = 30$) vs controls ($n = 30$) found that subjects with a forward head posture (found in the computer-based workers) had postural imbalance and impaired ability to regulate movements in forward and backward directions.[10]

# SOMATOSENSORY SYSTEM

Since the somatosensory system is responsible for a variety of sensory inputs, many tests are possible. Remember that the somatosensory system includes sensations of different types of touch (light, fluttering, vibration, and coarse), temperature, pain, pressure, joint position (proprioception), and movement (kinesthesia). We will not include tests of all of these but instead focus on those that are key inputs for the balance patient. For balance, we will examine touch, pressure, and proprioception.

## Light Touch

In evaluating light touch, you may decide to first do a quick screen of all limb dermatomes and then a more methodical exam if the screen indicates diminished light touch sensations. Where a neurologic pathology is suspected, you may wish to also check the face and trunk. For a quick screen of light touch, you quickly run a few fingers bilaterally along all dermatome of the arms and legs and ask the patient if the touch feels "the same or different" on each side, and if the sensation feels normal. If the patient indicates a presence of diminished sensations, you more slowly and deliberately check each dermatome. You may wish to check for gross sensation or have the patient close his or her eyes and report where he or she feels being touched by the examiner. This is also a good way to make sure that the patient is not reporting intact sensation inaccurately.

## Proprioception

Proprioception is the ability to use somatosensory input to know joint positions. We use proprioception to help us determine whether we are swaying while standing and allowing us to correct body position around the ankle joint. Therefore, it is an important sensation for the balance patient to have. Proprioception depends on stretch receptors in our soft tissues, like skin and joint capsules. There are also receptors that detect tension on the tendons as well as muscle spindle length.[11]

There are numerous tests of proprioception, including some of sensitivity and others of acuity. Some test motion sense while others test position sense. Currently there is little consensus about which method is best to use, with little guidance available from studies owing to mixed results.[12] Below we review 2 methods: threshold testing and joint matching.

### Discrimination Threshold Testing

Discrimination threshold testing involves passive movement of the patient's limb to 1 of 2 possible positions (eg, up or down)[13] and reflects the patient's proprioceptive acuity and processing of afferent sensory feedback.[12] In this example we will examine the ankle of a male patient, although this method may be applied to most joints.

**Test position:** The patient may be seated or lying.

**Demonstration:** Allow the patient to watch as you move the ankle into dorsi- and plantarflexion. As you move the ankle into dorsiflexion, you say, "This is up." As you move the ankle into dorsiflexion, you say, "This is down."

**Patient instructions:** Instruct the patient to close his or her eyes and indicate, when asked, whether the ankle is up (dorsiflexed) or down (plantarflexed).

**Test:** Hold the foot either on the lateral and medial edges or by carefully applying *equal pressure* with your grip on the dorsal and ventral surfaces of the foot. Remember that the patient may be able to use pressure to determine which way you are moving the foot, and we do not want the patient to use that information. Passively wiggle the ankle joint a few times into dorsi- and plantarflexion and then stop in either full dorsi- or plantarflexion. Then ask the patient to indicate the position of the foot (up or down) without looking. Repeat this at least 3 or more times, to make sure that the patient is not just guessing.

## Joint Position Matching

There are 2 methods of testing joint position matching: ipsilateral matching and contralateral matching.

You perform *ipsilateral matching* by passively moving a limb to the desired joint-angle test position and returning to the starting point. The patient must then actively move the same limb to the same joint-angle test position.

The second method is *contralateral matching*, where you passively move one limb to a desired joint-angle test position while the patient actively moves the contralateral limb to the same joint angle.[12] Let's review the steps of contralateral matching. For this method, we will use the knee joint as an example. You will test each limb separately. For example, you move the patient's right knee into 80 degrees of flexion. The patient should then move his or her left knee into 80 degrees of flexion to match. The difference between the 2 joint positions indicates the patient's proprioceptive acuity. You should do this a number of times on the same limb, each time choosing a different joint position. Repeat the test on the contralateral limb. This method not only assesses afferent proprioceptive feedback but, because of the active limb movement on the patient's part, it must use additional sensorimotor processes.[12]

# Pressure Sensations

For the balance patient, we want to check whether pressure sensations are intact on the feet. We use a monofilament as a tool to test these sensations, and there are a couple common methods. Most bedside tests use a 5.07 monofilament to check pressure on the foot. The phrase *protective sensations to the foot* indicates an intact ability to detect pressure on the foot, which is needed for balance planning.

Monofilaments are assigned numbers by the manufacturer indicating how stiff they are. Higher numbers indicate stiffer monofilaments that require more force to bend. Three monofilaments are commonly used to test for peripheral neuropathy: 4.17 (which requires 1 g of force to bend), 5.07 monofilament (which requires 10 g of force), and the 6.10 (which requires 75 g of force).[14] Several studies have support the use of the 5.07 monofilament to test for protective sensations of the feet.[15-18]

## The Monofilament Test[14]

While testing protective sensations of the foot using the Semmes-Weinstein test, the patient is usually sitting or lying with eyes closed, and is instructed not to watch as the test is administered. Push the tip of the monofilament against the foot perpendicular to the skin with enough force to make the monofilament bend. Hold it in that position for about 1 second. Test points usually include the first, third, and fifth metatarsal heads and distal pads of the digits, medial and lateral midfoot, and the pad of the heel. The American Diabetic Association promotes testing the metatarsal joints and the pads of the great toes. It also recommends testing vibration sensation with the monofilament to check for loss of protective sensations.[19] Various methods can be used in choosing which points to test. Many monofilaments even come with a map of the foot which shows the test points. During the test, the examiner pushes the monofilament against the patient's skin until the monofilament bends, or for 1 to 2 seconds, before releasing it. The patient is instructed to indicate when the monofilament is detected. Avoid asking, "Do you feel that?" as you press the monofilament against the test site, as it may lead the patient to respond that affirmatively even if no pressure is felt. Instead, instruct the patient to say the word *now* (or some similar word) when pressure is detected.

## Somatosensory Findings

The most common issues you will find will be lack of light touch or pressure sensations and reduced or absent proprioception. Different protocols are used with the monofilament test to check pressure sensations. The most conservative approach is to assume balance challenges if there is any loss of sensation.

Facial or extremity numbness or trigeminal neuralgia may indicate central pathologies.

# SOMATOSENSORY INTERVENTIONS

Studies have shown that there is a correlation between gait abnormalities, impaired balance, and increased risk of falling with the loss of distal sensations.[20] Training of proprioception is often called *neuromuscular exercise* or *training*. What constitutes a neuromuscular or proprioception exercise? Generally these are exercises that include joint movement. This is a very broad way to categorize these exercises; after all, we move our joints in walking, weight shifting, or weight lifting. It seems that proprioceptive exercises are those that include joint motion for the purpose of improving somatosensation. It may be argued that exercises that include joint motion for purposes other than increasing somatosensation (eg, balance exercises) are at the same time "working proprioception." Finding research on this subject is sometimes challenging for the simple fact that proprioception is not always measured or described in the same way. Results of various studies are mixed as to the efficacy of such exercises to improve proprioception. While proprioceptive (neuromuscular) exercises seem to have positive effects, they do not always have the effect that you would expect—that is, improving proprioception.

There have been a few studies showing improved somatosensation using proprioceptive exercises. While tai chi has been widely discussed in the literature as a balance exercise, it is not designed to be a proprioceptive exercise per se. However, owing to the constant weight shifting involving joint motion, weight bearing, and turning, it is a great proprioceptive exercise for the lower extremities by nature. One study of tai chi found, among other benefits, improved plantar sensation while studying its effects in a group of 25 subjects.[21] Other benefits of the intervention included Improved "Timed Up & Go" scores, and 6-minute walk times.

A different tai chi study compared proprioceptive exercises to the effects of tai chi on ankle strength and proprioception (ankle joint position sense). The proprioceptive exercise included both static and dynamic balance tasks and transitions. This study ($n = 60$) found that both proprioception exercises *and* tai chi significantly improved ankle proprioception in the elderly, with no significant difference between these groups.[22] As just discussed, given the constant weight bearing and shifting of the hip, knee, and ankle motions involved with tai chi, could it not already be classified as a proprioceptive exercise, at least in looked at from a western point of view? In a therapy scenario, we do not preform tai chi forms but rather incorporate the weight-shifting exercises and activities, which are integral components of tai chi, into our plans of care.

In a study of women with knee osteoarthritis[23] ($n = 66$), the subjects were divided into a group of that performed strengthening exercises and another that performed the same exercises plus kinesthesia and balance training. Outcomes were measured using the Western Ontario and McMaster University Osteoarthritis Index and the Medical Outcomes Study Short Form Health Survey before and after the 8-week trial. Other measures included isokinetic muscle strength of the quads and hamstrings, 10-minute walking time, 10 stairs climbing time, and sensation of proprioception at the knee (measured by absolute angle error for 10 different knee angles). The balance exercises included both static and dynamic exercises and gait under a variety of conditions. Outcomes of the 60 subjects who completed the trials found statistical improvements for both groups in all measures. While a 75% increase in proprioceptive sense accuracy was detected in both groups at postexercise vs preexercise, no differences were found between groups with respect to proprioceptive sense accuracy. It is interesting to note that observational fall risk assessments were not performed for this study.

In a different study of subjects who had total knee arthroplasty surgeries, 2 groups were compared: one with functional training and the other with functional training plus balance exercises. The study found that the addition of balance exercises improved gait speed and single-leg stance time.[24] The balance exercises are not well described and are included under "agility and perturbation techniques." It is difficult to say whether these exercises could be classified as proprioceptive.

Westlake et al examined sensory-specific balance training in older adults, who were randomized into either a balance-exercise group or a falls-prevention education group. Three proprioceptive measures were observed, including threshold to perception of passive movement, passive joint position sense, and velocity discrimination. Postintervention, there were improvements in the balance exercise group for velocity discrimination (measured at the ankle) but not movement and position sense.[25]

The improvement in the ability to discriminate between extents of movements into ankle inversion in subjects aged 65 and older has been demonstrated after a 5-week bobble-board exercise intervention in 20 subjects. Greater improvement in ankle movement discrimination was made in subjects who underwent bobble-board training vs subjects who did not. Active movements at the ankle were significantly better discriminated when subjects were wearing shoes than when barefoot.[26]

In short, some studies have demonstrated that proprioceptive exercises and exercises that incorporate active joint movements may increase the ability to discriminate joint movements, improve velocity discrimination at the ankle, improve plantar sensations, and improve scores of some standardized tests (Timed Up & Go, 6-minute walk, gait speed, single-leg stance time). We have looked at interventions directed at improving or measuring proprioception. However, we have not discussed the use of somatosensation as a tool during balance training. Earlier, we discussed how some elderly patients become visually dependent. Many patients who have balance deficits rely not only on vision to improve their balance but also actively seek increased somatosensory information through light touch. You may have had the experience of seeing a balance-impaired person touching anything within reach as he or she walks, such as furniture, walls, or other people. These people are not necessarily leaning on these objects but instead are collecting information through their hands to aid balance. When they touch the wall or furniture, for example, they have a reference to the location of the floor. This information helps to provide a frame of reference in which they can determine their own location in space and plan to balance against gravity. Studies have demonstrated that sensory input to the hand and arm through contact can reduce postural sway in people who do not have balance impairments as well as in those with vestibular deficits even when the contact is not used to physically support the body (that is, it is only for used for touch).[27]

The very act of touching things within reach while standing or walking is a red flag, letting you know that person likely does not have enough information with which to balance. How may this be useful? First, we know that some patients who are balance-compromised may benefit from the use of an assistive device. The added somatosensory information gained by touching a cane to the floor may be enough to increase function and decrease fall risk. Further, we may use the sense of touch during balance training. When a patient's ability to balance is compromised, we may choose to start balance interventions while allowing the patient to touch (not lean on) a counter, wall, chair, etc. The purpose would be to give him or her more somatosensory information to aid in training. As patients progress in their ability to balance (whether statically or dynamically), you may reduce touch information to increase the challenge of the balance intervention. For example, when you begin, the patient may be allowed to touch another object with both hands. Later, you may restrict his or her touch to only one hand. You may further challenge the patient by reducing the touching of a reference object to just 1 or 2 fingers. Ultimately you may wish to eliminate the allowance of using touch as a balance aid. Through this process, the patient can learn to use more information during balance training as well as having an increased sense of security.

In summary, proprioceptive interventions for the balance patient may include joint-specific proprioception exercises, such as wobble boards, to standing activities (both static and dynamic) that incorporate ankle, knee, and hip movements. Finally, we may use light touch as a somatosensory balance aid in retraining balance. Addressing muscle weakness and ROM limitations of the hips and lower extremities will improve the patient's stability.

If you plan to have strengthening-specific exercises in the same treatment session as functional or balance activities, perform the balance and functional interventions first, so you do not try to retrain balance and function with fatigued or overworked lower extremity muscles. If you are in an outpatient setting, plan for the patient to have a rest period after strengthening prior to leaving the clinic.

# CERVICAL VERTIGO, OR CERVICOGENIC DIZZINESS

This condition may be seen with neck pathology or following a neck injury. Symptoms usually include dizziness associated with neck movement, disequilibrium, ataxia, light-headedness, cervical pain, and limited cervical motion.[28,29] Ear pain may be present, but there should be no hearing symptoms. Diagnosis is difficult and at times controversial. The 2 recognized potential causes include vascular compression and abnormal proprioceptive information. Prior to treatment, the physician rules out other possible etiologies.[29]

On the basis of studies that have investigated whiplash-associated disorders, cervical injuries seem to have little effect on the oculomotor and vestibular systems but may lead to disturbances in postural control.[28]

In a review of studies of cervicogenic dizziness, Clendaniel and Landel described other studies of flexion-extension injuries that found vestibular signs and symptoms.[28] In one study of 262 patients, 63% had spontaneous nystagmus with central oculomotor findings of direction-changing nystagmus, saccadic smooth pursuit, and impaired visual suppression of the vestibule-ocular reflex.[30] Another study of 309 patients with flexion-extension injuries revealed that 57% had abnormal electronystagmography results and 51% had abnormal rotary chair findings.

While some authors recommend the testing of vertebrobasilar insufficiency using the vertebral artery compression test (full cervical rotation with full extension) or Wallenberg test, a study by Theil et al examined the blood flow of 30 subjects who displayed signs and symptoms of vertebral artery insufficiency while in the Wallenberg test position (supine with full cervical extension and rotation); these investigators found no support for the validity and reliability of that test.[31] Other studies have shown changes in blood flow (both reduced and increased flow) with patients in the test positions.[32]

You must use your clinical judgment to decide on the benefits or risks of using such tests. Clendaniel and Landel point to studies showing that bedside tests of vertebral blood flow do not have the needed sensitivity to rule out vertebral artery compromise.[28]

Treatment of the cervical spine should address restricted mobility, hypermobility, increased muscle tone, trigger points, poor cervical posture, and impaired cervical kinesthesia. Therapeutic treatments of the cervical spine may include cervical spine mobilization, ROM exercises, proprioception exercises, soft tissue mobilization, and therapeutic agents.[28]

Treatments of imbalance and dizziness for this population lack studies to help guide practice. Current trends are to treat known cervical limitations as well as employing vestibular exercises once the patient can tolerate head motion.

# REFERENCES

1. Harris-Love M. The manual muscle test: meeting the challenge of the therapeutic trail. Available at http://www.niehs.nih.gov/research/resources/assets/docs/the_manual_muscle_test_meeting_the_challenge_of_the_therapeutic_trial_508.pdf. Updated 2014. Accessed October 5, 2014.
2. Dutton M. Principles of manual muscle testing. Available at http://highered.mcgraw-hill.com/sites/0071474013/student_viewo/chapter8/manuaul_muscle_testing.html. Updated 2009. Accessed October 5, 2014.
3. Frese E, Brown M, Norton B. Clinical reliability of manual muscle testing: middle trapezius and gluteus medius muscles. *Phys Ther.* 1987;67:1072-1076.
4. Dutton M. Principles of goniometry. Available at http://highered.mcgraw-hill.com/sites/0071474013/student_viewo/chapter8/goniometry.html. Updated 2009. Accessed October 5, 2014.
5. Ramstrand N, Ramstrand S. AAOP state-of-the-science evidence report: the effect of ankle-foot orthoses on balance—a systematic review. *JPO.* 2010;22(4S):P4-P23.
6. Combs-Orteza L,Vogelbach WD, Denegar CR. The effect of molded and unmolded orthotics on balance and pain while jogging following inversion ankle sprain. *J Athl Train.* 1992;27(1):80, 82, 84.
7. Tzu-Hsuan Chen, Li-Wei Chou, Mei-Wun Tsai, Ming-Jor Lo, Mu-Jung Kao. Effectiveness of a heel cup with an arch support insole on the standing balance of the elderly. *Clin Interv Aging.* 2014;9:351-356.
8. Sweeting KR, Mock M. Gait and posture: assessment in general practice. *Aust Fam Physician.* 2007;36(6):398-401, 404-405.
9. Levi K. *Manipulative Theory in Rehabilitation of the Locomotor System.* Oxford, UK: Butterworth-Heinemann; 1999.
10. Kang JH, Park RY, Lee SJ, Kim JY, Yoon SR, Jung KI. The effect of the forward head posture on postural balance in long time computer based worker. *Ann Rehabil Med.* 2012;36(1):98-104.
11. Patton HD, Fuchs A. *Textbook of Physiology.* Vol. 1, 21st ed. Philadelphia: Saunders; 1989:301.
12. Elangovan N, Hermann A, Knoczak J. Assessing proprioceptive function: evaluating joint position matching methods against psychophysical thresholds. *Phys Ther.* 2013: Epub ahead of print.
13. Gescheider GA. *Psychophysics: Method, Theory, and Application.* 2nd ed. Mahwah, NJ: Lawrence Erlbaum Associates; 1985.
14. Mueller M. Identifying patients with diabetes mellitus who are at risk for lower extremity complications: use of Semmes-Weinstein monofilaments. *Phys Ther.* 1996;76(1):68-71.
15. Holewski JJ, Stress RM, Graf PM, Grunfeld C. Aesthesiometry: quantification of cutaneous pressure sensation in diabetic peripheral neuropathy. *J Rehabil Res Dev.* 1988;25:1-10.
16. Olmos PR, Cataland S, O'Dorisio TM, Casey CA, Smead WL, Simon SR. The Semmes-Weinstein monofilament as a potential predictor of foot ulceration in patients with noninsulin-dependent diabetes. *Am J Med Sci.* 1995;309(2):76-82.
17. Kumar S, Fernando DJ, Veves A, Knowles EA, Young MJ, Boulton AJ. Semmes-Weinstein monofilaments: a simple, effective and inexpensive screening device for identifying diabetic patients at risk of foot ulceration. *Diabetes Res Clin Pract.* 1991;13(1-2):63-67.

18. McNeely MJ, Boyko EJ, Ahroni JH, et al. The independent contribution of diabetic neuropathy and vasculopathy in foot ulceration: how great are the risks? *Diabetes Care.* 1995;18:216-219.
19. American Diabetic Association. Standards of medical care in diabetes—2013. *Diabetes Care.* 2013:S11-S66.
20. Alrwaily M, Whitney SL. Vestibular rehabilitation of older adults with dizziness. *Otolaryngol Clin N Am.* 2011;44:473-496.
21. Li L, Manor B. Long term tai chi exercise improves physical performance among people with peripheral neuropathy. *Am J Chin Med.* 2010;38(3):449-459.
22. Liu J, Wang XQ, Zheng JJ, et al. Effects of tai chi versus proprioception exercise program on neuromuscular function of the ankle in elderly people: a randomized controlled trial. *Evid Based Complement Alternat Med.* 2012:265486.
23. Diracoglu D, Aydin Baskent A, Celik A. Effects of kinesthesia and balance exercises in knee osteoarthritis. *J Clin Rheumatol.* 2005;11(6):303-310.
24. Piva SR, Gil AB, Almeida GJM, et al. A balance exercise program appears to improve function for patients with total knee arthroplasty: a randomized clinical trial. *Phys Ther.* 2010;38(3):880-894.
25. Westlake KP, Yushiao W, Culham EG. Sensory-specific balance training in older adults: effect on position, movement, and velocity sense at the ankle. *Phys Ther.* 2007;87:560-568.
26. Waddington GS, Adams RD. The effect of a 5-week wobble-board exercise intervention on ability to discriminate different degrees of ankle inversion, barefoot and wearing shoes: a study in healthy elderly. *J Am Geriatr Soc.* 2004;52(4):573-576.
27. Jeka JJ. Light touch contact as a balance aid. *Phys Ther.* 1997;77:476-487.
28. Clendaniel R, Landel R. Non-vestibular diagnosis and imbalance: cervicogenic dizziness. In: Herdman S, ed. *Vestibular Rehabilitation.* 3rd ed. Philadelphia: FA Davis; 2007:467-484.
29. Hain T. Cervical vertigo. Available at http://american-hearing.org/disorders/cervical-vertigo/. Updated 2012. Accessed October 5, 2014.
30. Oosterveld W, Kortschot H, Kingma G, et al. Electronystagmographic findings following cervical whiplash injuries. *Acta Otolaryngol.* 1991;111:201.
31. Thiel H, Wallace K, Donat J, Yong-Hing K. Effect of various head and neck positions on vertebral artery blood flow. *Clin Biomech.* 1994;9:105-110.
32. Stevens A. Functional Doppler sonography of the vertebral artery and some considerations about manual techniques. *J Manual Med.* 1991;6:102-105.

# 8

# Central Processing, Memory, and Cognition

## CEREBELLUM

The cerebellum is responsible for the accuracy and coordination of movements. Since part of the cerebellum (the vestibulocerebellum) is responsible for calibrating and processing the vestibular system, a problem in the cerebellum may present in a variety of ways. The principal signs of cerebellar dysfunction are ataxia, hypotonia, tremor, gait abnormalities, and oculomotor abnormalities.[1]

Bedside tests of the cerebellum include tests of tone, gait, accuracy, and coordination. In addition, neurologists use heel-to-toe walking. Patients may not be "positive" for all cerebellar screens just because they are positive for one. Effects of cerebellar dysfunction on abilities and reflexes depend on the location and extent of cerebellar damage. Therefore, you should use more than one cerebellar test, include tests of

Plishka CM.
*A Clinician's Guide to Balance and Dizziness:*
*Evaluation and Treatment* (pp 249-268).
© 2015 Taylor & Francis Group.

**Figure 8-1.** Point-to-point 1.

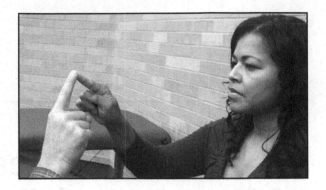

both the upper and lower extremities, and make sure to screen for both *accuracy* and *coordination* of movements. There is no one overriding precedent for how many or which to perform. Let's review various tests of cerebellar function.

Tests using the upper extremities include the following:

- Finger-to-nose (tests accuracy movements)
- Point-to-point, also known as *finger-nose-finger* (accuracy)
- Diadochokinesia (coordination)
- Hand clapping (coordination)

Tests using the lower extremities (accuracy) include the following:

- Heel-knee
- Heel-shin

## Accuracy of Movement Tests

### Point-to-Point Test

Instruct the patient to alternately touch the tip of his or her nose using the pad of the index finger and then to touch the pad of the examiner's extended finger with the pad of his or her own index finger. Have the patient do this as rapidly as possible. Repeat this test of accuracy several times. Some examiners keep their fingers (targets) stationary during the test while others reposition their finger targets between touches. The examiner observes the repetitive accuracy of finger placement on the alternating targets. Describe consistently missing the target as *dysmetria*. Also document if the patient demonstrates an intention tremor. Intention tremors increase as the finger approaches the target (Figures 8-1 and 8-2).

### Finger-to-Nose Test

With eyes open, the patient (sitting or standing) extends his or her upper extremity laterally (shoulder at 90 degrees of abduction) and is instructed to touch the tip of the nose using the pad of his or her index finger. After each touch of the target (nose tip), the patient returns to the starting position with the arm abducted to 90 degrees. Repeat this several times using each hand and arm. Then repeat the test on each side

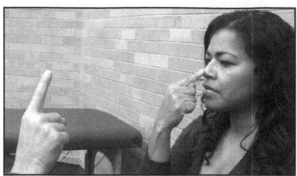

**Figure 8-2.** Point-to-point 2.

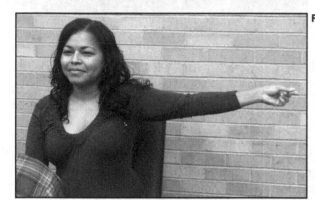

**Figure 8-3.** Finger-to-nose 1.

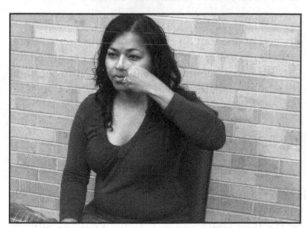

**Figure 8-4.** Finger-to-nose 2.

with the patient's eyes closed.[2] The examiner observes the repetitive accuracy and smoothness of movement of finger placement on the target (Figures 8-3 and 8-4). Tests are positive when the patient consistently misses the target or has intention tremors. Positive tests indicate cerebellar dysfunction.

**Figure 8-5.** Heel to knee 1.

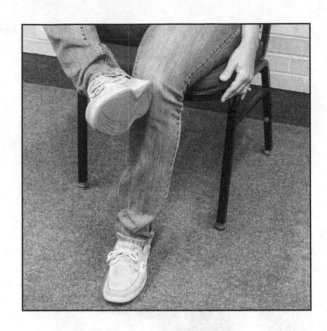

### Heel-Knee Tap Test

The heel of one foot taps the contralateral patella gently and repetitively. Each leg swing toward and away from the patella should be large (about 2 feet, or 60 cm) (Figure 8-5). Note any abnormalities of force or rhythm. Test each side.[1]

### Heel-Shin Slide Test

Instruct the patient to slide the heel of one foot down the shin of the contralateral leg from knee (just distal to the patella) to ankle. The heel should stay exactly on top of the shin (midline) and move in a slow and controlled manner down to the shin. Observe and report any side-to-side (mediolateral) leg tremors during the slide[1] (Figures 8-6 and 8-7).

## Coordination of Movement Tests

### Diadochokinesia

Instruct the patient to perform rapid alternating movements bilaterally. Typically this involves supinating and pronating the hands (palm up and then palms down), then slapping the hands against the thighs just proximal to the knees repetitively and as rapidly as possible. Repeat several times. The examiner observes if both hands move with equal speed, timing, force, and range of movement. Compare the quality of movement side to side (Figures 8-8 and 8-9). If the patient is unable to perform rapid alternating movements, report *dysdiadochokinesia*.

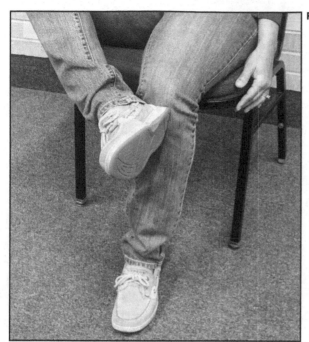

**Figure 8-6.** Heel to shin 1.

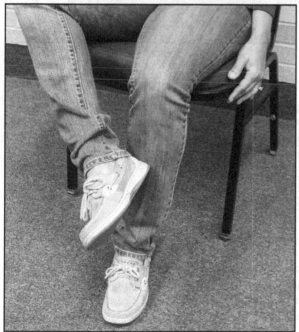

**Figure 8-7.** Heel to shin 2.

**Figure 8-8.** Diadochokinesia 1.

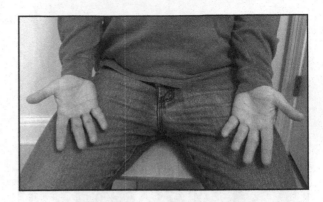

**Figure 8-9.** Diadochokinesia 2.

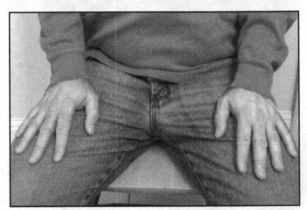

## Hand Clapping

Instruct the patient to clap both hands together with equal motion, distance, speed, and force. The clinician demonstrates and then asks the patient to replicate the hand clapping. The clinician observes for symmetry and coordination of motions (Figures 8-10 and 8-11).

# CENTRAL FINDINGS

## *Central Versus Peripheral Etiology*

There are central causes of dizziness, nystagmus, and imbalance that mimic peripheral causes. Without diagnostic testing, a bedside clinician cannot be 100% sure if causes are central (brain) or peripheral (outside of the central nervous system [CNS]). However, there are some clues to help suggest which case is likely. Table 8-1 contains pathologies that can cause dizziness and disequilibrium.[3,4]

Central vertigo may be accompanied by motor or sensory deficits, hyperreflexia, extensor plantar response, dysarthria, or limb ataxia.[5]

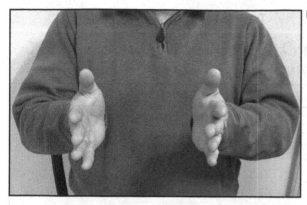

**Figure 8-10.** Hand clap 1.

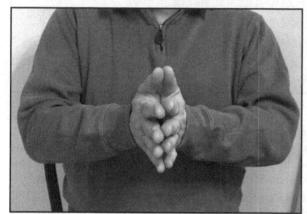

**Figure 8-11.** Hand clap 2.

## Coordination and Accurate Movements

During our examination, we checked for coordinated movements such as hand clapping, tapping the feet, and rapid alternating motions (diadochokinesia). We also examined motions requiring accuracy, such as having the patient touch the distal pad of his or her index finger to the tip of the nose, tapping the heel directly on the patella, or sliding the heel of one foot along the shin of the contralateral leg. If the patient is unable to perform these motions synchronously, you may suspect cerebellar dysfunction. During your examination, if time permits, include tests that use both the upper and lower extremities.

## Central Positional Vertigo

Symptoms of central positional vertigo (CPV) include vertigo (movement sensations) as soon as the patient is put in a provoking position, which persists as long as the patient remains in this position, and which may or may not be accompanied by nystagmus.[6]

## TABLE 8-1

# COMMON CENTRAL AND PERIPHERAL PATHOLOGIES CAUSING DIZZINESS AND IMBALANCE

| CENTRAL | PERIPHERAL |
|---|---|
| Brainstem strokes | Benign paroxysmal positional vertigo (BPPV) (vestibular) |
| Cerebellar degeneration | Tumors of the cerebellopontine angle |
| Head trauma | Labyrinthitis (vestibular) |
| Migraine-related | Ménière's disease |
| Multiple sclerosis | Postsurgical (labyrinthectomy) |
| Parkinson's disease | Post-trauma |
| Vestibulopathy | Schwannomas |
|  | Dehiscence of the superior canal (vestibular) |
|  | Vestibular neuritis |

CPV can occur in various disorders affecting the brainstem, such as infarct, tumors, and multiple sclerosis.[6-8] A small cerebellar hemorrhage, especially around the vermis, sometimes causes isolated dizziness with positional nystagmus.[9,10] This condition does not respond to canalith repositioning maneuvers or habituation.[6]

CPV (sometimes referred to as *central paroxysmal positional vertigo*, or CPPV) presents much like BPPV, with position changes of the patient causing vertigo and nystagmus. Not surprisingly, CPPV is sometimes misdiagnosed as BPPV.[11] When central issues cause nystagmus, the nystagmus is often (but not always) pure up- or downbeating, or pure torsional. If, during testing for BPPV, you see nystagmus that lacks both torsion and the vertical (up or down) component, you need to consider that the nystagmus may be central in origin. If you are not using equipment such as Frenzel or infrared goggles, these motions may be too subtle to see with the naked eye. In the absence of other central signs, you may try canalith repositioning. If the patient does not respond to this within a few sessions, consider referring him or her for further testing, such as an electronystagmography/audiography or even computed tomography (CT)/ magnetic resonance imaging (MRI).

Small cerebellar hemorrhages sometimes cause CPPV, as reported by Johkura.[11] He believes that CPPV has been underdiagnosed owing to an influx of BPPV information. In his facility, of patients who presented to the emergency room over a 2-year period with isolated acute-onset dizziness ($n$ = 1332), only 1.7% were found to have cerebrovascular disease while 53% were diagnosed with BPPV. Johkura points out that while cerebellar hemorrhage, ischemia to the posterior inferior cerebellar artery (PICA), and BPPV may cause nystagmus, he believes that in those with PICA ischemia the nystagmus is "obscure in comparison to imbalance" and that this may help differentiate central causes of dizziness from BPPV.

Watch for brainstem and cerebellar signs[12]: paralytic strabismus, trigeminal hypesthesia (reduced touch sensation)/pain, facial or tongue paralysis, dysphagia (difficulty swallowing), hoarseness, gaze-evoked nystagmus, jerky pursuit eye movements, ataxia (lack of coordination), or dysarthria (impaired speech or articulation).

## Mild Head Injury

Head trauma may cause CNS symptoms, labyrinthine concussion, a neck injury, or some combination of these,[3] which can produce dizziness resulting from cerebral or brainstem injuries. Dizziness of central origin after mild head injury may occur because of damage to the brainstem, cerebral or cerebellar connections, or pathways of the peripheral vestibular organs. Peripheral structures which, when injured, can cause dizziness include cranial nerve VIII, the semicircular canals, the otolith organs, and the bone surrounding the labyrinth. Whitney et al, based on previous studies, report that brain disruption in the area of the posterior fossa and brainstem, usually including the vestibular nucleus, can cause CNS vestibular dysfunction, with symptoms that are often unrecognized and can persist for years before medical or therapeutic intervention.[13] Symptoms may include dizziness, vertigo, balance difficulties, ataxia, episodic unilateral hearing loss, and tinnitus. Patients may also complain of difficulty reading, watching television, and walking. Other indications of a central problem following a head injury include confusion, weakness, or incoordination.[13]

## Multiple Sclerosis

MS affects the brain, spinal cord, and optic nerves; it is an abnormal immune response directed against the CNS.[14] Episodes of inflammation damage the myelin sheath surrounding nerve fibers in the white matter of the brain and spinal cord, causing scars called *plaques*. The plaques disrupt nerve transmission along these nerves and produce the symptoms, which vary from person to person depending on the location and extent of scarring.[15] MS is more common further from the equator, and having a first-degree relative (parent, sibling) with MS increases an individual's risk of developing the disease.[16] Women are about twice as likely as men to develop MS, and Caucasians whose families originated in northern Europe are at highest risk.[17]

While individuals with MS are not necessarily sedentary, few may achieve daily levels of recommended physical activity.[18] Symptoms may include fatigue, motor weakness, paresthesia, unsteady gait, double vision, tremor, and electric shock sensations with certain head motions, as well as slurred speech and dizziness.[15,17] People with MS have balance impairments characterized by increased sway in quiet stance, delayed responses to postural perturbations, and a reduced ability to move toward their limits of stability.[19]

Factors associated with falls in persons with MS are similar to those of other neurologic diseases. The majority of persons with MS fall at least once annually,[20] with many studies reporting that greater than 50% of persons with MS fall more than 2 times annually.[21-24] Despite the high incidence of falls in this population, fewer than 50% of patients receive information about fall prevention from a health care professional.[25] In a study of 575 community-dwelling people with MS by Matsuda et al, about 62% reported having concerns about falling and about 67% reported activity restrictions related to these concerns, even if they had not experienced falls.[21] The association of fall status with mobility function did not appear to be linear. Fall risk increased with declining mobility; however, at a certain threshold, further declines in mobility were associated with fewer falls. This is probably due to reduced fall risk exposure by limited functional mobility.

Recommendations by the Medical Advisory Board of the National Multiple Sclerosis Society, detailed in an expert opinion paper,[26] include referring patients to rehabilitation professionals when there is an abrupt or gradual worsening of function or an increase in impairment that has a significant impact on the individual's mobility, safety, independence, and/or quality of life. Maintenance therapy includes rehabilitation interventions designed to preserve the current status of ADL, safety, mobility, and quality of life and to reduce the rate of deterioration and development of complications. The opinion paper also highlights a number of studies that outline positive outcomes of rehabilitation in this population.

## Parkinson's Disease

Parkinson's disease (PD) is a progressive brain disorder that results from the reduction in the number of cells in the substantia nigra that produce the neurotransmitter dopamine, which helps to coordinated muscle movements. According to the National Parkinson Foundation, the motor symptoms of PD appear after damage to 60% to 80% of dopamine-producing cells has occurred.[27] PD affects approximately 1% of individuals older than 60 years of age.[28]

There are 4 primary symptoms:
1. Tremor
2. Rigidity
3. Bradykinesia
4. Postural instability[29]

Impairments may include[30] cataracts, vestibular hair cell loss, and slowed transmission times of somatosensory messages. The patient becomes vision-dominant for balance and has restricted limits of stability. The ankle strategy becomes dominant, and the patient's movements become bradykinetic (slow). Co-contraction and rigidity are common. Other common signs and symptoms include decreased extremity and trunk strength as well as moderately impaired endurance. Over time, the patient will adopt a flexed posture in the neck, trunk, and hips. Bilateral ankle plantarflexor contractures may limit ankle range of motion. There is a decrease in posture and balance reactions and a severe decrease of trunk rotation.

Other symptoms may include[31] akinesia (a lack of motion) and freezing, tremor, postural instability, gait abnormalities, perceptual and attentional deficits, cognitive deficits, sleep disturbances, and autonomic dysfunction (eg, bowel and bladder problems, sweating, libido changes), and dizziness.

# Progressive Supranuclear Palsy

Progressive supranuclear palsy (PSP) is a rare brain disorder but one that you will be asked about if you work a lot with dizziness and balance. The National Institute of Neurologic Disorders and Stroke (part of the US National Institutes of Health) describes PSP as causing progressive problems with gait and balance as well as problems of complex eye motions and thinking. The incidence is 1:100,000 people over the age of 60, with middle-aged or elderly people affected (men more than women). Symptoms include loss of balance while walking, unexplained falls, stiffness, and awkward gait. Early symptoms, which vary with different people, may include irritability, forgetfulness, laughing or crying for no reason, and angry outbursts. Later symptoms may include blurred vision, difficulty with downward voluntary gaze, trouble maintaining gaze—for example, while making eye contact—prolonged or infrequent blinking, slurred speech, and difficulty swallowing. The etiology is unknown.[29]

# Stroke

The 2 main categories of strokes are ischemic stroke and hemorrhagic stroke. Ischemic strokes, as the name implies, result from a lack of oxygen to the brain due to blocked arteries (eg, secondary to atherosclerosis or emboli). Hemorrhagic strokes are due to sudden bleeding in the brain, which can cause swelling and pressure in the skull and damage to the brain.[32] Stroke is the most common cause of long-term disability,[33] with impaired balance early after stroke being strongly associated with compromised future function and recovery.[34,35] Disabilities from strokes may include paralysis or motor control problems, sensory disturbances, aphasia, cognition and memory impairments, and emotional disturbances.[36]

Red flags for stroke probably include a history of dizziness over weeks or months; auditory symptoms; and headache, neck pain, or recent trauma.[37]

# Acute Vestibular Syndrome

When patients reporting to an emergency room complain of dizziness lasting longer than 24 hours—that is, patients presenting with acute vestibular syndrome—there is a quick bedside test battery detailed by Kattah[38] that may help to determine whether the problem is a stroke vs a peripheral vestibular problem. This procedure uses the HINTS and INFARCT acronyms, outlined below, to guide testing.

Kattah suggests that when a patient presents with acute vestibular syndrome, it may be possible to determine whether they are having a stroke by using the following tests as a battery:

HINTS

HI: head impulse test

N: nystagmus

T: tests of skew

In using this battery, look for any of the following signs that may indicate stroke.

INFARCT

IN: (head) impulse normal

Or

FA: fast-phase alternating (nystagmus) (eg, direction-changing nystagmus)

Or

RCT: refixation on cover test (eg, vertical skew during the alternating cover test)

Results from the study ($n$ = 100): The presence of normal horizontal head impulse tests, direction-changing nystagmus with eccentric gaze, or vertical skew deviation was 100% sensitive and 96% specific for stroke. Twelve percent of initial MR diffusion-weighted imaging was falsely negative, with all MRI obtained less than 48 hours after symptom onset. The study concludes that in acute vestibular syndrome, the 3-step bedside exam appears to be more sensitive for stroke than early MRI.[38]

# COGNITION AND MEMORY

Cognitive impairment has been associated with increased fall risk as well as deficits in physical function.[39-44] Even mild declines in cognitive function are importantly associated with falling.[45] A decrease in the volume of gray matter in the middle and superior frontal gyri of the brain has been associated with falls in the older adult with mild cognitive impairment.[44]

If you suspect that your patients have memory or cognitive issues, you should screen them, because defective memory and cognition can impact functional mobility and increase fall risk. There are a variety of screens available; some commonly used tests include the Mental Status Assessment of Older Adults (Mini-Cog), Montreal Cognitive Assessment (MoCA), and Mini-Mental State Examination (MMSE) (also known as the *Folstein test*).

The Mini-Cog is a composite of 3-time recall and clock drawing. It was developed as a brief test for discriminating demented from nondemented persons. It takes approximately 3 minutes to administer and there are no test forms. In a study of 129 subjects, it had a sensitivity[46] of 99%. Other authors report sensitivity ranging from 76% to 99% and specificity[47] ranging from 89% to 93%. The test protocol is as follows:

- Instruct the patient to listen to and remember 3 words and to repeat them.
- Instruct the patient to draw a clock with the time of 11:10.
- Finally, instruct the patient to once again repeat the 3 words he or she was given initially.

A total score of 5 points is possible. Test interpretation[47]: One point is given for each recalled word after the Clock Drawing test for a total possible score of 3. Next, the Clock Drawing test is scored 2 if normal, with no points given if the clock is incorrectly drawn. Adding the recalled word score to the Clock Drawing score yields the total test score. The patient is positive for dementia for scores of 0 to 2 and negative for scores of 3 to 5.

The MoCA is a cognitive screening test designed to help health professionals detect mild cognitive impairment. This test may be reproduced for clinical and educational uses without permission; however, uses in research require permission from the author. Test domains include visuospatial/executive skills, language, memory, conceptual thinking, calculations, and orientation. Time to administer is approximately 10 minutes. It is a 30-point test with impairment noted for mild cognitive impairment or Alzheimer's disease for scores of 25 or less (a score of 26 or above is considered normal).[48]

The MMSE is a 30-point questionnaire. According to the publisher of this test, it is a test of cognitive function. The "standard" edition of the test is appropriate for ages 18 to 85 years of age; it takes 10 to 15 minutes to administer and an additional 5 minutes to score. Test books and forms are available at the publisher's website. There is a second edition of the test (MMSE-2) that is reported to be appropriate for ages 18 to 100; it takes up to 20 minutes to administer and an additional 5 minutes to score.[49]

# RESEARCH FINDINGS

## Central Disorders

### Stroke

There is conflicting evidence as to whether the location of the lesion is associated with functional outcome, but the size of the lesion has a significant impact on recovery.[50] Bayona et al found that severe strokes fail to exhibit the same degree of recovery owing to significant widespread damage to both the primary and the adjacent brain areas and that age is an inconsistent predictor of recovery, since both older and younger stroke patients benefit from rehabilitation.

Tyson et al studied the frequency of balance disability by looking at 75 people with first-time anterior circulation stroke and found that 83% of the subjects had a balance disability poststroke. Subjects with more severe balance disability had more severe strokes, impairments, and disabilities. Weakness and sensation were associated with balance disability. Subject demographics, stroke pathology, and visuospatial neglect were not associated with balance disability.[51]

### Acute Stroke and Dizziness Versus Peripheral Etiology

In the United States, 10 million ambulatory visits per year occur due to complaints of dizziness,[52] with about 25% of these to emergency rooms.[53] Of those presenting to the ER, 6% are diagnosed with a peripheral vestibular diagnosis (vestibular labyrinthitis or neuritis), 4% receive a cerebrovascular diagnosis, and 22% leave without a causal diagnosis and receive a diagnosis of dizziness or vertigo.[53,54] Best evidence suggests that nearly two-thirds of patients with stroke lack focal neurological signs that would be readily apparent to a non-neurologist, and one third lack signs that would be readily apparent to a neurologist.[37] Fewer than half of acute vestibular syndrome presentations include limb ataxia, dysarthria, or other obvious neurological features.[55]

Acute vestibular syndrome is dizziness that develops acutely, along with nausea or vomiting, unsteady gait, nystagmus, and intolerance to head motion. Symptoms persist for a day or more, with vestibular neuritis and ischemic stroke in the brainstem or cerebellum being the most common causes.[37] While vestibular neuritis is probably the most common cause, Tarnutzer et al point out that vertebrobasilar ischemic stroke may mimic a peripheral vestibular disorder, with focal neurological signs absent in more than half of those presenting with acute vestibular syndrome due to stroke.[37]

What bedside tests are useful in determining central vs peripheral causes of acute vestibular syndrome? Tarnutzer et al suggest the following:

- Vestibulo-ocular reflex (VOR) function using the Head Impulse test (also known as the *Head Thrust test*): A normal Head Impulse test of VOR function was the single best bedside predictor of peripheral vs central causes of acute vestibular syndrome. The Head Impulse test has a sensitivity for detecting stroke essentially matching that of diffusion-weighted MRI; it also has comparable specificity.[38] More common infarctions of the posterior inferior cerebellar artery generally affect only the cerebellum or lateral medulla, sparing structures needed for an intact VOR.[38,56]

  There are other causes of stroke, such as those involving the anterior inferior cerebellar artery, as well as other central etiologies that may cause an abnormal Head Impulse test, leading the examiner to suspect a peripheral cause other signs are not taken into consideration, such as eye (oculomotor) findings.[37]

  Stenosis of the basilar artery near the origin of the anterior inferior cerebellar artery causes an infarction of the labyrinth; such a patient may present with an abnormal head impulse test, new unilateral hearing loss, and other subtle oculomotor signs, such as direction-changing nystagmus or skew deviation. These oculomotor signs should be present when the brainstem or cerebellum is affected.[37]

- Gaze-evoked nystagmus: Direction-changing horizontal nystagmus on lateral gaze generally reflects dysfunction of gaze-holding structures in the brainstem and cerebellum.[57] This type of eye movement correctly identified central causes of acute vestibular syndrome with 92% specificity but a low sensitivity of 38%.[37]

- Ocular alignment: Skew deviation (vertical ocular misalignment) during the Alternate Cover test was found the be 98% specific but only 30% sensitive in predicting central causes of acute vestibular syndrome.[37] With rare exceptions, vertical skew deviations are generally of central origin.[58]

## Chronic Stroke

Harris et al[59] examined the relationship between balance/mobility and fall incidence in 99 community-dwelling subjects with chronic stroke; they report that impaired cognition/mood,[60,61] balance,[62,63] and ADL[61-63] increased fall risk in this population. The investigation found 49 subjects in their study (50%) experienced at least one fall over a 6-month period, with 56% of the falls occurring indoors, and of those 62% were within the home. The most frequent activity at the time of the fall was walking (51%). Of those who fell, 41% reported an injury, and 85% of those sought medical attention.[59] Further, those in this study who used a 4-wheel walker had a low fall incidence (equal to or less than 1%), while those who used a cane had 2 or more falls.

Another study in the chronic stroke population ($n = 20$) found that subjects with poststroke hemiparesis exhibited greater trunk repositioning error than age-matched controls.[64] As trunk control is key for other functions, the authors suggest using weight-shifting exercises to help address this issue.

In a study of acute stroke patients who incorporated optokinetic stimulation as an intervention, the authors concluded that optokinetic stimulation was effective in restoring voluntary movements, postural control, and mobility.[65]

Vestibular therapy is effective with central vestibular disorders, including stroke.[66] In a large study of 6342 hospitalized patients, the use of physical therapy increased the probability of discharge to home.[67] Important changes in balance performance can be achieved in participants in the chronic stage poststroke, even if they are more than 10 years poststroke.[35] What is the best way to train balance poststroke? Good question! We don't have any evidence that currently points toward a best practice. We know from animal studies dating more than 10 years back that repetition of motor activities alone does not produce reorganization of cortical maps. Instead, research suggests that the acquisition of motor skills (ie, motor learning) drives plasticity.[68] If we follow this concept, performing functional motions and activities should drive plasticity.

Examining the effects of physical therapy for central vestibular dysfunction, Brown et al assessed 48 subjects using the Activities-Specific Balance Confidence Scale, the Dizziness Handicap Inventory, the Dynamic Gait Index, the Timed Up & Go test, and the Five Times Sit-to-Stand. Physical therapy programs were customized for each patient for a mean of 5 visits over an average of 5 months. Significant differences were demonstrated between initial evaluation and discharge in each of the assessment measures for the entire group. The patients improved in both subjective and objective measures of balance after physical therapy intervention.[66]

### Therapy Frequency—Stroke

There currently is a wide-variety of methods used as interventions for patients who are poststroke, but there is a surprising lack of large studies to guide practice. While case studies abound, it is difficult to recommend (much less find) protocols based on large studies. We may gain helpful information by comparing the various studies.

A systematic review of research between January 2006 and February 2010 by Lubetzky-Vilnai and Kartin[35] found that there is wide diversity among balance rehabilitation programs with regard to interventions. Some interventions cited as efficacious include the following:

- Acute stage: There is moderate evidence to suggest that balance can improve with training for patients who are in acute stages poststroke.

- ◦ Exercising for 90 minutes or more for 5 sessions per week may be excessive and may be more likely to cause adverse effects compared with less demanding programs.[30,69]
- ◦ Intensive balance training performed 2 or 3 times per week may be sufficient to improve balance performance.[70-72]
- Subacute and chronic stages
  - ◦ Balance can be improved with intensive individualized training[73-75] as well as group exercise performed 2 times per week.[76-81]
  - ◦ Limited evidence indicates that balance performance late after stroke might deteriorate in the absence of an intervention.[78,79]

There was a poster presentation from 2006 that made a very interesting comparison between the practice habits of physical therapy and occupational therapy treatments and clinical studies looking at neuroplasticity. The poster made the point that in inducing neuroplastic changes in stroke models, animals often perform 200 to 400 repetitions of a single task. Healthy adults in motor learning studies often perform 100 to 500 repetitions of a task to be learned. However, when the investigators observed 36 treatment sessions, they found that far fewer repetitions were used during interventions. In sessions that addressed the lower extremity, the average task repetition per session was 33 for active movements, 6 for passive movements, and 8 for purposeful movements. The average number of steps taken was 292, and the average number of transfers was 11. Clearly this was a small sample, but the information provided compared with the research is shocking and leads us to wonder whether we are not pushing patients hard enough during treatment sessions to induce neuroplastic changes once these patients are past the acute stage.[82]

### Postural Responses

A small study ($n = 32$) by Gray et al of patients with hemiparesis poststroke noted that postural responses are impaired after stroke, with reduced or delayed muscle activity in the muscles of the paretic leg. They found that exercises emphasizing speed of movement, such as protective stepping to avoid a fall, and also quick standing squats (about 30 degrees of knee flexion), improved postural responses to internal perturbations. Also noted was improved weight bearing on the paretic leg to become more symmetrical in weight-bearing stance.[83]

## Cerebellar Disorders

Patients who have either acute or chronic cerebellar lesions may improve in postural stability following vestibular rehabilitation.[84,85] While improvement in patients with cerebellar disorders is possible, one researcher has reported that of all central disorders, cerebellar disorders improved the least after vestibular rehabilitation.[66]

## Concussion

There is a lot of research regarding concussion, and the topic merits further review beyond the scope of this book. Alsalaheen et al state that vestibular rehabilitation in both young and older persons postconcussion may speed recovery.[84,86] Alsalaheen et al concluded that vestibular therapy should be considered in the management of individuals postconcussion who have dizziness, gait, and balance dysfunctions that do not resolve with rest.[86]

## Supranuclear Palsy

Zampieri and Di Fabio examined the effects of balance training complemented by oculomotor exercises and visual awareness training vs balance training alone in patients with PSP ($n = 19$). They found that gaze control after balance and eye-control exercises improved; there was no significant improvement in the control group.[87]

# REFERENCES

1. Lichstein PR. Clinical methods: The history, physical, and laboratory examinations. 3rd ed. In: Walker H, Hall W, Hurst J, eds. *Clinical Methods: The History, Physical, and Laboratory Examinations.* 3rd ed. Boston, MA: Butterworths; 1990. http://www.ncbi.nlm.nih.gov/books/NBK349.
2. Scifers J. *Special Tests for Neurologic Examination.* Thorofare, NJ: SLACK, Inc; 2008.
3. Furman J, Whitney S. Central causes of dizziness. *Phys Ther.* 2000;80(2):179-187.
4. Bhattacharyya N, Baugh RF, Orvidas L, et al. Clinical practice guideline: benign paroxysmal positional vertigo. *Otolaryngol Head Neck Surg.* 2008;139(5 Suppl 4):S47-S81.
5. Greenberg D, Aminoff M, Simon R. Disorders of equilibrium. In: Greenberg D, Aminoff M, Simon R, eds. *Clinical Neurology.* 8th ed. New York: McGraw Hill Medical; 2012:187-218.
6. Herdman S. Treatment of benign paroxsymal positional vertigo. *Phys Ther.* 1990;70:381-388.
7. Fisher C. Vertigo in cerebrovascular disease. *Arch Otolaryngol.* 1967;85:529-537.
8. Troost T. Diziness and vertigo in vertebrobasilar disease: I. Central causes and vertebrobasilar disease. *Curr Concepts Cerebrovascr Dis Stroke.* 1979:413-415.
9. Watson B, Barber H, Deck J, Terbrugge K. Positional vertigo and nystagmus of central origin. *Can J Neruol Sci.* 1981;8:133-137.
10. Brandt T. Positional and positioning vertigo and nystagmus. *J Neurol Sci.* 1990:3-28.
11. Johkura K. Letters to the editor: central paroxysmal positional vertigo: isolated dizziness caused by small cerebellar hemorrhage. *Stroke.* 2007;38:e26-e27.
12. Bronstein A, Lempert T. *Dizziness: A Practical Approach to Diagnosis and Management.* Cambridge, UK: Cambridge University Press; 2007.
13. Whitney S, Unico J. Vestibular disorders in mild head injury. *Athl Ther Today.* 2001:33-39.
14. National Multiple Sclerosis Society. Definition of MS. Available at http://www.nationalmssociety.org/What-is-MS/Definition-of-MS. Updated 2014. Accessed October 5, 2014.
15. Frankel D. Mulitple sclerosis. In: Umphred D, ed. *Neurologic Rehabilitation.* 5th ed. St. Louis: Mosby Elsevier; 2007.
16. National Multiple Sclerosis Society. What causes MS? Available at http://www.nationalmssociety.org/What-is-MS/What-Causes-MS. Updated 2013. Accessed October 5, 2014.
17. Mayo Clinic. Multiple sclerosis risk factors. Available at http://www.mayoclinic.com/health/multiple-sclerosis/DS00188/DSECTION=risk-factors. Updated 2014. Accessed October 5, 2014.
18. Cavanaugh JT, Gappmaier VO, Dibble LE, Gappmaier E. Ambulatory activity in individuals with multiple sclerosis. *J Neurol Phys Ther.* 2011;35(1):26-33.
19. Cameron MH, Lord S. Postural controls in mulitple sclerosis: implications for fall prevention. *Curr Neurol Neurosci Rep.* 2010;10(5):407-412.
20. Dibble LE, Lopez-Lennon C, Lake W, Hoffmeister C, Gappmaier E. Utility of disease-specific measures and clinical balance tests in prediction of falls in persons with mulitple sclerosis. *J Neurol Phys Ther.* 2013;37:99-104.
21. Matsuda PN, Shumway-Cook A, Ciol MA, Bombardier CH, Kartin DA. Understanding falls in multiple sclerosis: association of mobility status, concerns about falling, and accumulated impairments. *Phys Ther.* 2012;92:407-415.
22. Cattaneo D, De Nuzzo C, Fascia T, Macalli M, Pisoni I, Cardini R. Risks of falls in subjects with multiple sclerosis. *Arch Phys Med Rehabil.* 2002;83(6):864-867.
23. Peterson EW, Cho CC, von Koch L, Finlayson ML. Injurious falls among middle aged and older adults with multiple sclerosis. *Arch Phys Med Rehabil.* 2008;89(6):1031-1037.

24. Fjeldstad C, Pardo G, Bemben D, Bemben M. Decreased postural balance in multiple sclerosis patients with low disability. *Int J Rehabil Res.* 2011;34(1):53-58.
25. Matsuda PN,Shumway-Cook A, Bamer AM, Johnson SL, Amtmann D, Kraft GH. Falls in mulitple sclerosis. *PMR.* 2011;3(7):624-632.
26. National Clinical Advisory Board of the National Multiple Sclerosis Society. Expert opinion paper. Available at http://ftp.nmss.org/casadmin/programs_services/professional_tool_kit/Expert_Opinion_Papers/Rehab_Recommendations.pdf. Updated 2006. Accessed October 5, 2014.
27. National Parkinson Foundation. What is Parkinson's disease? Available at http://www.parkinson.org/Parkinson-s-Disease/PD-101/What-is-Parkinson-s-disease. Updated 2014. Accessed October 6, 2014.
28. Hauser R, Lyons K, McClain T, Pahwa R. Parkinson disease. Available at http://emedicine.medscape.com/article/1831191-overview. Updated 2013. Accessed October 6, 2014.
29. National Institute of Neurological Disorders and Stroke. NINDS Parkinson's disease information page. Available at http://www.ninds.nih.gov/disorders/parkinsons_disease/parkinsons_disease.htm. Updated 2014. Accessed October 6, 2014.
30. Allison L, Fuller K. Balance and vestibulalr disorders. In: Umphred D, ed. *Neurological Rehabilitation.* 5th ed. St. Louis: Mosby Elsevier; 2007:732-774.
31. Melnick M. Metabolic, hereditary, and genetic disorders in aduts with basal ganglia movement disorders. In: Umphred D, ed. *Neurological Rehabilitation.* 5th ed. St. Louis: Mosby Elsevier; 2007:775-811.
32. National Institute of Health. Stroke causes. Available at http://www.ninds.nih.gov/disorders/psp/detail_psp.htm. Updated 2014. Accessed October 6, 2014.
33. Wolfe CDA. The impact of stroke. *Br Med Bull.* 2000;56(2):275-286.
34. Tyson S, Hanley M, Chilala J, Snelly A, Tallis R. The relationship between balance, disability, and recovery after stroke: predictive validity of the Brunel balance assessment. *Neurorehabil Neural Repair.* 2007;21(4):341-346.
35. Lubetzky-Vilnai AKD. The effect of balance training on balance performance in individuals poststroke: a systematic review. *JNPT.* 2010;34:127-137.
36. US Department of Health and Human Services. Post-stroke rehabilitation. NIH.gov website. http://www.ninds.nih.gov/disorders/stroke/Post-Stroke%20Rehabilitation.pdf. Updated 2011. Accessed April 1, 2015.
37. Tarnutzer A, Berkowitz A, Robinson K, Hsieh YH, Newman-Toker D. Does my dizzy patient have a stroke? A systematic review of bedside diagnosis in acute vestibular syndrome. *CMAJ.* 2011;183(9):E571-E592.
38. Kattah J, Talkad A, Wang D, et al. HINTS to diagnose stroke in the acute vestibular syndrome: three-step bedside oculomotor examination more sensitive than early MRI diffusion-weighted imaging. *Stroke.* 2009;40:3504-3510.
39. American Geriatric Society, British Geriatric Society, American Academy of Orthopaedic Surgeons Panel on Falls Prevention. Guideline for the prevention of falls in older persons. *J Am Geriatr Soc.* 2001;49(5):664-672.
40. Bueno-Cavanillas A, Padilla-Ruiz F, Jimenez-Moloen JJ, Peinado-Alonso CA, Glavez-Vargas R. Risk factors in falls among the elderly according to extrinsic and intrinsic precipitating causes. *Eur J Epidemiol.* 2000;16(9):849-859.
41. van Doorn C, Gruber-Baldini A, Zimmerman S, et al. Dementia as a risk factor for falls and fall injuries among nursing home residents. *J Am Geriatr Soc.* 2003;51(9):1213-1218.
42. van Dijk PT, Meulenberg OG, van de Sande HJ, Habberna JD. Falls in dementia patients. *Gerontologist.* 1993;33(2):200-204.
43. Tinetti ME, Speechley M, Ginter SF. Risk factors for falls among elderly persons living in the community. *N Engl J Med.* 1988;319(26):1701-1707.
44. Makizako H, Shimada H, Doi T, et al. Poor balance and lower grey matter volume predict falls in older adults with mild cognitive impairment. *BMC Neurol.* 2013;13(102).
45. Anstey KJ, von Sanden C, Luszcz MA. An 8-year prospective study of the relationship between cognitive performance and falling in very old adults. *J Am Geriatr.* 2006;54(8):1169-1176.
46. Borson S, Scanlan J, Brush M, Vitaliano P, Dokmak A. The mini-cog: a cognitive "vital signs" measure for dementia screening in multi-lingual elderly. *J Geriat Psychiatry.* 2000;15(11):1021-1027.
47. The Hartford Institute for Geriatric Nursing. Mental status assessment of older adults: the minicog. Available at http://consultgerirn.org/uploads/File/trythis/try_this_3.pdf. Updated 2013. Accessed October 5, 2014.

48. Nasreddine Z. Welcome page. Available at www.mocatest.org. Updated 2013. Accessed October 5, 2014.

49. Doerflinger Carolan D. Mini-mental state examination. Available at http://www4.parinc.com/Products/Product.aspx?ProductID=MMSE-2#Items. Updated 2013. Accessed October 5, 2014.

50. Bayona N, Bitensky J, Foley N, Teasell R. Intrinsic factors influencing post stroke brain reorganization. *Top Stroke Rehabil.* 2005;12(3):27-36.

51. Tyson SF, Handley M, Chillala J, Selley A, Tallis R. Balance disability after stroke. *Phys Ther.* 2006;86(1):30-38.

52. Kruschinski C, Hummers-Pradier E, Newman-Toker D, et al. Diagnosing dizziness in the emergency and primary care settings [letter]. *Mayo Clin Proc.* 2008;83:1297-1298.

53. Newman-Toker DE, Hsieh YH, Camargo CA Jr, et al. Spectrum of dizziness visits to US emergency departments: cross-sectional analysis from a nationally representative sample. *Mayo Clin Proc.* 2008;83:765-775.

54. Newman-Toker DE, Camargo CA Jr, Hsieh YH, et al. Disconnect between charted vestibular diagnoses and emergency department management decisions: a cross-sectional analysis from a nationally representative sample. *Acad Emerg Med.* 2009;16:970-977.

55. Newman-Toker D, Kattah J, Alvernia J, et al. Normal head impulse test differentiates acute cerebellar strokes from vestibular neuritis. *Neurology.* 2008;70:2378-2385.

56. Edlow JA, Newman-Toker DE, Savitz SI. Diagnosis and intial management of cerebellar infarction. *Lancet Neurol.* 2008;5:951-964.

57. Baier BDM. Incidence and anatomy of gaze-evoked nystagmus in patients with cerebellar lesions. *Neurology.* 2011;76:361-365.

58. Brodsky M, Donahue S, Vahiades M, et al. Skew deviation revisited. *Surv Ophthalmol.* 2006;51:105-128.

59. Harris J, Eng J, Marigold D, Tokuno C, Louis C. Relationship of balance and mobility to fall incidence in people with chronic stroke. *Phys Ther.* 2005;85:150-158.

60. Jorgensen L, Engtad T, Jacobsen B. Higher incidence of falls in long-term stroke survivors than in populuation controls: depressive symptoms predict falls after stroke. *Stroke.* 2002;33:542-547.

61. Hyndman D, Ashburn A, Stack E. Fall events among poeple with stroke living in the community: circumstances of falls and characteristics of fallers. *Stroke.* 2002;83:165-170.

62. Lamb S, Ferrucci L, Volapto S, et al. Risk factors for falling in home-dwelling older women with stroke: the women's health and aging study. *Stroke.* 2003;10:494-501.

63. Hyndman DAA. People with stroke living in the community: attention deficits, balance, ADL ability, and falls. *Disabil Rehabil.* 2003;83:817-822.

64. Ryerson S, Byl N, Brown D, Wong R, Hidler J. Altered trunk position sense and its relation to balance functions in people post-stroke. *JNPT.* 2008;32:14-20.

65. Chitambira B. Use of an optokinetic chart stimulation intervention for restoration of voluntary movement, postural control and mobility in acute stroke patients and one post intensive care polyneuropathy patient: a case series. *Neurorehabilitation.* 2011;28(2):99-104.

66. Brown K, Whitney S, Marchetti D, Wrisley D, Furman J. Physical therapy for central vestibular dysfunction. *Arch Phys Med Rehabil.* 2006;87:76-81.

67. Freburger J. An analysis of the relationship between the utilization of physical therapy services and outcomes for patients with acute stroke. *Phys Ther.* 1999;10:906-918.

68. Plautz EJ, Milliken GW, Nudo RJ. Effects of repetitive motor training on movement representations in adult squirrel monkeys: role of use versus learning. *Neruobiol Learn Mem.* 2000;74(1):27-55.

69. English C, Hillier S, Stiller K, Warden-Flood A. Circuit class therapy versus individual physiotherapy sessions during inpatient stroke rehabilitation: a controlled trial. *Arch Phys Med Rehabil.* 2007;88(8):955-963.

70. Langhammer B, Stanghelle J, Lindmark B. Exercise and health-realated quality of life during the first year following acute stroke. A randomized controlled trial. *Brain Inj.* 2008;22(2):135-145.

71. Hidler J, Nicholas D, Pelliccio M, et al. Multicenter randomized clinical trial evaluating the effectiveness of the Lokomat in subacute stroke. *Neurehabil Neural Repair.* 2009;23(1):5-13.

72. Chan D, Chan C, Au D. Motor relearning programme for stroke patients: a randomized controlled trial. *Clin Rehabil.* 2006;20(3):191-200.

73. Olawale OA, Ogunmakin OS. The effect of exercise training on balance in adult patients with post-stroke hemiplegia. *Int J Ther Rehabil.* 2006;13(7):318-322.

74. Fritz S, Pittman A, Robinson A, Orton S, Rivers E. An intense intervention for improving gait, balance, and mobility for individuals with chronic stroke: a pilot study. *J Neurol Phys Ther.* 2007;31(2):71-76.

75. Gok H, Geler-Kulcu D, Alptekin N, Dincer G. Efficacy of treatment with a kinaesthetic ability training device on balance and mobility after stroke: a randomized controlled study. *Clin Rehabil.* 2008;22(10/11):922-930.
76. Bayouk J, Boucher J, Leroux A. Balance training following stroke: effects of task-oriented exercises with and without altered sensory input. *Int J Rehabil Res.* 2006;29(1):51-59.
77. Leroux A, Pinet H, Nadeau A. Task-oriented intervention in chronic stroke. *Am J Phys Med Rehabil.* 2006;85(10):820-830.
78. Huijbregts MPJ, McEwen S, Taylor D. Exploring the feasibility and efficacy of a telehealth stroke self-management programme: a pilot study. *Physiother Can.* 2009;61(4):210-220.
79. Stuart M, Benvenuti F, Macko R, et al. Community-based adaptive physical activity program for chronic stroke: feasibility, safety, and efficcay of the Empoli model. *Neurrehabil Neural Repair.* 2009;23(7):726-734.
80. Huijbregts M, Myers A, Streiner D, Teasell R. Implementation, process, and preliminary outcome evaluation of two community programs for persons with stroke and their care partners. (grand rounds). *Top Stroke Rehabil.* 2008;15(5):503-518.
81. Macko R, Benvenuti F, Stanhope S, et al. Adaptive physical activity improves mobility function and quality of life in chronic hemiparesis. *J Rehabil Res Dev.* 2008;45(2):323-328.
82. Lang CE, MacDonald JR, Gnip C. Counting reps: an observational study of outpatient day treatment for people with hemiparesis. *JNPT.* 2006;30(4):209.
83. Gray V, Juren L, Ivanova T, Garland S. Retraining postural responses with exercises emphasizing speed poststroke. *Phys Ther.* 2012;92:924-934.
84. Alghadir A, Iqbal Z, Whitney S. An update on vestibular physical therapy. *J Chinese Med Assoc.* 2013;76(1):1-8.
85. Gil-Body KM, Popat RA, Parker SW, Krebs DE. Rehabilitation of balance in two patients with cerebellar dysfunction. *Phys Ther.* 1997;77:534-552.
86. Alsalaheen BA, Mucha A, Morris LO, et al. Vestibular rehabilitation for dizziness and balance disorders after concussion. *J Neurol Phys Ther.* 2010;34:87-93.
87. Zampieri C, Di Fabio RP. Improvement of gaze control after balance and eye movement training in patients with progressive supranuclear palsy: a quasi-randomized controlled trial. *Arch Phys Med Rehabil.* 2009;90(2):263-270.

# 9

# Evidence-Based Practice

## CHAPTER GOALS

1. List the types of research design.
2. Describe best practice guidelines.
3. Explain the differences between qualitative and quantitative research designs.
4. Explain the difference between experimental, quasi-experimental, and non-experimental research designs.
5. Name standardized tests commonly used with the balance patient population.
6. Explain the difference between reliability and validity.

Many authors describe evidence-based practice as the conscientious and judicious use of current best evidence in conjunction with clinical expertise and patient values to guide health care decisions.[1,2] When enough scientific evidence is available, best practice methods are guided by research and clinical expertise. Evidence used to guide best practice may come from a variety of sources, including randomized controlled trials, case reports, descriptive and qualitative research, and information from case reports, scientific principles, and expert opinion. When research is not

Plishka CM.
*A Clinician's Guide to Balance and Dizziness: Evaluation and Treatment* (pp 269-279).
© 2015 Taylor & Francis Group.

available, practice decisions are derived from non-research sources of expert opinion and scientific principles.[3] Clinical practice guidelines can focus on the following[4]:

- The management of a diagnosis or condition
- The measurements of a condition
- Interventions needed for a condition

## RESEARCH DESIGN FEATURES

There are different types of research designs. Table 9-1 outlines some of the general features.[1,5]

## UNDERSTANDING BEST PRACTICE GUIDELINES

How can you implement best practices using research? A guideline to develop practice guidelines for physical therapy has been outlined by Kaplan et al,[4] but the structure can easily be applied to other disciplines. Detailed steps to creating practice guidelines are beyond the scope of this chapter, but an overview of the process will help outline how such guidelines are created and why they are helpful in guiding clinical practice.

Generally there is a question in response to a patient's or client's problem or concern that needs to be solved; using evidence of research to answer the question, not *tradition*, represents evidence-based practice.[5] For example, we could ask, "What is the best way to treat benign paroxysmal positional vertigo?" Once you choose the subject, you need to find sources of valid and reliable research. Many health care professional associations provide such research to their membership. If you cannot find such materials, enlist the help of a medical reference librarian. Many teaching hospitals and medical schools have medical libraries whose staff will be willing to help you find relevant research. By routinely searching for new research, you will help to keep your clinical practice on the cutting edge; this should also help to guide your choice of tests and interventions for the best possible patient outcomes. Obviously the patient has a vital role in participation. A noncompliant patient can derail even the best plan. However, by actively reading research we can at least *have* the best plan.

It is important to realize that the mere existence of a relevant research article doesn't mean that the data it provides will be valid or reliable. You need to analyze each study critically to determine how trustworthy or strong its evidence really is. In reading reviews of research studies, you will find that the studies are assigned "levels" to indicate the quality of their evidence. Once you have a list of criteria, or critical components that should be included in each study, you can analyze the study and assign it a level. Based on the components comprised by a research study,[5] you can create list of questions to use in analyzing it. Some questions might be as follows:

- Were the subjects randomized?
- Does the sampling procedure reduce bias?

| TABLE 9-1 |
|-----------|
| **FEATURES OF RESEARCH DESIGNS** |

| DESIGN TYPE | DESCRIPTION |
|-------------|-------------|
| Quantitative | • Uses objective numerical data measures under standardized conditions. |
| Qualitative | • Data are subjective and described narratively.<br><br>• Data are obtained under less structured conditions, such as using open-ended questions, interviews, and observations. |
| Experimental | • Uses subjects who are randomly assigned to 2 or more groups.<br><br>• Purposely manipulates one or more variables and observes the resulting variation in the other variables.<br><br>• Searches for cause and effect. |
| Quasi-experimental | • Subjects are not randomly assigned to groups or there is only one group.<br><br>• Variables are purposely manipulated. |
| Nonexperimental | • Subjects are not randomly assigned to group, or there is only one group.<br><br>• Observation are made without manipulation of variables. |

- Were information collectors blinded?
- Is the study prognostic?
- Were all subjects accounted for?
- Did subjects in each group have similar backgrounds?
- Were the subjects treated equally?
- Were groups compared?
- What types of statistics were used?
- Was the minimally clinically important difference reported?

Once you establish your criteria and questions and *critically analyze* your study against them, you can assign a *level of evidence* to the study. A software called BRIDGE-Wiz (http://gem.med.yale.edu) provides one such scale. It can be used to assign a level of evidence—ranging from I to V—to describe the quality of evidence provided by a study. Refer to Table 9-2 for definitions of these levels.[4]

| | |
|---|---|
| **TABLE 9-2** | |
| **BRIDGE-Wiz Levels of Evidence** | |
| **LEVEL** | **CRITERIA** |
| I | Evidence obtained from high-quality diagnostic studies, prognostic or prospective studies, cohort studies or randomized controlled trials, meta-analyses, or systematic reviews (critical appraisal score >50% of criteria) |
| II | Evidence obtained from lesser-quality diagnostic studies, prognostic or prospective studies, cohort studies or randomized controlled trials, meta-analyses, or systematic reviews (eg, weaker diagnostic criteria and reference standards, improper randomization, no blinding, <80% follow-up) (critical appraisal score <50% of criteria) |
| III | Case-controlled studies or retrospective studies |
| IV | Case studies and case series |
| V | Expert opinion |

By reading the criteria to obtain each level, you can see that level I represents the highest level of evidence available. Ideally you would use level I evidence to choose your practice guidelines.

Once you assign the evidence a level of quality, you can give the defined practice guideline a *grade* based on the levels of evidence of the supporting studies that were used to create it. Table 9-3 shows the BRIDGE-Wiz recommended grades as listed by Kaplan et al.[4]

# STANDARDIZED TESTS

Up to this point we have looked at the physical aspects of balance. We have examined the systems that contribute to a person's ability to balance and move as desired. We use standardized tests to quantify the person's ability to move, balance, function, and measure risk of falling. As an industry, we are moving away from subjective scales that use terms like *good, fair,* and *poor.* Instead we try to quantify by using numerical scales, scores, and measures in an effort to be more objective and standardized. Such tests also tend to improve interrater reliability.

Common standardized tests used for the balance patient include tests for activities of daily living (ADL), instrumental activities of daily living (IADL), fall risk, gait, and cognition and memory. ADLs are self-care things you typically do when you get out of bed (such as bathing, grooming, dressing, toileting, eating, etc), while IADLs are things you do that are not directly self-care and involve planning, such as using the phone, planning a meal, shopping, and balancing the checkbook.[6]

Some commonly used standardized tests include those shown in Table 9-4.

| | TABLE 9-3 | |
|---|---|---|
| | **BRIDGE-WIZ RECOMMENDED GRADES** | |
| LEVEL | QUALITY OF EVIDENCE | SOURCES OF EVIDENCE |
| A | Strong | A preponderance of level I studies but at least one level I study directly on the topic supports the recommendation. |
| B | Moderate | A preponderance of level II studies but at least one level II study directly on the topic supports the recommendation. |
| C | Weak | A single level II study with a less than 25% critical appraisal score or a preponderance of level III and IV studies, including statements of consensus by content experts support the recommendation. |
| D | Theoretical/ foundational | A preponderance of evidence from animal or cadaver studies, conceptual/theoretical models/ principles, basic science/bench research, or from published expert opinions in peer-review journals supports the recommendation. |
| P | Best practice | Recommended practice based on current clinical practice norms; experimental situations where validation studies have not or cannot be performed; where there is a clear benefit, harm, or cost; and/ or the clinical experience of the guideline development group. |
| R | Research | There is an absence of research on the topic, or higher-quality studies conducted on the topic disagree with respect to their conclusions. The recommendation is based on these conflicting or absent studies. |

Table 9-5 shows interpretations of common tests for fall risk.

To understand why standardized tests are important, we need to understand what they are. Standardization of any process or procedure means that rules are in place for everyone to follow. These rules make sure that we all perform the process or procedure in the same way. In the case of clinical tests, this means the clinicians should be able to perform the tests in the same manner, ask the same questions, and score the patient in the same way. This does not guarantee that every clinician will arrive at the exact same score for the same patient, but scores should be similar enough that everyone would classify functional ability with very little difference.

| TABLE 9-4 | |
|---|---|
| **COMMONLY USED STANDARDIZED TESTS** | |
| **CATEGORY** | **STANDARDIZED TEST** |
| Fall risk | • Dynamic Gait Index |
| | • Functional Reach test |
| | • Four Square Step test |
| | • Gait Speed |
| | • Performance Oriented Mobility Assessment (also known as *Tinetti Gait & Balance*) |
| | • Timed Up & Go test |
| ADL | • Activities of Daily Living Scale |
| | • Barthel Index of Activities of Daily Living |
| | • Physical Performance test |
| IADL | • Frenchay Activities Index |
| | • The Lawton Instrumental Activities of Daily Living Scale |
| Cognition & Memory | • The Montreal Cognitive Assessment |
| | • Mini-Cog |
| | • Mini-Mental State Examination |

How is this helpful? Let's use an example. We may send 2 clinicians to evaluate a patient's risk of falling. If the therapists are not using standardized tests, they may choose to assess the patient very differently. One therapist may simply ask the patient questions like, "Do you fall often?" "Do you have any problems with your balance?" or "Do you need a walker?" Personal and social situations will affect your patients' responses. If they are afraid they may be placed in a retirement home owing to difficulties with balance and walking, they may report that "all is fine." Patients may tell their clinicians that they have no difficulty walking if, for example, they are embarrassed at being seen using a cane or walker. If the clinician takes patient reports at face value but never actually observes the patient's functional motion, the accuracy of any assessment regarding the patient's safety and ability must be called into question.

The second therapist actually asks the patient to get up from the chair and walk, observing the patient's ability to transfer, balance, and ambulate. This therapist, however, uses a scale that is subjective, meaning that how well the patient functions and balances will be a report of that therapist's opinion. Typically, subjective scales use words such as *poor, fair,* and *good.* The problem with these types of subjective descriptions is that their meanings may be interpreted differently by clinicians. What one clinician calls *fair* may be reported as *good* by someone else. It is hard to get

TABLE 9-5

# Score Interpretations of Common Tests for Fall Risk

| CATEGORY | TEST | SCORE INTERPRETATION |
|---|---|---|
| Balance and/ or fall risk | Activity-Specific Balance Confidence Scale[7] | < 50: low level of physical functioning. 51 to 80: moderate level of physical functioning. 81 to 100: highly functioning. |
| | Berg Balance Scale[8,9] | 56: functional balance. < 45: risk for multiple falls. ≤ 40: Almost 100% risk of falling. |
| | Dynamic Gait Index[9] | < 19 indicates fall risk. |
| | Falls Efficacy Scale[10] | > 80 indicates increased fall risk. > 70 indicates a fear of falling. |
| | Functional Reach test | Frail elderly: < 7.28 inches indicates fall risk. Parkinson's disease: < 12.5 inches indicates fall risk. Most healthy with adequate balance: ≥ 10 inches.[11] |
| | Four Square Step test[12-15] | Older adults: > 15 seconds indicates fall risk. Patients with vestibular problems: > 12 seconds indicates fall risk. Acute stroke: failed attempt or > 15 seconds indicates increased risk for falls. Transtibial amputees: > 24 seconds indicates fall risk. |
| | Functional Gait Assessment (FGA)[16,17] | Older adults: ≤ 22 indicates fall risk. Parkinson's disease: ≤ 15 indicates fall risk. |

*(continued)*

| TABLE 9-5 (CONTINUED) | | |
|---|---|---|
| SCORE INTERPRETATIONS OF COMMON TESTS FOR FALL RISK | | |
| CATEGORY | TEST | SCORE INTERPRETATION |
| | Gait Speed[18] | Those doing < 100 cm/s are 28% more likely to fall than those doing better than 100 cm/s. Those doing < 70 cm/s are 54% more likely to fall than those doing better than 100 cm/s. Every 10 cm/s decrease in gait speed is associated with 7% increase in fall risk. |
| | Tinetti Performance-Oriented Mobility Assessment[19] | < 19: high fall risk 19 to 24: moderate fall risk 25 to 28: less likely to fall |
| | Timed Up & Go test[20] | Community-dwelling adults: > 13.5 seconds indicates fall risk |

consistent reports or to know how much fall risk, or function, is actually involved if different clinicians using subjective scales are seeing the same patient.

Now, let's discuss how *standardized tests* help this situation. Standardized tests typically have set questions or detailed directions of how to take a measure. These tests are scored or timed and avoid subjective ratings like poor, fair, and good. Anyone administering a standardized test follows directions, so they administer the test in the same way as anyone else administering the test. In this way it is more likely that different clinicians will reach the same conclusion and measure of a patient's abilities and risks. There are many tests that can help us to measure human function, and we need to review the research studies to choose tests that are both *valid* and *reliable*.

# RELIABILITY

A reliable test is one that will consistently yield the same result. Different types of reliability are referred to in scientific studies.[21] A couple types commonly referred to in discussing tests of function or fall risk include these:

1.  **Test-retest reliability** describes how reliable a test is when administered twice over a period of time to the same group of subjects.

    A simple example would be using a thermometer. Imagine that you have a cup of hot coffee and assume, for this example, that the temperature of the coffee doesn't change. You put the thermometer in the cup and take a measurement and the coffee is at 158 degrees. If you were to measure the coffee's temperature again, you should again get the same temperature. If you do, then the thermometer is *reliable*. If the thermometer gives a different temperature each time you take a measurement, then it is not reliable. For test of human function, does a given test yield the same results within a given range of allowed variability if you administer the test twice?

2. **Interrater reliability** measures the degree to which different raters agree in their assessment. If 2 different clinicians performed a Timed Up & Go test on the same patient, how similar would the test scores be?

# VALIDITY

A valid test is one that actually assesses what it says it intends to assess and does not inadvertently measure something else. Commonly discussed types of validity in scientific research include[21] the following:

1. **Face validity** describes the situation where a test appears to be assessing the intended subject (construct) of interest. At face value, does the test measure what we want to measure?

2. **Construct validity** assesses if the construct (test or measure) actually tests or measures the intended variable and no other variables. For example, let's say you want to measure a patient's right shoulder abduction using a goniometer and you follow a protocol of written instructions of how to take the measurement. As you are taking the measurement, the patient leans to the left in an attempt to raise the right arm higher. If you follow the directions in your protocol that tells you how to place the goniometer and how to read it, would you actually be measuring shoulder abduction or would you also unintentionally capture trunk side flexion in your measurement? Construct validity would measure if the directions you used captured just the intended measurement of shoulder flexion or if your directions were insufficient, as they unintentionally include a measurement of trunk flexion. Construct validity can be applied to any test or measure you use, whether it is a questionnaire or a test of function.

There are a great many standardized tests in use, and we do not need to use them all. However, it is good practice to use more than one, especially in assessing fall risk. Not all tests of fall risk measure exactly the same things, and they test patients in different ways. A study looking at fall risk in the Parkinson's patient population found that to accurately identify a patient as *not* being at risk of falling, we need to use between 2 and 4 *different* tests.[22] A patient may be able to pass one balance test but still be at risk of falling if that test did not address the specific aspect of balance in which that patient has a deficit. For example, the Timed Up & Go test is both valid and reliable to identify some patients as being at risk for falling. In this test, the time taken on command to stand from a chair, walk about 10 feet, return to the chair, and sit is measured. While the test requires the patient to turn around and return to the chair, it does not specifically require patients to turn their heads on the body. As a result, patients with a partially compensated vestibular loss may pass the Timed Up & Go test but fail a test that requires them to turn their heads as they walk.

Which tests are better? It would seem, based on some research studies, that the answer may vary depending on the patient's diagnosis. For example, in a study by Dibble et al, 38 community-dwelling persons with MS were examined using 5 balance tests (Activities-Specific Balance Confidence, Berg Balance Scale, Functional Reach, Timed Up & Go, and Dynamic Gait Index) and then followed for 1 year to record fall incidence. At the 12-month follow-up, 61% were classified as "fallers," but only the Berg Balance Scale, Dynamic Gait Index, and Activities-Specific Balance Confidence demonstrated useful levels of accuracy and distinguished between fallers and nonfallers.[23] This does not at all mean that the other tests are not valid or accurate. However, for this particular patient population, this study found that some tests were more useful.

In evaluating the usefulness of a test for your particular patient population, see whether the test was valid and reliable in a similar patient population. You may do this by searching for studies on the test you wish to use. There is a very useful website—www.rehabmeasures.org—that lists reliable and valid tests for use in the older adult population. This database outlines the studies that support the uses of these tests and describes the patient populations evaluated by each test. The website is available through a collaboration between the Center for Rehabilitation Outcomes Research at the Rehab Institute of Chicago and the Department of Medical Social Sciences Informatics group at Northwestern University Feinberg School of Medicine. It is a free resource.

## SUMMARY

To embrace evidence-based practice, we need to have a basic understanding of research and how it is useful in guiding our choices of tests, measures, and interventions. Find sources of information that provide you with the research addressing the questions or practice needs specific to your practice and then routinely analyze the research that applies to your patient population.

## REFERENCES

1.  Portney LG, Watkins MP. *Foundations of Clinical RESearch: Applications to Practice.* 3rd ed. Upper Saddle River; NJ: Pearson/Prentice Hall; 2009.
2.  Agency for Healthcare Research and Quality. *Patient Safety and Quality: An Evidence-Based Handbook For Nurses.* Available at http://www.ahrq.gov/professionals/clinicians-providers/resources/nursing/resources/nurseshdbk/index.html. Updated 2008. Accessed October 6, 2014.
3.  Titler MG, Kleiber C, Steelman VJ, et al. The Iowa model of evidence-based practice to promote quality care. *Crit Care Nurs Clin North Am.* 2001;13(4):497-509.
4.  Kaplan SL, Coulter C, Fetters L. Developing evidence-based physical therapy clinical practice guidelines. *Pediatr Phys Ther.* 2013;25(3):257-270.
5.  Jewell DV. *Guide to Evidence-Based Physical Therapy Practice.* 2nd ed. Boston: Jones and Bartlett; 2011.
6.  Cohen HS. Assessment of functional outcomes in patients with vestibular disorders after rehabilitation. *NeuroRehabilitation.* 2011;29(2):173-178.

7. Powell LE, Myers MA. The activities-specific balance confidence (ABC) scale. *J Gerontol A Biol Sci Med Sci.* 1995;50(1):M28-M34.

8. Berg KO, Maki BE, Williams JI, Holliday PJ, Wood-Dauphinee SL. Clinical and laboratory measures of postural balance in an elderly population. *Arch Phys Med Rehabil.* 1992;73(11):1073-1080.

9. Shumway-Cook A, Baldwin M, Polissar NL, Gruber W. Predicting the probability for falls in community-dwelling older adults. *Phys Ther.* 1997;77(8):812-819.

10. Tinetti M, Richmand D, Powell L. Falls efficacy as a measure of fear of falling. *J Gerontol.* 1990;45(6):P239-243.

11. Duncan PW, Weiner DK, Chandler J, Studenski S. Functional reach: a new clinical measure of balance. *J Gerontol.* 1990;45(6):M192-7.

12. Dite W, Temple VA. A clinical test of stepping and change of direction to identify multiple falling older adults. *Arch Phys Med Rehabil.* 2002;83(11):1566-1571.

13. Whitney SL, Marchetti GF, Morris LO, Sparto PJ. The reliability and validity of the four square step test for people with balance deficits secondary to a vestibular disorder. *Arch Phys Med Rehabil.* 2007;88(1):99-104.

14. Blennerhassett JM, Jayalath VM. The four square step test is a feasible and valid clinical test of dynamic standing balance for use in ambulant people poststroke. *Arch Phys Med Rehabil.* 2008;89(11):2156-2161.

15. Dite W, Connor HJ, Curtis HC. Clinical identification of multiple fall risk early after unilateral transtibial amputation. *Arch Phys Med Rehabil.* 2007;88(1):109-114.

16. Wrisley DM, Kumer NA. Functional gait assessment: concurrent, discriminative, and predictive validity in community-dwelling older adults. *Phys Ther.* 2010;90(5):761-773.

17. Leddy AL, Crowner BE, Earhart GM. Functional gait assessment and balance evaluation system test: reliability, validity, sensitivity, and specificity for identifying individuals with Parkinson disease who fall. *Phys Ther.* 2011;91(1):102-113.

18. Verghese J, Holtzer R, Lipton RB, Wang C. Quantitative gait markers and incident fall risk in older adults. *J Gerontol.* 2009;64A(8):896-901.

19. Tinetti ME. Performance-oriented assessment of mobility porblems in elderly patients. *JAGS.* 1986;34:119-126.

20. Shumway-Cook A, Brauer S, Woollacott M. Predicting the probability for falls in community-dwelling older adults using the timed up & go test. *Phys Ther.* 2000;80(9):896-903.

21. Phelan C, Wren J. Exploring reliability in academic assessment. Available at http://www.uni.edu/chfasoa/reliabilityandvalidity.htm. Updated 2014. Accessed October 6, 2014.

22. Dibble LE, Christensen J, Ballard DJ, Foreman KB. Diagnosis of fall risk in Parkinson disease: an analysis of individual and collective clinical balance test interpretation. *Phys Ther.* 2008;3:323-332.

23. Dibble LE, Lopez-Lennon C, Lake W, Hoffmeister C, Gappmaier E. Utility of disease-specific measures and clinical balance tests in prediction of falls in persons with mulitple sclerosis. *J Neurol Phys Ther.* 2013;37:99-104.

# 10

# Medications

It is a rare occurrence to evaluate an adult patient who is not taking medications. The increasing understanding of pharmaceuticals has dramatically improved and extended lives. While medications are useful to address problems, they may also have unintended side effects involving other systems or functions. We do not all need to be pharmacists, but we should be familiar with the more common medications that affect the balance/dizziness patient for good or ill.

Plishka CM.
*A Clinician's Guide to Balance and Dizziness:*
*Evaluation and Treatment* (pp 281-287).
© 2015 Taylor & Francis Group.

## TABLE 10-1
## COMMON MEDICATION TREATMENTS OF VERTIGO/DIZZINESS

| CAUSE/CONDITION | MEDICATIONS USED |
|---|---|
| Acute vertigo/dizziness[1] | • Antiviral medications<br>• Antiemetic medications<br>• Vestibular suppressants<br>• Steroids for selected patients |
| Peripheral dizziness (non-BPPV)[2] | • A brief course of an antiemetic and a vestibular suppressant.<br>• Corticosteroids may improve long-term outcomes. |
| Peripheral dizziness (BPPV)[3] | • The most effective treatment is canalith repositioning.<br>• Medications may be used for short-term symptom relief but are not effective in long-term treatment. |
| Ménière's disease[1] | • Conservative: salt-restricted diet and diuretics.<br>• Disabling vertigo: gentamicin chemical labyrinthectomy. |

# MEDICATIONS USED TO
# TREAT SYMPTOMS OF DIZZINESS

Medications are commonly used to treat symptoms of dizziness. As there are a variety of medications, there are different treatment options based on the etiology. Table 10-1 outlines some of these medication choices.[1]

Three classes of medications are commonly used to suppress symptoms of dizziness: antihistamines, benzodiazepines, and anticholinergic agents. Table 10-2 lists some commonly prescribed medications used to control dizziness.[4]

Physicians prescribe these agents to reduce symptoms because they are sedating to the vestibular system and CNS or increase tolerance to motion. Often, however, one or more of these medications are prescribed for chronic use. As people take medications for different reasons, it is important to identify the reason for their use and assess the impact they have on the patient's function. Do not assume that a patient is taking a medication for its primary indication.

Sometimes it is helpful for the patient to take medications for their symptoms of dizziness if their symptoms interfere with their exercises. A good example of this is

| TABLE 10-2 MEDICATIONS COMMONLY USED TO CONTROL DIZZINESS |||
| --- | --- | --- |
| MECHANISM | CLASS OF DRUG | SAMPLE DRUG |
| Vestibular suppression | Antihistamines | Dimenhydrinate |
| | | Meclizine |
| | Benzodiazepines | Diazepam |
| | | Lorazepam |
| | | Clonazepam |
| | Anticholinergics | Scopolamine |
| | | Meclizine |
| | | Promethazine |

when we are teaching vestibular exercises to those with inner ear deficits or habituation exercises for central dizziness. If the dizziness and nausea are too bothersome during the intervention, they may interfere with the patient's ability or willingness to participate. It will also reduce compliance with home exercises. When this is the case, it may be beneficial for the patient to take a medication that will reduce symptoms to a level where the intervention is tolerable.

Sedating medications may prolong the adaptation or habituation process, which means that the patient may need therapy for a longer period of care than if he or she were not taking the medication. However, this is a small price to pay to resolve symptoms if the alternative is to be chronically sedated. For these patients, medications may reduce symptoms, anxiety, or fear and thereby allow greater participation, which, in turn, will lead to improved compensation and function. Later in the treatment period, when the brain has begun its adaptation/habituation, the medications may be weaned or eliminated under the care of the referring clinician.

If you are scheduled to evaluate a patient who is complaining of balance or dizziness problems, it is helpful to get hold orders for medications that are sedating, as they may hide symptoms. If you cannot get these medications held for medical reasons or physician choice, then clearly document which medications the patient was taking when he or she was evaluated (or if they are being taken during interventions) along with an explanation indicating that these medications may have altered your findings.

# MEDICATIONS THAT COMMONLY CAUSE DIZZINESS

Now let's look at medications that commonly *cause* dizziness. When we hear patients complain of dizziness, medications that can change blood pressure, heart rate, and blood sugar come to mind. This is especially true when these types of medications have recently been added or adjusted. However, there are other types of medications that frequently cause patients to feel dizzy[5,6]; these include anticonvulsants, antidepressants, anxiolytics, sedatives (including hypnotics), strong analgesics, muscle relaxants, and antiarrhythmic agents. This would seem to present a problem, as some medications used to treat dizziness belong these classes. Realize that just because someone is taking one of these medications, it may not be causing their dizziness. However, if such medications were recently added or adjusted and symptoms seem to coincide with their use, then they move up the list of possible or likely causes. Also, when all other tests have failed to identify an etiology, a closer review of current medications may be revealing.

In evaluating a patient complaining of dizziness and/or balance issues, you should clearly list in your report any medications that are being used to treat symptoms of dizziness or that may cause dizziness/imbalance.

A benefit to obtaining orders for electronystagmography (ENG), oculomotor battery, and audiography (hearing) tests is that the audiologist will have the patient hold sedating medications prior to being examined. If needed, the patient may be placed on a weaning schedule with guidance from a physician. This will give a better picture of true vestibular and oculomotor function, and help screen for central pathologies.

A real-life example will help to highlight this point. A female patient was referred to a balance clinic by a neurologist to address falls and balance problems. The patient was dependent on her husband for walking and sitting balance. She needed 24-hour supervision and even needed help to remain seated on the commode. She was being treated by other medical professionals for clinical depression and anxiety as well as hypertension. As a result, she was taking mood-altering medications and anxiety medications as well as a medication to control her blood pressure. The patient failed every balance test given; she had abnormal smooth pursuit, gaze nystagmus, and saccades as well as post-head-shake nystagmus and orthostatic hypotension. She could not sit on the exam table without verbal cues to keep her from falling over. Electronystagmography/audiography was ordered to help in the differential diagnosis. It took a couple of weeks, with the assistance of the physician, to wean the patient from all medications that might have impaired the test results. The results of the audiology test were that vestibular function was normal and there were only minor oculomotor findings. However, given the patient's history, the audiologist recommended a head scan based on the abnormal oculomotor findings. The head scan was ordered and results were all within normal limits. It was concluded that the medications were the primary cause of the patient's complaints of disequilibrium and dizziness. The patient still needed the psychiatric medications to keep a stable mood, allowing for normal social function, and she still needed medication to control her hypertension. With a combination of the physician adjusting medication dosages and continued therapy to retrain balance, the patient was ultimately discharged with a good outcome and normal balance test scores. She no longer was a fall risk according to multiple standardized tests and could ambulate independently. The moral of the story is that one should not discount the possibility that a patient's medications might be involved in his or her symptomology. Also, a team approach helped not only to discover the cause of the problem, but also to recover the patient's motor function.

# MEDICATION EFFECTS ON RECOVERY OF VESTIBULAR LOSS

There is evidence that medications that are sedating to the CNS and vestibular system slow the progress of recovery during adaptation. Shepard et al examined the extent of this interference and found that patients taking vestibular suppressants, antidepressants, tranquilizers, and anticonvulsants ultimately achieve the same level of compensation as those who are not taking such medications, but that the length of therapy is significantly longer.[7-9]

# RESEARCH OF MEDICATIONS VERSUS VESTIBULAR REHABILITATION

It is not at all uncommon for physicians to prescribe sedating medications for patients who have vestibular deficits to help control their symptoms of dizziness. Often they do not refer these patients to therapy. According to research, compared with medications, vestibular rehabilitation was superior to medication in improving subjective reports of dizziness in people with unilateral peripheral vestibular dysfunction.[10,11]

Vestibular rehabilitation was found to be more effective than betahistine for the treatment of BPPV.[11,12]

Comparing vestibular rehab to medications (diazepam and meclizine) and "general exercise" in patients with chronic vestibular symptoms, a study by Horak et al found that all groups reported reduced symptoms of dizziness, but only the vestibular rehabilitation group showed significant objective improvement in scores obtained from the sensory organization test and other standing balance tests.[10]

# MEDICATION TREATMENT FOR BENIGN PAROXYSMAL POSITIONAL VERTIGO

Patients with BPPV often go to the emergency room owing to their sudden symptoms of vertigo and are often treated with vestibular suppressants, antiemetic agents (anti-nausea and anti-vomiting medications), or medications to improve blood flow.[13]

There is no evidence to support the use of medications in the treatment of BPPV.[3] That is to say, medications will not resolve BPPV. According to Halker et al, BPPV can be quickly and effectively treated using canalith repositioning maneuvers. Hence pharmacological therapies such as antihistamines or benzodiazepines are not recommended for the treatment of BPPV.[14]

| TABLE 10-3 FREQUENCY OF ATTACKS OF VERTIGO AFTER TREATMENT WITH BETAHISTINE DIHYDROCHLORIDE | | | | |
|---|---|---|---|---|
| | LOW DOSE (16-24 MG T.I.D.) | | HIGH DOSE (48 MG T.I.D.) | |
| | Initial | 12 months | Initial | 12 months |
| Mean | 7.6 | 4.4 | 8.8 | 1.0 |
| Median | 4.5 | 2.0 | 5.5 | 0.0 |

Vestibular suppressants are not recommended for patients with a diagnosis of BPPV. However, the treatment of nausea symptoms to improve patient tolerance of repositioning maneuvers can help a great deal. If you are treating a patient who becomes overly nauseous during repositioning, anti-nausea medications often allow for interventions without having the patient's symptoms stop the intervention sessions. If you are a therapist, consult with the referring physician to obtain orders and make sure that the patient has someone else available to drive him or her to and from the clinic for repositioning. If you are a home health practitioner, once the patient has received orders and anti-nausea medications, call the patient prior to arriving to allow sufficient time for the medication to be at a therapeutic level by the time you arrive.

## MÉNIÈRE'S DISEASE AND BETAHISTINE

Compared with placebo, betahistine dihydrochloride at a dosage of 16 mg twice daily for 3 months had a significant effect on the frequency, intensity, and duration of vertigo attacks in 144 subjects.[15]

For patients with Ménière's disease, betahistine is frequently ordered as part of their medication regimen. In a 2008 study of 112 patients, it was concluded that higher doses of betahistine dihydrochloride (48 mg tid) and a long-term treatment of 12 months seems to be more effective than a low dosage (16 to 24 mg tid) and short treatment (Table 10-3).[16]

## REFERENCES

1.  Samy HM, Hamid MA, Friedman M, Mandolidis S. Dizziness, vertigo, and imbalance treatment & management. Available at http://emedicine.medscape.com/article/2149881-treatment. Updated 2013. Accessed October 8, 2014.
2.  Walker MF. Treatment of vestibular neuritis. *Curr Treat Options Neurol.* 2009;11(1):41-45.
3.  Fife T, Iverson D, Lempert T, et al. Practice parameter: therapies for benign paroxysmal positional vertigo (an evidence-based review). Report of the quality standards subcommittee of the American Academy of Neurology. *Neurology.* 2008;70(22):2067-2074.

4.  Hain T. Drug treatment of vertigo. Available at http://dizziness-and-balance.com/practice/drugrx.html. Updated 2014. Accessed October 4, 2014.
5.  Lawson B. Dizziness in the older person. *Rev Clin Gerontol.* 2005;15:187-206.
6.  Furman J, Raz Y, Whitney S. Geriatric vestibulopathy assessment and management. *Curr Options OtolaryngolHead Neck Surg.* 2010;18:386-391.
7.  Shepard N, Telian S, Smith-Wheelock M. Habituation and balance retraining therapy: a retrospective review. *Neurol Clin.* 1990;8(2):459-475.
8.  Shepard NT, Telian SA. Programmatic vestibular rehabilitation. *Head Neck Surg.* 1995;112:173-182.
9.  Shepard NT, Telian SA, Smith-Wheelock M, Raj A. Vestibular and balance rehabilitation therapy. *Ann Otol Rhinol Laryngol.* 1993;102(3 Pt 1):198-205.
10. Horak F, Jones-Rycewicz C, Black F, Shumway-Cook A. Effects of vestibular rehabilitation on dizziness and imbalance. *Otolaryngol Head Neck Surg.* 1992;106(2):175-180.
11. Hillier SL, McDonnell M. Vestibular rehabilitation for unilateral peripheral vestibular dysfunction. *Cochran Database Syst Rev.* 2011;16(2):CD005397. doi: 10.1002/14651858.CD005397.pub3.
12. Kulcu D, Yanik B, Boynukali S, Kurtais Y. Efficacy of a home-based exercise program on benign paroxysmal positional vertigo compared with betahistine. *Otolaryngol Head Neck Surg.* 2008;37(3):373-379.
13. Do Y-K, Kim J, Yang H-S, et al. The effect of early canalith repositioning on benign paroxysmal positional vertigo on recurrence. *Clin Exp Otorhinolayngol.* 2011;4(3):113-117.
14. Halker R, Barrs D, Wellik K, Wingerchuck D, Demaerschalk B. Establishing a diagnosis of benign paroxysmal positional vertigo through the Dix-Hallpike and side-lying maneuvers. *The Neurologist.* 2008;14:201-204.
15. Guidetti ME, Ghilardi L, Fattori B, et al. Betahistine dihydrochloride in the treatment of peripheral vestibular vertigo. *Eur Arch Otorhinolaryngol.* 2003;260(2):73-77.
16. Strupp M, Huppert D, Frenzel C, et al. Long-term prophylactic treatment of attacks of vertigo in Ménière's disease: comparison of a high with a low dosage of betahistine in an open trial. *Acta Otolaryngol (Stockh).* 2008;128:620-624.

# 11

# Balance Interventions

## CHAPTER GOALS

1. Define sensory reweighting.
2. List interventions for balance.
3. Name 3 things described by Shumway-Cook that influence movement.
4. Discuss researched interventions for balance deficits.
5. Explain how to advance a balance program to increase difficulty level.

## SENSORY REWEIGHTING

Sensory reweighting is the process by which the brain places relative importance on the information coming from each input system. Since we use this information for balance and functional motion, the weighting strategy chosen will dictate which input system's information dominates the formation of balance strategies. Sensory reweighting occurs after vestibular loss. Research evidence shows that an increase in muscle spindle input occurs following a unilateral vestibular loss. It is hypothesized that this change occurs so as to increase somatosensory information, which may be used to substitute for the missing vestibular input.[1] If such changes to nonvestibular regions of the brain are possible with reduced information to one sensory system

Plishka CM.
*A Clinician's Guide to Balance and Dizziness:*
*Evaluation and Treatment* (pp 289-314).
© 2015 Taylor & Francis Group.

(vestibular), then perhaps challenging other deficient sensory systems may also have a similar effect, inducing changes to aid in substitution and compensation.

How can we use this research? Many elderly patients are visually dependent for balance. That is, they rely mostly on visual cues to get information for balance. This does not necessarily mean that their other input systems do not work. What it does mean is that, for whatever reason, they have learned to trust their visual cues, and the brain puts more importance on this information and less on information from other input systems (eg, somatosensory, vestibular). When such patients are in dark environments, their ability to balance is compromised since the main system they use (vision) to gather information and form a balance strategy cannot gather enough useful information. Some balance-impaired patients have reduced input information secondary to damaged somatosensation or vestibular system loss. These patients will balance best in well-lit environments owing the use of visual information. They also likely perform better on firm, flat surfaces. How might we train such patients to use (and not ignore) somatosensory and vestibular cues? One way is to reduce or eliminate visual cues during the balance training session. Deprive these patients of the visual information they are used to using and force them to rely on information from other inputs (eg, proprioceptive and vestibular). For a visually dependent patient, an example of a balance intervention to help drive sensory reweighting (ie, teaching the brain to give more attention and importance to other inputs) would be to have the patient perform balance exercises in darker environments or in complete darkness. You may do this by reducing the lighting in the room or by having patients close their eyes during balance training. When you reduce or eliminate visual cues, patients are deprived of information they prefer and must learn to use sensory information from other systems in order to accomplish the task of balancing.

# BALANCE INTERVENTIONS

Many systems can impact a person's balance. Deficits to any system used to gather needed information, process that information, or carry out the intended movement or muscle activity may adversely impact balance. The more systems that are affected, the more likely disequilibrium becomes. We have looked at ways to assess each system that contributes to functional motion and how to address deficits in each. Now we will look at the methods used to train balancing motions and postures.

Gatekeepers (MDs, DOs, NPs, PAs) have an opportunity to refer patients who are at risk of falling to therapy to reduce that risk. The office nurse or nurse's aide is often the first person who has the opportunity to make observations that identify patients at risk for falling. Patients who shuffle or take small steps, touch walls or furniture while walking, or those who need help to get on and off of the office's scale or in and out of a chair should have a fall risk assessment. Those who are already using an assistive device but have not had any interventions in a while or those who have a very slow gait may benefit from an evaluation and possible interventions. For elderly patients, an annual balance test may detect problems that could place them at risk for falling. Often there are easily correctable issues that, if detected, can reduce the patient's fall risk.

The physical therapist can provide balance retraining, while the occupational therapist can apply controlled movement to functional activities. There are cross-over responsibilities between these 2 disciplines regarding balance interventions. While audiologists treat balance as it relates to the vestibular system, they should refer patients to physical and occupational therapists when comorbidities beyond the vestibular system are involved or when a patient has functional deficits. The team approach typically yields the best outcomes for functional movement.

It is common to find interventions addressing balance that recommend progressions from stability to mobility. There are some particular interventions that are specific to different diseases, which we will discuss. First let's look at general balance training.

In designing a balance intervention program, it is very important to keep each individual patient's needs in mind. The 90-year-old patient's balance needs are, not surprisingly, different from those of the college or professional athlete. By considering the individual functional needs of each patient, it becomes easier to choose the appropriate interventions, activities, and exercises.

In the case of the geriatric patient, a helpful strategy is to start with basic stability exercises, such as standing postures with a variety of feet positions. From there you can move to reaching, weight-shifting activities, trunk sways, stepping, and then more dynamically moving activities. Patients with significant balance impairments often stand with a wide base of support and may even walk with a wide base (feet wide apart). Others forms of balance compensation include touching nearby pieces of furniture or walls in an attempt to gain more proprioceptive information through the hands in order to plan more stable movements. For the patient whose balance is very unstable, we can use these more stable strategies as a starting point. That is to say, we may choose to begin with exercise or activities that allow for a wide-based stance or touching a supporting surface for proprioceptive input. This will help patients feel safe as well, and we can then advance them into more challenging positions, such as having the feet closer together or reducing the amount of touching they are allowed to do for balance assistance.

For athletes, treatment focus depends upon whether they are patients or clients. When they have been injured, treatment will first have to address the physical impairments and deficits and later progress to more dynamic interventions. For clients, we perform a physical assessment to test their abilities, and plan training strategies around any deficiencies or the athlete's sport or position within a sport.

## Varying Conditions

According to Shumway-Cook, 3 things influence our movement: the individual, the task, and the environment.[2] By changing one or more of these, the exercise or activity may require more concentration or the recruitment of different systems in order to complete the task at hand. By varying the conditions or tasks, we challenge the body to respond and perform under a wider variety of circumstances requiring balance. The take-home message is that you can avoid repetitiously using the same exact interventions by varying the conditions and in the process challenge the body in new and different ways. As patients progress with their abilities to succeed with one intervention or task, you may vary the environment, task, or person to further challenge the body to improve. Ways to advance an intervention include the following:

- Varying environments (eg, standing surface, noise, light)
  - We may change the environment by varying the surface the patient is standing on. For example, more firm surfaces (such as wood, tile, or concrete) are generally easier to stand on because they are stable and noncompliant (ie, they do not deform under the patient's weight). A softer, more compliant surface—such as a thick carpet or grass outdoors—provides a greater challenge. Even more compliant surfaces such as high-density foam or unstable surfaces such as rocker boards add maximal challenges.
- Varying tasks (eg, static vs dynamic, stability vs mobility)
  - We may vary the way in which the patient performs a task. Stable tasks may use a wider base of support or allow for additional proprioceptive input by allowing the patient to touch a wall, counter, or assistive device. We may increase the challenge provided to the patient during a task by reducing the allowance to use the hands for added touch proprioception or by reducing the base of support. Further progression may lead to moving or reaching tasks within and then outside of the base of support.
  - For upper extremity tasks performed while standing, we may change the task by changing the objects to be manipulated (eg, using a variety of object contact surfaces: slippery, smooth, coarse, etc). The weight or size of objects can also be varied.
  - For upper extremity use while in standing, we may vary the angle to which the patient must reach (eg, overhead, lower than the waist, or movements that require trunk rotation).
- Varying something about the individual (eg, single- vs dual-task concentration)
  - Consider the patient's cognition, attention, motivation, emotion, and the sensory and motor abilities of the individual.
  - Adding a mental task to the physical task is an example of dual tasking. We are asking the patient to do 2 or more things at once, such as balancing on a piece of high-density foam while counting backward by twos. Another example of dual tasking combines changing the individual and the task by having the patient carry an object while walking or move objects from one pants pocket to another while walking. When we divide concentration between more than one task, patients are challenged. There may be times when we decide that dual-tasking is a beneficial activity, and at other times we may instruct the patient to *avoid* dual tasking, as it may prove to be too challenging and thus present a safety hazard. A commonly seen example is that some elderly patients lack sufficient cognition to safely talk while walking. When they do attempt this, you notice that their steps become smaller

and some may even stumble. Use your clinical judgment to decide when dual tasking is appropriate as an intervention or when you should advise against it.

Here are some general progression strategies for balance training. Not everyone starts at the same level. Your assessment will provide you with a list of physical and functional problems that will help guide your choice of interventions. Remember, you can change any of these exercises by varying the task, environment, or individual.

## Force Plate and Biofeedback

There are studies that both support and refute the benefits of force-plate platforms as interventions over traditional vestibular therapy. A study by Geiger involved a comparison of patients trained with force plates and biofeedback vs patients treated without this intervention. The results showed no additional benefits from the use of the first intervention over other forms of physical therapy.[3]

Supporting studies outlined by Herdman[4] include the following:

- Nardone et al[5] compared Cawthorne-Cooksey exercises with an intervention using an oscillating force platform; both interventions improved balance and decreased subjective ratings of disequilibrium.
- Winkler and Esses[6] found that adding platform perturbation with changes in foot position to other exercises that included visual cues, habituation, and gaze stabilization resulted in greater improvement than gaze stabilization and habituation alone.

## Sitting Balance

Most therapists are very familiar with training sitting balance, from managing sitting on a firm to soft surface and then reaching within and outside of the base of support. Vary the sitting surface from a firm chair to a soft bed. You may further challenge balance as a progression by removing a foot surface—that is, do not let the patient's feet touch the floor. You may choose to start with added stability by allowing the patient to use his or her hands to help maintain seated balance or to touch a reference object. Later, you may limit or eliminate the use of the upper extremities for the assistance in sitting balance.

For more advanced sitting balance challenges, you may wish to incorporate sitting on a wobble board or inflatable therapy ball. Once patients have acquired the skill to sit on unstable surfaces, they may further be challenged by adding reaching tasks or seated marching while sitting on such surfaces. The patient should be wearing a gait belt and guarded against falling.

### Sitting Balance and Central Nervous System Damage

There seems to be an association with the side of stroke and sitting balance ability. In a study of 105 patients there was a statistically significant difference between the 2 sides, with patients who had left hemiparesis being more likely to have difficulty with independent sitting.[7]

Sitting balance ability has long been associated with outcomes of rehabilitation following stroke. Patients with improved sitting balance had higher Barthel Index scores compared with a group of patients whose sitting balance did not improve.[8] Similarly, for patients who suffered brain injury, impairments in sitting balance appear to have a significant impact on functional outcome.[9]

Using reaching activities beyond the patient's arm length is an effective way to improve reach speed and distance as well as increasing load through the affected foot and activation of the affected leg muscles, as shown in one study when compared with the control group.[10]

# Standing Balance

Different standing balance interventions are available. They are in order from *more stable* to *less stable* or *more mobile*.

## Static Standing

- Static standing on a firm surface (wider base → narrow base) → static standing with eyes closed → standing eyes open/closed on a soft surface
  - Typically wider bases of support are easier to maintain. As the patient becomes more skilled at balancing with a certain stance width, you may make the task or exercise more challenging by narrowing the base of support used while performing it. Many therapists also have patients stand in tandem (heel to toe) or partial tandem stance (feet closely side by side with one foot somewhat advanced). This may occur within the same treatment session or over numerous sessions.
  - Standing with eyes closed removes a lot of information used to balance and also simulates balance in low-light environments. You may time the patient's ability to perform these tasks to show how long he or she can stand with eyes closed. Documenting these times will help show the patient's progress in balance ability.
  - Standing on high-density balance foam simulates standing on other compliant or unstable surfaces, such as thick carpeting, grass, or gravel. Patients who have difficulty standing on balance foam will likely have difficulty while standing on these real-life examples. Since the task of standing on foam is similar to standing on these other environments, there will be cross over improvement for balancing on them when you train the patient on foam.

## Standing With Some Movement

Using the variations from the "static standing" list, we can begin challenging standing-moving tasks by using different techniques, such as trunk sways, weight shifting, balance challenges, balancing while performing an upper extremity task such as reaching within and outside of the limits of stability, and adding unilateral stance activities.

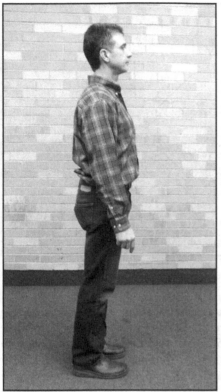

**Figure 11-1.** Trunk sway 1.

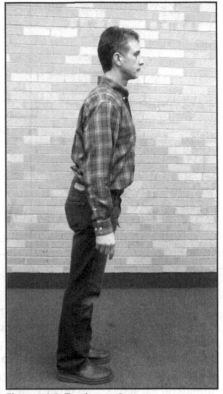

**Figure 11-2.** Trunk sway 2.

 *Trunk Sways*

Trunk sways are a great starting place for those who are challenged by activities of daily living (ADL) that require standing, such as grooming, brushing teeth at the sink, cooking at the stove, standing at the bus stop, etc. While using trunk sways as an intervention, the patient is instructed to stand with feet together or with a close-stance width. While performing the trunk sway, do not allow bending at the waist in any direction (eg, no forward flexing or side-bending), and instruct the patient to stand as straight as possible. Instruct trunk sways to the furthest point of trunk excursion possible as long as the patient's feet (heels or toes) do not lift from the floor.

You may actually assess balance control and limits of stability by instructing the patient to use trunk sways to trace a box pattern around the base of support. As he or she moves the trunk (again, without bending at the waist) observe any areas around the base of support the patient avoids. You may also use trunk sways as a balance exercise, swaying toward areas the patient has less control over, to improve stability through practice and strengthening while performing this intervention. Examples of anteroposterior trunk sways are shown in Figures 11-1 through 11-3.

As if looking down from above, use Figure 11-3 as a guide for trunk sways, prompting the patient to sway to different points around the limits of stability.

**Figure 11-3.** Trunk sway chart.

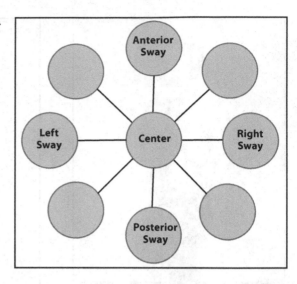

### Unilateral Stance

Unilateral stance is needed to perform many functional movements, from putting a leg through a pant leg while getting dressed to bearing weight on one limb while stepping into a bathtub or up a stair step. How many activities can you imagine with which to practice unilateral weight-bearing stance? You may simply challenge your patients to stand on one foot while being timed. To keep patient interest, incorporate unilateral leg stance into other games or activities. One example is to draw a large number pad (as on a phone) and place it on a step. While the patient stands on one leg, he or she is instructed to type out numbers with the contralateral foot (eg, phone numbers of friends or family, birth dates of family members, etc). When the activity is meaningful in some way, the patient will be more interested in participating.

### Foam Standing

Changing the surface on which a patient stands challenges balance. Standing on compliant foam presents a similar condition as standing on other soft, unstable, or uneven surfaces, such as thick carpeting, grass, or gravel. Changing the surface on which your patients stand challenges their balance. Standing on compliant foam presents a similar condition as standing on other soft, unstable, or uneven surfaces, such as thick carpeting, grass, or gravel. Patients may be further challenged by changing stance width, or adding a secondary task while standing on the foam. For example, you may ask them to perform upper extremity tasks such as reaching (both inside and outside of the base of support), toss a ball or hitting a balloon, performing a mental task (eg, counting backwards by 3s), or further changing the environment by having them close their eyes to eliminate visual input. For more advanced exercises, you may include stepping on and off of the foam.

## Standing With Dynamic Movement

When the patient is ready to perform more challenging interventions, we introduce more dynamic movement activities such as weight shifting diagonally, stepping

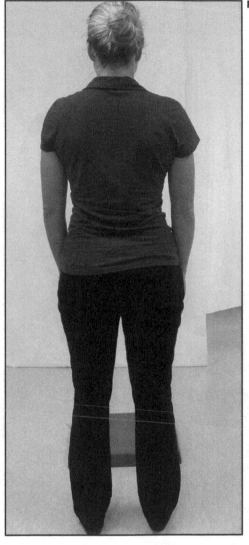

**Figure 11-4.** Weight shift center.

up/down movements, or walking activities that incorporate head turns or dual tasking. For athletes you may incorporate running with varying head and body positions and progress to tossing/catching a ball while the patient is performing these motions.

 *Weight Shifting*

Patients may be taught awareness and control of their centers of gravity by performing lateral and diagonal weight shifting. Weight shifting challenges the patient to transfer, in a controlled manner, weight from one supporting foot to the other. For lateral weight shifting, begin with the feet close together but not touching (or wider if the patient is unable to perform this with a closer stance width) while the weight is shared equally between the feet (Figure 11-4).

**Figure 11-5.** Weight shift asymmetrical stance.

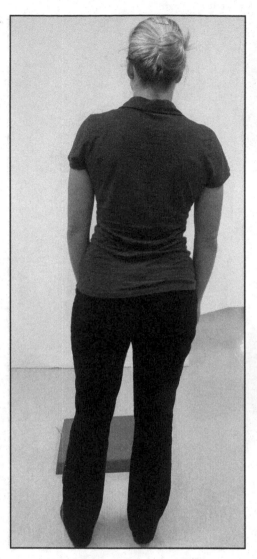

Begin by instructing a patient to stand with the center of gravity directly over the base of support. Next, instruct a weight shift to place more weight through one foot (called *asymmetrical stand*). This asymmetrical stance position is held for a few seconds, and the therapist should count out loud, after which the patient returns to a more symmetrically balanced stance. This technique is the same for lateral and diagonal weight shifts, as if taking a step forward or back (Figure 11-5).

When first performing lateral weight shifts, patients with poor balance will usually avoid asymmetrical stance, preferring instead to keep either hips or head closer to the base of support. For example, while performing lateral weight shifting,

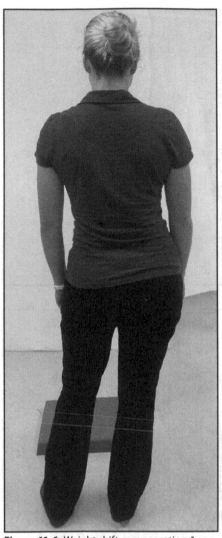
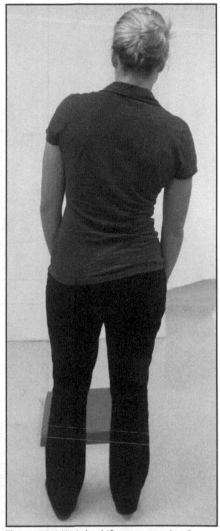

**Figure 11-6.** Weight shift compensation 1.          **Figure 11-7.** Weight shift compensation 2.

balance-impaired patients typically either lean their heads sideways (trunk side flexion) while keeping the hips centered, or they keep their heads centered over the base of support while pushing their hips out sideways in an attempt to perform the weight-shifting tasks as instructed. These patients do not realize they are making these compensatory movements; therefore, the therapist needs to use verbal, visual, and tactile cues to draw attention to and correct these compensations. For the first few treatment sessions, a full-length mirror is a helpful way to provide visual feedback; however, do not overly use this during your intervention, as the goal is for the patient to begin relying more on proprioceptive feedback for trunk position and not too much on vision for balance. Examples of compensations are shown in Figures 11-6 and 11-7.

**Figure 11-8.** Diagonal shift 1.

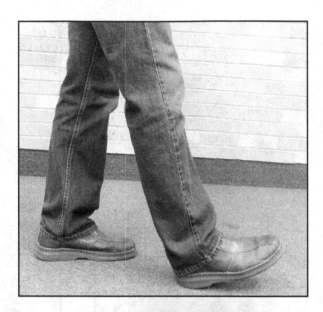

**Figure 11-9.** Diagonal shift 2.

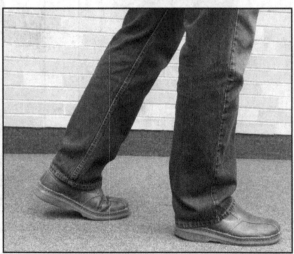

If needed, allow the patient to touch the wall or some other support surface such as a chair back, countertop, or even you for proprioceptive feedback. Patients are not allowed to lean on support surfaces, but just to touch them. As they improve their ability to weight shift from one foot to the other while maintaining good posture (ie, without excess leaning to compensate for a lack of control), begin limiting or removing the support surfaces.

During diagonal weight shifting, begin with the patient placing most of the weight on the back foot while placing the contralateral foot in a simulated heel strike (Figure 11-8). As the patient shifts to bear weight primarily on the front (advanced) foot, the heel of the back foot lifts off the ground, as in the toe-off position of gait (Figure 11-9).

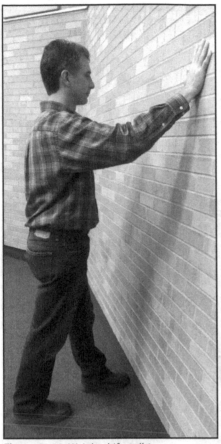

**Figure 11-10.** Weight shift wall 1.

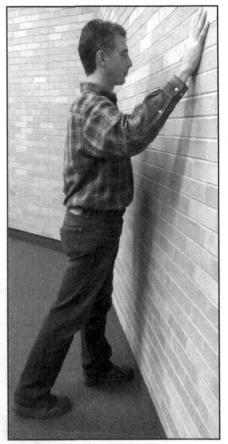

**Figure 11-11.** Weight shift wall 2.

It is common for patients to avoid shifting completely to the advanced front foot in first attempting this exercise. They typically shift part way, leaving their center of gravity directly between the 2 feet, and then lean the trunk forward over the front foot. They are usually not even aware they are doing this until the therapist tactilely cues their hips and torso to line up over the front foot.

Examples of using support surfaces for proprioceptive feedback may be seen in Figures 11-10 through 11-12.

In this example (Figures 11-13 and 11-14), the therapist instructs the patient to place his or her hands on either the therapist's forearms or hands for proprioceptive feedback. Next, the therapist instructs the patient to step and shift weight (one step at a time) with constant verbal cues for step length and body position.

### Step-Ups

There are a variety of ways to perform stepping activities to incorporate weight shifting. For example, you may have the patient step up and down from a stair step or balance platform while cueing deliberate weight shifts, first laterally and then

**Figure 11-12.** Weight shift with chair.

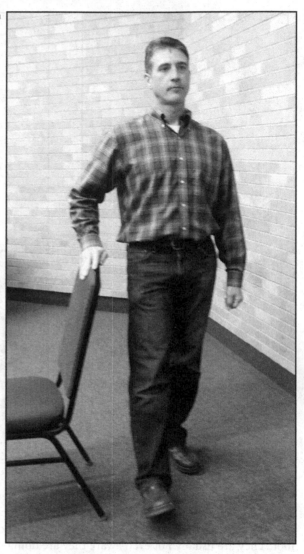

diagonally. Correct any excessive leaning laterally past the supporting foot while shifting laterally. Do not allow patients to perform compensatory motions such as attempting to move quickly and "power" their way while stepping or changing positions. Instead, cue controlled and deliberate movements. Let's review a series of figures that demonstrate this exercise (Table 11-1).

To return to standing on the floor, perform the same motions given to step up, only in reverse order. Repeat this activity by alternately stepping up with each leg. Repeat alternating steps several times as tolerated.

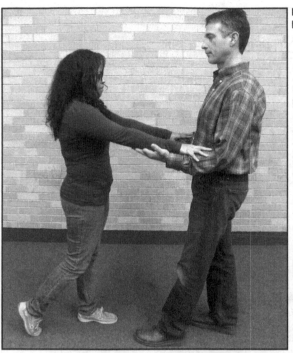

**Figure 11-13.** Weight shift hand held 1.

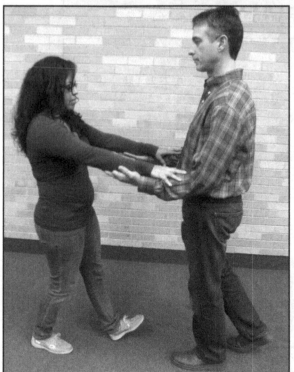

**Figure 11-14.** Weight shift hand held 2.

## TABLE 11-1
## STEP-UP EXERCISE

| | |
|---|---|
| Begin in centered stance and then move to an asymmetrical stance over one foot. | 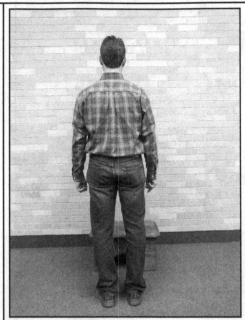<br>**Figure 11-15.** Step centered stance. |
| | 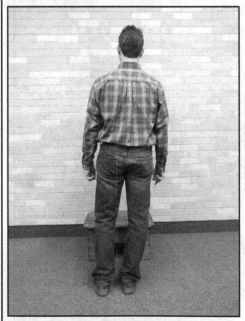<br>**Figure 11-16.** Step weight shift R. |

(continued)

### TABLE 11-1 (CONTINUED)
## STEP-UP EXERCISE

| | |
|---|---|
| Next, place the unweighted foot on the step and perform a diagonal shift onto the step. | 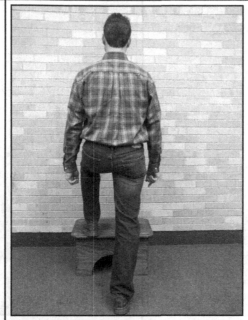 **Figure 11-17.** Step up with L. |
| Once you are bearing weight on the advanced foot (keeping head and hips over that foot), place the unweighted foot on the step. | 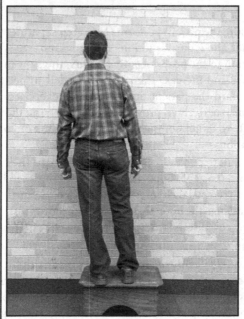 **Figure 11-18.** Step asymmetrical L. |

*(continued)*

| TABLE 11-1 (CONTINUED)<br>STEP-UP EXERCISE | |
|---|---|
| Now perform a lateral shift back to center. | 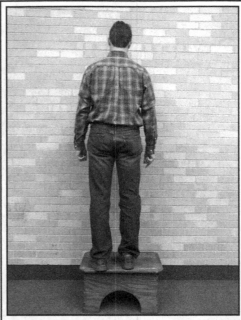<br>**Figure 11-19.** Step shift center. |

Make sure the patient performs each step separately in a slow and controlled manner. Do not allow quick motions for this exercise. While the patient is learning to pay attention to the proprioceptive inputs, the slow movements also help strengthen the muscles and increase the stability needed to perform these motions. Use a gait belt and guard the patient during balance exercises. Verbally and tactilely cue the patient constructively to provide feedback during the motions. The feedback should be accurate to either commend correct motions or correct undesired movements or compensations.

You will notice that during each weight shift, the head and hips are over the supporting foot (base of support). Weight-shifting exercises and activities should form the core of your balance interventions. Increase difficulty levels as tolerated to constantly challenge the body to improve. Track progress of balance improvements using timed and scored standardized balance or fall-risk tests.

### Other Dynamic Balance Exercises

Once patients gain control over weight shifting, you may progress them to more dynamic exercises and activities. Some examples include side-stepping, backwards walking, stepping up/down from a raised surface, stepping in a variety of directions, or stepping while performing other tasks (eg, turning the head, carrying an object, or performing mental tasks).

In performing side-stepping, make sure to prevent compensatory movements of trunk/hip rotation or external leg rotation and flexion. An easy way to do this is to use a gait belt to physically restrain the patient from rotating the hips during the side-step. Perform this exercise/activity at both a comfortable patient-selected pace and also a quick pace to help train quicker reactions that guard against falling. It is an exercise as it strengthens hip abductors and an activity used in ADL and also protective responses.

Backward walking is a very dynamic and difficult activity, especially if performed slowly. Typically the patient will need some tactile assistance or guarding as well as verbal cues when first attempting this activity. For the balance-impaired patient, perform each step deliberately and slowly. Athletes involved in more advanced training may actually run backward as part of their training.

Perturbations are another way to add balance challenges. In terms of balance, a perturbation occurs when we introduce an external force like a nudge or pull to move the patient's center of gravity away from the base of support. The patient's task is to regain control of the center of gravity. You may use perturbations during sitting, standing, or walking balance tasks.

Reaching activities challenge balance control in sitting and standing. These activities may be as simple as reaching within the base of support or more challenging by reaching outside of the base to touch or grasp an object. The following are some examples of reaching activities:

- Reaching (sitting or standing) to hit a balloon back and forth to the therapist
- Reaching to move items along a counter from one side of the patient to the other
- Picking up objects from the floor
- Removing items placed on an overhead shelf
- Performing a ball toss

Sometimes, having the patient perform an ADL in standing challenges balance, such as the following:

- Grooming in front of a mirror
- Performing upper and lower body dressing while standing

If you want to further challenge the patient, remember to vary the "individual, task, or environment." While the physical therapist may instruct weight shifting as an exercise to improve control of balance, proprioceptive awareness, and lower extremity strength, the occupational therapist may have the patient perform the same weigh shifts while performing functional activities, such as putting dishes in a cupboard, getting clothes out of the closet, or stepping into a bathtub. This would not be a duplication of service, since each discipline is performing the weight shift for different reasons.

### Optokinetics

As discussed earlier, optokinetic stimulation is achieved by creating a moving environment across the visual field by moving the actual visual target or environment, by moving the observer, or by moving both. The use of optokinetic stimulation may be used to treat the optokinetic system itself to address a deficit, to address a deficient vestibular system, or as part of a treatment regimen that includes other types of balance interventions. Customized vestibular rehab that incorporates opto-kinetic stimuli is more beneficial than rehab without it for improving dizziness and postural instability.[11] Optokinetic stimulation may be "full field," which means that the entire visual environment is used as a stimulus. One way to achieve this is to use a disco-ball in a dark room. Optokinetic stimulation may also be "less than full field" by using a striped piece of paper as was described in Chapter 6.

# BALANCE RESEARCH

Here are some studies that look at different aspects of balance interventions. These are not critical reviews of these articles but a sample of some published studies that discuss balance and stimulate further discussion or review.

## Computer Games

In a study of 30 community-dwelling patients with balance impairments who attended a day program, the subjects were randomized into a control group that received balance and gait training and an experimental group that received graded dynamic balance exercises on different surfaces coupled with computer games requiring the subject to stand and perform weight-shifting tasks. Both the control and experimental groups exhibited significant improvements in Berg Balance Scale scores. Analysis of change scores revealed that while there was no significant effect on the Timed Up & Go (TUG) scores, the improvements in Berg Balance Scale scores, Loss of Balance count, and Activity-Specific Balance Confidence scores were significantly greater for the experimental group compared with the controls.[12]

## Weight Shifting and Gaze Stability

Marioni et al[13] demonstrated that gaze stability and weight-shifting exercises with biofeedback resulted in improved stability compared with no treatment.[4]

## Dual-Task Training

Dual-task training involves simultaneously performing more than one physical task, such as walking while carrying an object, or adding a cognitive task to a physical task. An example of adding a cognitive task is having the patient count backwards, name words that begin with a specified letter, naming as many objects as they can which are red, etc. In a 23-subject study, dual-task training was effective in improving balance under dual-task conditions in elderly patients with balance impairments. The authors also noted that training under single-task conditions may not generalize to balance control during dual-task contexts.[14]

# Tai Chi for Balance

Tai chi is a Chinese martial art that is often practiced in western cultures for exercise and balance maintenance. It involves dynamic weight shifting with slow and controlled movements. It challenges the practitioners balance, strength, and endurance. Studies of tai chi for therapeutic purposes have had mixed results. In a study of 25 subjects using tai chi as an exercise, Li and Manor found that participants improved outcomes measured by the 6-Minute Walk test, TUG, and leg strength.[15] Tai chi has been found to improve strength and flexibility,[16,17] and balance.[18,19] In these studies, the subjects were "robust elderly." However, in a study of "transitionally frail elderly," tai chi reduced fall risk to a degree that was clinically important but not statistically significant.[19]

# Parkinson's Disease

Many therapists are at a loss when treating the patient with Parkinson's disease. Owing to the lack of research to guide us as to what interventions are best at each stage of the disease, this is not surprising. A 2013 Cochrane study reviewed[20] physical therapy versus placebo or no intervention in the Parkinson's disease patient population with a literature search that included 39 published randomized controlled trials of 1827 patients through the end of January 2012. The authors do note that there is a mixed risk of bias with the studies. Outcome measures were recorded for gait speed, Freezing of Gait questionnaire, TUG test, Functional Reach test, Berg Balance Scale, and the United Parkinson's Disease Rating Scale (UPDRS). While a wide range of therapy interventions were used across studies, there was no evidence of difference in treatment effect between different interventions. The authors of the review point out that differences between interventions were made with indirect comparisons and limited data within each intervention, so caution needs to be used in interpreting the data.

The researchers were not able to identify a best practice pattern from these studies and mention the need for large, randomized controlled trials to demonstrate long-term efficacy and best practice. However, what they were able to conclude is that, in the short term (less than 3 months), most measures support the use of physical therapy in the Parkinson's disease population. Improvements were noted in walking speed, walking endurance, and freezing of gait. Mobility and balance also improved, demonstrated with the TUG test, Functional Reach, and Berg Balance Scale. Clinician-rated disability was improved using the UPDRS as a measure. Interestingly, fear of falling did not change between test groups (using the Falls Efficacy Scale as a measure). Few trials assessed actual numbers of falls, and there was a trend toward a reduction in the number of falls with physical therapy intervention but with no differences between treatment arms of the study. ADL scores were improved with therapy interventions as measured by the UPDRS. No significant benefits were noted for quality-of-life measures using the Parkinson's Disease Questionnaire (PDQ-39).

In 2009, Dibble et al[21] performed a systematic review of the literature using the keywords *Parkinson's disease* and *exercise*. They concluded that despite some studies showing improvements in postural stability and balance task performance, the optimal delivery and content of exercise interventions (dosing, component exercises) at different stages of the disease are not clear.

Here are some research examples (without critically reviewing each) that show some efficacy for the Parkinson's disease population:

- Vestibular therapy reduced the risk of falling and improved gait velocity, balance, and ability to perform ADL.[22]
- Fuzhong et al[23] compared the effects of tai chi, resistance training, and stretching in a 24-week study including twice-weekly interventions. Subjects had mild to moderate Parkinson's disease as rated by the Hoehn and Yahr scale. Primary outcomes were limits of stability. Secondary outcomes included measures of gait, strength, and scores of Functional Reach, TUG, UPDRS motor scores, and number of falls. Intervention in the tai chi group included selected movements used in tai chi, including symmetrical movements, diagonal movements, weight shifting, controlling displaced center of mass over the base of support, ankle sways, and anteroposterior and lateral stepping. The results showed that subjects in the tai chi group consistently performed better than resistance training and stretching groups in maximal excursion of limits of stability. They outperformed the stretching group in all secondary outcomes and had better stride length and functional reach than the strength training group. Tai chi movements lowered the incidence of falls as compared with stretching but not as compared with resistance training. These beneficial effects of tai chi movement training were maintained for 3 months after intervention ceased.

## Peripheral Neuropathy

With the use of tai chi for 24 weeks as an intervention, plantar sensation was improved in patients who had peripheral neuropathy.[24]

## Stroke

The use of ankle-foot orthoses improved symmetry in quiet and dynamic standing balance and increased speed and cadence in subjects with hemiparesis of short duration. Effectiveness was minimal for those with hemiparesis of long duration.[25]

## Multiple Sclerosis

Even in the early stages of the disease, MS may affect balance and gait. Kalron et al studied 52 subjects who were asked to ambulate under 3 conditions: normal, fast, and at normal pace while performing the modified Word-List-Generation test. The combined walking and cognitive task was expressed in prolonged double support (gait cycle) and reduced velocity in MS patients. Since in early MS gait-cognitive dual tasking may lead to an increased risk of falling, the author suggests that it should be addressed by physical rehabilitation as an intervention.[26]

There are some indications that strength training alone will not improve balance and functional motion in the MS population. In a small study of 19 subjects, Hayes et al[27] found that the addition of eccentric training and standard exercises did not result in significantly greater gains of strength in the lower extremities, nor was it effective as standardized exercise alone in improving balance or the ability to ascend/descend stairs. It is noted that the small sample size makes it difficult to detect strength differences between groups. Further, no significant time effects were noted for the TUG test, 10-Meter Walk test (self-selected and maximal pace), time to ascend/descend one flight of stairs, or the 6-Minute Walk test.

In a 14-week, single-blinded, stratified blocked randomized controlled trial of 38 subjects by Hebert et al,[28] the experimental group underwent vestibular rehabilitation, an exercise group performed bike endurance and stretching, and a waitlist group received usual medical care. Primary measures included the Modified Fatigue Impact Scale, posturography balance measures, and the 6-Minute Walk test. Secondary measures included the Dizziness Handicap Inventory, and the Beck Depression Inventory-II. The vestibular rehabilitation group's protocol included postural control exercises of (a) standing, (b) static body position—half-kneeling, and (c) static body position—standing. Exercises in these protocols included standing with eyes open or closed on both firm and foam surfaces while performing various tasks, standing on a trampoline while performing various tasks, half-kneeling on a tilt board performing various tasks, Walking heel to toe, walking while tossing a ball, walking while turning 180 degrees upon command, and finally performing eye (oculomotor) and vestibular exercises. The results showed that the vestibular exercise group, which participated twice-weekly for 6 weeks in the intervention, had greater improvements in fatigue, balance, and disability due to dizziness or disequilibrium compared with the other groups. Minimal changes were noted at a 4-week follow-up.

Balance exercises in the MS patient population have also been shown to have beneficial effects. In a pilot study on the effects of balance exercises in 44 MS patients, Cattaneo et al[29] randomized subjects into 3 intervention groups: balance rehab to improve motor and sensory strategies, balance rehab to improve motor strategies, and finally a group whose treatments were not specifically aimed at improving balance. Outcome measures included the Berg Balance Scale, Dynamic Gait Index, Activities-Specific Balance Confidence, and the Dizziness Handicap Inventory. They concluded that balance rehabilitation appeared to be useful in reducing fall rates and improving balance skills in subjects with MS. Also, they reported that exercises in different sensory contexts may have an impact in improving dynamic balance.

For MS patients who have foot drop, a study using a Odstock dropped foot stimulator was found to have improved scores on the Canadian Occupational Performance Measure (an ADL measure), improved satisfaction scores on identified ALD problems, and demonstrated fewer falls than for the control group who received physical therapy (without a foot drop stimulator).[30]

# PROGRESSION OF EXERCISES

The progression of exercises varies depending the individual patient's needs. However, in general there are 3 things we can typically change to increase the difficulty of any exercise routine: the person, the environment, and the activity.[31]

We may change the person by adding a secondary mental task (dual task), such as counting backward, to an activity or exercise. Even with this, you can increase difficulty by asking a patient to count backward, then by 2s, then by 3s, starting at 95, etc. We can change the environment by changing the surface on which the patient is sitting or standing, by changing the lighting in the room, or even by adding or removing background noise (eg, turning on/off a TV or radio). We may change the activity itself by changing the body position in which the patient performs the activity. Or we can simply change to a different activity altogether.

Feedback is very important. Using operant conditioning, we can provide verbal feedback. When possible, incorporate a reward for completion of a task or exercise.[31] You accomplish this by making the exercise or activity goal-oriented and meaningful. For example, when training gait, try to avoid walking up and down a hall without a purpose. Instead, walk somewhere that has a goal. For example, walk to the kitchen to get a drink or walk to the mailbox to check for mail, etc. Whenever we can make an activity or exercise meaningful in some way, the patient has more "buy in," is more compliant, and is more engaged in the plan of care. How can you make 10 reps of a strengthening exercise meaningful? Sometimes you can, as in performing hip extensor strengthening and using sit-stand transfers as your exercise. But we can all recognize that sometimes you just have to perform an exercise for strengthening or range of motion.

Feedback should be accurate. Avoid saying "good job" all time, especially if the patient did not properly perform the desired movement.[31] Offer encouragement in a positive manner. You may say, for example, "Good effort!" or "You are working hard, that's great!" These are motivating but not reinforcing an incorrect movement pattern. Be sure to include instructions of how to improve the movement patterns.

Occupational therapists should avoid meaningless activities such as digging things out of buckets of rice or using the plastic tube arch to move rings around. Do we sometimes need the rice for tactile desensitization or hand strengthening? Sure. But this probably will not be most of your patient population unless you are in a specialty clinic. How can we perform hand or arm motions that are meaningful? Typically by performing actual ADL. Vary the patient's position (eg, sitting vs standing) when appropriate to further challenge function and balance.

General progression of exercises for balance typically progress from *very stable* positions to *moving*. The most stable positions, such as lying or sitting, are typically the easiest to maintain. If the patient can stand, the stable position is standing with both feet on the floor, shoulder-width apart (or slightly wider if needed), while standing on a solid surface (hard floor). You may even increase stability by allowing the use of one or both hands to touch a reference surface such as a countertop or wall to add somatosensory input. You may advance this patient by reducing stance width and

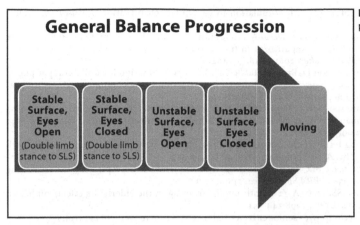

**Figure 11-20.** Balance progression.

reducing or eliminating use of hands for feedback. To advance the patient who starts on a solid and stable surface, we can change the surface to carpet, grass, or balance foam. When appropriate, add dual tasking, such as having a patient name objects that begin with a particular letter while performing the balance exercise. You may further change the environment by turning the lights down or turning a radio on. Using similar environments, you may change the activity/task entirely. Figure 11-20 lists a common balance exercise progression.

While documenting your interventions, make sure to include any changes to person, task, or environment and explain how this increases the difficulty level of the intervention. You may use the patient's abilities to perform activities under these "easier to harder" conditions to show progression toward goals.

# REFERENCES

1. Strupp M, Arbusow V, Dieterich M, et al. Perceptual and oculomotor effects of neck muscle vibration in vestibular neuritis. Ipsilateral somatosensory substitution of vestibular function. *Brain.* 1998;121:677-685.
2. Shumway-Cook A, Woollacott MH. *Motor control: Translating Research into Clinical Practice.* 3rd ed. Philadelphia: Williams & Wilkins; 2007.
3. Geiger R, Allen J, O'Keefe J, Hicks R. Balance and mobility following stroke: effects of physical therapy interventions with and without biofeedback/forceplate training. *Phys Ther.* 2001;81:995-1005.
4. Herdman S. Vestibular rehabilitation. *Curr Opin Neurol.* 2013;26(1):96-101.
5. Nardone A, Godi M, Aruso A, et al. Balance rehabilitation by moving platform and exercises in patients with neuropathy or vestibular deficit. *Arch Phys Med Rehabil.* 2010;91:1869-1977.
6. Winkler PA, Esses B. Platform tilt perturbation as an intervention for people with chronic vestibular dysfunction. *J Neurol Phys Ther.* 2011;35:105-115.
7. Bohannon RW, Smith MB, Larkin PA. Relationship between independent sitting balance and side of hemiparesis. *Phys Ther.* 1986;66:944-945.
8. Sandin KJ, Smith BS. The measure of balance in sitting in stroke rehabilitation prognosis. *Stroke.* 1990;21:82-86.
9. Black K, Zafonte R, Millis S, et al. Sitting balance following brain injury: does it predict outcome? *Brain Inj.* 2000;14(2):141-152.
10. Dean CM, Shepard RB. Task-related training improves performance of seated reaching tasks after stroke. *Stroke.* 1997;28(4):722-728.

11. Pavlou M. The use of optokinetic stimulation in vestibular rehabilitation. *J Neurol Phys Ther.* 2010;34(2):105-110.

12. Szturm T, Betker AL, Moussavi Z, Desai A, Goodman V. Effects of an interactive computer game exercise regimen on balance impairment in frail community-dwelling older adults: a randomized controlled trial. *Phys Ther.* 2011;91:1449-1462.

13. Marioni G, Fermo S, Zanon D, Broi N, Staffieri A. Early rehabilitation for unilateral peripheral vestibular disorders: a prospective, randomized investigation using computerized posturography. *Eur Arch Otorhinolaryngol.* 2013;270(2):425-435.

14. Silsupadol P, Shumway-Cook A, Lugade V, et al. Effects of single-task versus dual-task training on balance performance in older adults: a double-blind, randomized controlled trial. *Arch Phys Med Rehabil.* 2009;90(3):381-387.

15. Li L, Manor B. Long term tai chi exercise improves physical performance among people with peripheral neuropathy. *Am J Chin Med.* 2010;38(3):449-459.

16. Hong Y, Li JX, Robinson PD. Balance control, flexibility and cardiorespiratory fitness among older tai chi practitioners. *BR J Sports Med.* 2000:29-34.

17. Lan C, Lai LS, Chen SS, et al. A 12-month tai chi training in the elderly. Its effects on health fitness. *Med Sci Sports Exerc.* 1998:344-351.

18. Yan J. Tai chi practice improves senior citizens' balance and arm movement control. *J Aging Phys Perform.* 1998;6:271-294.

19. Wolf SL, Sattin RW, Kutner M, O'Grady M, Greenspan A, Gregor RJ. Intense tai chi exercise training and fall occurrences in older, transitionally frail adults: a randomized, controlled trial. *J Am Geriatr Soc.* 2003;51:1693-1701.

20. Tomlinson CL, Patel S, Meek C, et al. Physiotherapy versus placebo or no intervention in Parkinson's disease (review). *Cochrane Database Syst Rev.* Epub 2013;9:321-340.

21. Dibble L, Addison O, Papa E. The effects of excersice on balance in persons with Parkinson's disease: a systematic review across the disability spectrum. *J Neurol Phys Ther.* 2009;33:14-26.

22. Rossi-Izquierdo M, Soto-Varela A, Santos-Pérez S, et al. Vestibular rehabilitation with computerised dynamic posturography in patients with Parkinson's disease: improving balance impairment. *Disabil Rehabil.* 2009;31(23):1907-1916.

23. Fuzhong L, Harmer P, Fitgerald K, et al. Tai chi and postural stability in patients with Parkinson's disease. *N Engl J Med.* 2012;366:511-519.

24. Li L, Manor B. Long term tai chi exercise improves physical performance among people with peripheral neuropathy. *Am J Chin Med.* 2010;38(3):449-459.

25. Wang RY, Yen L, Lee CC, Lin PY, Wang MF, Yang YR. Effects of an ankle-foot orthosis on balance performance in patients with hemiparesis of different durations. *Clin Rehabil.* 2005;19(1):37-44.

26. Karlon A, Dvir Z, Achiron A. Walking while talking—difficulties incurred during the initial stages of multiple sclerosis disease process. *Gait Posture.* 2010;32(3):332-335.

27. Hayes HA, Gappmaier E, LaStayo PC. Effects of high-intensity resistance training on strength, mobility, balance, and fatigue in individuals with multiple sclerosis: a randomized controlled trial. *J Neurol Phys Ther.* 2011;35:2-10.

28. Herbert J, Corboy J, Manago M, Schenkman M. Effects of vestibular rehabilitation on multiple sclerosis-related fatigue and upright postural control: a randomized controlled trial. *Phys Ther.* 2011;91:1166-1183.

29. Cattaneo D, Jonsdottir J, Zocchi M, Regola A. Effects of balance exercises on people with multiple sclerosis: a pilot study. *Clin Rehabil.* 2007;21(9):771-781.

30. Esnouf JE, Taylor PN, Mann GE, Barrett CL. Impact on activities of daily living using a functional electrical stimulation device to improve dropped foot in people with mulitple sclerosis, measured by the Canadian occupational performance measure. *Mult Scler.* 2010;16(9):1141-1147.

31. Shumway-Cook A, Woollacott MH. *Motor control: Translating research into clinical practice.* 3rd ed. Philadelphia: Williams & Wilkins; 2007.

**Please visit www.routledge.com/9781617110603 to access additional material.**

# 12

# Plan of Care and Examples of Documentation

Clinical documentation tells the story of your patient, and you are the author. Anyone reading your documentation should be able to identify why the patient needed a skilled clinician, identify (and, when possible, understand) test results, and be able to duplicate any interventions that were provided. These components are part of recording your management of the patient. Throughout your documentation you need to show clinical problem solving, provide proof of medical necessity, proof of skilled care, and the resulting outcome.[1] The examples listed will be in SOAP format. SOAP is the acronym that stands for Subjective, Objective Assessment, and Plan. These parts of the clinical document will be briefly explained. This chapter is not an all-inclusive discussion of documentation, as there are entire books on the subject. Instead, it discusses those parts of the clinical documentation that are pertinent to the patient with balance deficits and/or dizziness.

Plishka CM.
*A Clinician's Guide to Balance and Dizziness:*
*Evaluation and Treatment* (pp 315-327).
© 2015 Taylor & Francis Group.

Many payer sources, such as the government and private insurance providers as well as professional associations, publish their own documentation standards.[2-4] These documents outline the general expectations of the payer for medical records created by the provider. Medical records should be clearly organized and in chronological order. All medical records should be out of reach and view of unauthorized people who are not part of the medical team.

Clinicians new to vestibular rehab are often challenged over how to document findings and interventions for this patient population. In this chapter, commonly used terminology for these patients will be used in examples of documented tests and interventions. As you will see, you do not need to write a great deal if you know which terms to use.

# SOAP Notes

## Subjective

The clinician should document those subjective comments of the patient that pertain to the condition/reason for which he or she is seeking help from a medical/health care professional. These patient complaints/remarks may describe and give insight into the current problem/complaint as well as the patient's medical/social history. A skilled clinician, through careful questioning, may elicit helpful subjective patient information. An example given earlier in the book is getting the patient to explain what he or she means by "dizzy." Other helpful subjective comments will describe provoking and relieving situations, frequency, duration, history, and descriptions of symptoms. After the initiation of interventions, the patient's subjective remarks may reflect his or her functional progress, changes in symptomology, and responses to previous interventions. Be careful not to be leading. You may need to prompt the patient for this information. Clinicians and their assistants should compare subjective remarks made during interventions with those reported during the initial evaluation/encounter to help assess the patient's progress.[1]

Here are a few examples of undesirable subjective statements:

- I had a great dinner last night.
- There was a nice movie on TV last night.
- Back in 1966, my husband had knee surgery.

For these examples, we are assuming they are not evidence of some improved function that was lacking. They are generally irrelevant to the patient's history or current condition. When patients provide these types of answers, you will need to redirect them to focus on the desired subject.

## Objective

Under the "Objective" category, you will record the data you collect through observation, tests, measures, and reviews of body systems. For the patient with complaints of dizziness and imbalance, a careful examination of the systems used for balance is imperative, including the visual/oculomotor, vestibular, somatosensory, cerebellar, and musculoskeletal systems. Further, you should include standardized tests of function and balance that are valid and reliable.

Another part of this section describes any interventions that were provided or prescribed. You should include the name of the exercise or activity, number of repetitions, or time performed and the number of cues (verbal or tactile) or level of assistance the patient needed for successful performance. Remember, you need to show proof of *skilled care* for each intervention. Record any observed deficits, motion or muscle substitutions, or signs. For tests and measures, record any changes from previous trials.

## Assessment

The assessment summarizes the patient's status, provides a diagnosis, and presents a potential prognosis and measurable goals. It is also used to associate the identified impairments with the functional deficits that the patient demonstrates. This section should answer the question of "why" your interventions and skilled services are/were medically necessary.[1] The assessment also includes your diagnosis, and explains the need for skilled care. The implementation of ICD-10 diagnostic codes increases the number of diagnoses and procedure codes from about 13,000 to more than 141,000. The addition of more codes provides more detail regarding the patient and patient care.[5]

## Plan

The plan lists the treatments and interventions you plan to employ; they should reflect and address findings recorded in your evaluation. The creation of a plan of care is a relatively simple process if you have done a thorough evaluation. When you are first implementing the multisystem evaluation approach advocated by this book, you will find it helpful to make lists of your patients' subjective complaints and physical/functional deficits. These lists help guide your clinical (and critical) thinking regarding your patient. They also serve as checklists against which you may compare your interventions to make sure you are addressing everything you possibly can to reduce the patient's limitations. First, list the patient's complaints. During your physical examination, you looked at each system that might contribute to functional mobility and balance, so next you may list examination findings and the physical deficits that you have found for each system. List the functional impairments resulting from these deficits. Do the physical deficits explain the functional impairments? Do either of these explain subjective patient complaints? If not, do you need to have other tests ordered? Finally, list the exercises, activities, pharmacological choices, and any other treatment interventions you have available to address the physical deficits, functional deficits, impairments, and patient complaints. These available treatment options will form your *plan of care.*

In many vestibular and balance cases you may be able to use the identified impairments as interventions. For example, if the patient has impaired saccades, you may choose to use saccades as an intervention. If the vestibular system is not working at

100%, you may choose to use the vestibulo-ocular reflex (VOR) as an intervention. Let's see how this works by examining Table 12-1, which lists a variety of deficits common to the balance-impaired patient. You can see how making a list will aid in the creation of the plan of care and also help you avoid missing a piece of the puzzle. The more deficits you can address, the better the chance that your patient will have to improve.

In 2001 The World Health Organization implemented the International Classification of Functioning, Disability and Health (ICF) to measure health and disability at both individual and population levels by use of a 2-list classification system. If you prefer a more standardized way to classify patients, you may wish to explore the ICF. One list describes body functions and structures, while the other describes activity and participation. Qualifiers are used to describe a person's performance in an environment and his or her ability to execute a task or action. The ICF also contains a list of environmental factors. While the International Statistical Classification of Diseases and Related Health Problems (ICD-10) classifies by etiology of diseases, disorders, and other health conditions, the ICF classifies by function and disability associated with health conditions.[6]

A plan of care that includes *vestibular rehabilitation therapy*, or *vestibular rehab* for short, encompasses more than just interventions for an impaired vestibular system. It includes interventions that address *any system* that contributes to balance and functional movement. The patient in vestibular rehab may have interventions for any of the systems of balance (oculomotor, vestibular, somatosensory, cerebellar, and musculoskeletal). He or she may have interventions that address specific functional limitations or activities (eg, gait, activities of daily living [ADL], etc). The goal of these interventions is ultimately to return the patient to improved function or to reduce symptoms that may impair function. Sometimes these interventions induce changes in the system that is targeted by the exercise, while at other times they act as a stimulus forcing the patient to find different ways to collect/process information or perform a given task when a particular system is deficient.

# EXAMPLES OF DOCUMENTATION FOR BALANCE

## Balance and Gait

Record observations of the patient's posture, balance, and stability in the section of the evaluation labeled "Objective."

Observations made during interventions or evaluation should lead to the documentation of any deficiencies, limitations, or substitutions. Descriptions of gait should describe any problems observed during the gait cycle, such as step length, lack of heel strike or toe off, etc.

For therapists documenting balance and gait interventions, remember to show the skill involved. Simply describing the exercise or activity is not enough. After noting your intervention, exercise, or activity, ask yourself if it is something your nonclinical neighbor could have done. If it is, you probably need to add phrases to show the skill

TABLE 12-1

## CREATION OF THE PLAN OF CARE

| SYSTEM | FUNCTIONAL IMPAIRMENTS AND COMPLAINTS | TEST/ ASSESSMENT FINDINGS | PHYSICAL DEFICIT | PHYSICAL IMPAIRMENTS | POSSIBLE INTERVENTION(S) |
|---|---|---|---|---|---|
| Oculomotor | • Blurred vision<br>• Dizzy<br>• Impaired balance | • Saccadic smooth pursuit<br>• Hypometric saccades | • Oculomotor function | • Smooth pursuit<br>• Saccades | • Refer for tests<br>• Oculomotor exercises |
| Vestibular | • Impaired balance<br>• Impaired gait<br>• Fear of falling | • Positive head-thrust or head-shake test | • Impaired vestibular function | • Impaired VOR<br>• Symptoms of nausea and dizziness | • Refer for electronystagmogram/audiogram<br>• Therapy: VOR exercises, optokinetic stimulation,<br>• Balance & Gait Training<br>• Antiemetic meds<br>• Vestibular suppressants |
| Somatosensory | • Impaired balance<br>• Trips frequently | • (+) 5.07 monofilament test with decreased plantar pressure sensation | • Decreased plantar pressure sensation | • Lack of protective sensation of the feet | • Therapy: weight shifting,<br>• Home exercise: tai chi, weight shifting |

*(continued)*

TABLE 12-1 (CONTINUED)
## CREATION OF THE PLAN OF CARE

| SYSTEM | FUNCTIONAL IMPAIRMENTS AND COMPLAINTS | TEST/ ASSESSMENT FINDINGS | PHYSICAL DEFICIT | PHYSICAL IMPAIRMENTS | POSSIBLE INTERVENTION(S) |
|---|---|---|---|---|---|
| Cerebellar | • Impaired balance and/or coordination<br>• Reduced ability for visual tracking | • Impaired cerebellar screens for accuracy, coordination, muscle tone | • Unknown cerebellar dysfunction | • Reduced movement accuracy and coordination of limbs and possibly eyes | • Refer for tests<br>• Accuracy and coordinated activities<br>• Therapy: oculomotor, balance, gait<br>• Medications |
| Musculoskeletal | • Functional activities: gait, transfers, ADLs | • Manual muscle tests and goniometry reveal reduced strength and range of motion | • Weakness, short/tight or contracted muscles, overstretched/ weak muscles | • Insufficient strength or range of motion to perform activities | • Therapy: strengthening and stretching, • Functional activities |

you provided to instruct or improve the patient's ability to ambulate. Some examples include the following:

*Verbal cues were needed to*

- Improve step length
- Increase heel strike
- Narrow stance width

*Tactile cues were needed to*

- Recover loss of balance
- Correct placement of walker
- Initiate hip abductor activation

Let's look at an example of documentation reflecting gait training.

**Therapist's note:** *Ambulated 150 feet x 2, min assist with rolling walker.*

Looking at this example, we need to ask ourselves if the neighbor could ambulate with the patient for 150 feet. He or she probably could. The phrase "Min assist" does not by itself show skill. Could the neighbor offer min assist to the patient? No skill is evident in this example. Next, is 150 feet significant in some way? Does the patient need to walk 150 to be functional within his or her environment? Finally, a description of the gait mechanics is missing, as well as any instruction that improved it.

There are a couple of things that could improve in this note. First, if the patient needs the skill of a therapist in order to improve, your documentation needs to indicate how. How do you show skill during gait training? Helpful phrases such as "Verbal cues needed for…" and "Tactile cues needed to…" help you show that you have provided professional skill that will improve the patient's condition.

**Improved example:** *Ambulated 150 feet x 2 (Distance from bedroom to kitchen) using a rolling walker. Verbal cues were needed to increase knee extension in terminal swing phase and to increase heel strike. Tactile cues were needed to instruct proper advancement and placement of the walker.*

Next, if this is a patient who needs gait training and not just aerobic exercise, there should be a description of the gait pattern. Sometimes the description of the need for cues implies the deficit, such as "Verbal cues were needed to increase step length."

Now let's look at an example of a balance exercise. Like the first example, it will not be ideal, and we will use this as a way to highlight ways to document meaningful exercises.

**Therapist's note:** *Performed balance exercise x 15.*

Can you identify what is missing in this example? Which balance exercise? What were the deficiencies during patient performance that required the skill of a therapist? What skilled interventions were provided during the exercise? What does 15 represent—time or repetitions? Remember, the exercise should address a deficit you record in your evaluation or add to the plan of care later. If the exercise or activity does not reflect the evaluation findings or plan of care, a reviewer may question its need.

## Example of Improved Balance

*Diagonal weight shifting x 15 reps (holding each 3 seconds) to an advanced right foot. Tactile cues needed for instructing positioning of the center of gravity over the base of support and for proprioceptive cues to maintain balance while in asymmetrical stance. Loss of balance x 3 was corrected with minimal tactile cues during the exercise.*

# DOCUMENTATION OF VESTIBULAR FINDINGS

In documenting a vestibular test, document the name of the test, which ear was tested, any modifications you made, and findings. For cases of BPPV, describe:

- The test used
- The involved ear
- The involved canal
- Classification of canalithiasis vs cupulolithiasis
- Which canalith repositioning maneuvers were performed

The plan of care should list *canalith repositioning* as the intervention when you plan to use repositioning maneuvers. Avoid naming maneuvers, such as "the Epley maneuver," in your plan of care, as this will limit your choice of interventions. By using the broad category of *canalith repositioning*, you may use any number of maneuvers that you will describe in your treatment documentation.

## Tests for Benign Paroxysmal Positional Vertigo

### Example of a Canalithiasis Evaluation

*Positive Dix-Hallpike for right posterior canal canalithiasis.*

The use of the word *positive* indicates the presence of BPPV. Next, the name of the test that was employed is documented, "Dix-Hallpike." The words *right posterior canal* indicate that the involved canal and the ear that was tested. The use of *canalithiasis* indicates loose crystals, that observed nystagmus lasted less than 1 minute, and that it had a latency prior to onset.

While it is not required, you could further describe the nystagmus. Using the above example, we could add the following information:

*Positive Dix-Hallpike for right posterior canal (canalithiasis), with right-torsional and upbeating nystagmus. Latency ~5 seconds, duration <30 seconds.*

If you are sending a report to another clinician who may not have a lot of vestibular patients or experience reading reports regarding vestibular tests, it is often helpful to include this added information.

### Example of an Intervention

*Performed canalith repositioning maneuvers for the treatment of BPPV, including the modified Epley x 2, Semont-liberatory x 1. Minimal nausea reported. Negative Dix-Hallpike following repositioning.*

Your plan for this patient would include retesting for BPPV at the next clinical visit.

## Example of a Cupulolithiasis Evaluation

*Positive Dix-Hallpike for right posterior canal cupulolithiasis.*

This note indicates that

- The test used was the Dix-Hallpike.
- The right ear was tested.
- BPPV was found (ie, the test was positive).
- The involved canal was the posterior.

"Cupulolithiasis" implies an immediate onset of nystagmus that lasted longer than a minute and that crystals were either stuck to the cupula or trapped in the short arm of the canal.

While not required, you could write a more descriptive note describing the latency and duration of nystagmus. The term *cupulolithiasis* already implies this information, but sometimes it is good to describe, depending on the intended audience of the note.

### A More Descriptive Example

*Positive Dix-Hallpike for right posterior canal cupulolithiasis with right-torsional and upbeating nystagmus. Latency: none; duration >60 seconds. The patient was taken out of the test position after 60 seconds.*

# Tests of Vestibular Function

These examples review how to describe positive bedside tests of the VOR and oculomotor observations and tests. Descriptions reflect positive test results. Negative tests indicate normal function.

## Vestibulo-ocular Reflex Function Test

We will use a patient who has a left unilateral vestibular loss for our examples.

**Example:** Positive left Head Thrust test indicating possible left unilateral vestibular weakness.

**Example:** Positive Head Shake test with right-beating post-head shake nystagmus, indicating a possible left unilateral vestibular weakness.

Remember, if you find positive tests of VOR function, to recommend further testing, such as an electronystagmography/audiography to help confirm vestibular loss and rule out central pathologies.

# OCULOMOTOR FUNCTION TEST EXAMPLES

## Fixation

Document any inability to maintain fixation.

## Gaze Nystagmus

**Example:** Positive right-gaze nystagmus at 45 degrees with increased quick phases with rightward gaze, indicating a possible vestibular asymmetry (eg, left unilateral vestibular loss).

**Example:** Positive right-gaze nystagmus at end-range (>3 beats observed), indicating a possible vestibular asymmetry (eg, left unilateral vestibular loss). No other gaze nystagmus noted.

Remember, if you find positive gaze nystagmus, to recommend further testing, such as an electronystagmography/audiography, to help confirm vestibular loss and rule out central pathologies.

## Smooth Pursuit

When patients lack smooth pursuit, they will use saccades (if available) to substitute. In a positive test, the patient is unable to generate smooth tracking motions and you will see a series of saccades. Document this as positive saccadic smooth pursuit.

## Saccades

Deficiencies you will record are:
- **Hypometric saccades,** which are undershooting saccades; thus more than 2 are required to reach targets held within the patient's visual field.
- **Hypermetric saccades,** which are overshooting saccades; thus a corrective saccade in the reverse direction is required after the eyes pass the target.

## Ocular Range of Motion

Document any loss of range, such as:
- Limited upward gaze
- Inability to perform upward gaze
- Limited left gaze to the left eye—does not move left past primary gaze position

## Vergence

Vergence limitations are noted at bedside usually by a limitation of binocular fusion during convergence. Measure the distance from the tip of the patient's nose to the point where he or she loses fusion.

**Example:** Vergence to 25 cm

**Example:** Convergence insufficiency to 25 cm

## Cover Tests

Terminology of eye motions and positions can be intimidating, especially when not used routinely. Recall that the unilateral cover test checks for heterotropia (also known as *manifest strabismus*), which is an abnormal eye deviation. Document

- Any corrective eye motion during testing of the uncovered eye
- The eye position noted during the Unilateral Cover test: Exotropia, Esotropia, Hypertropia, Hypotropia
- The eye position noted during the Alternating Cover test: Exophoria, Esophoria, Hyperphoria, Hypophoria
- Which eye is involved or if both are positive

**Example:** Positive esotropia during Unilateral Cover test of the right eye

**Example:** Positive hypophoria during the alternating cover test

If you cannot recall these terms, use the word *strabismus*, which is a general term describing improper alignment of the eyes, and include if the eyes were moving laterally or vertically. Recall that vertical skews are significant central findings.

**Example:** Positive unilateral cover test with a left lateral strabismus

**Example:** Positive alternating cover test with vertical strabismus bilaterally

This general description is enough for an oculomotor specialist, such as a neurologist; neurotologist; or ear, nose, and throat doctor to understand what you observed in the patient's eye motions. Vertical corrective eye motion requires further examination by one of these specialists.

## VESTIBULAR REHAB EXERCISE EXAMPLES

In general, describe or name the exercise/activity, time or repetition performed, patient tolerance, *and the skill involved.*

**Example:** *Performed VOR x 1, 2 x 1 min with verbal cues needed to keep frequency of head motion >0.5 Hz. The patient became slightly nauseous and required 2 minutes to recover after exercise.*

**Example:** *Performed motion habituation exercise of seated left-ear to left knee x 15 reps with verbal cues for timing and head position. Positions were held until dizziness symptoms lessened (less than 40 seconds were required for each repetition).*

For therapists, in documenting exercises and interventions, it is extremely important to include the skill that was used. This is easy to do if you get used to including phrases like, "Verbal cues needed for…" and "Tactile cues needed to…" Without an explanation of the clinician's skill, many insurance companies refuse to pay for the service. Read your clinical note and ask yourself if the described intervention could be performed by the patient's neighbor.

# GOAL SETTING FOR THERAPISTS

A goal should be measurable and have a time frame associated with it to detail when the achievement of the goal is expected. Your goals should reflect functional activity and *not a test score* or performance of an exercise. Use the test scores or performance descriptions as part of the goal to quantify the improvement toward the desired functional activity. Another thing to keep in mind is that you do not have to write a goal for every intervention you are using. Test scores may be used to show that the functional goal was reached. In writing goals for the balance patient, you *should not* have goals such as these:

- Improve Tinetti Score to 22/25.
- Perform 5 repetitions of the motion sensitivity exercise.
- Ambulate 200 feet.

These examples lack the functional component that insurance adjusters want to see. Remember, *you* may know that an improved Tinetti score is likely associated with an increase in function and decreased fall risk, but the people who review your notes for reimbursement often do not.

In writing goals for balance, the goal should be *improved balance, decreased fall risk*, or increase *the ability to perform some functional task*. The test scores help to support the fact that these things are improving.

## Improved Balance Goals

- Decrease fall risk, as evidenced by an increase in the Tinetti score from 19/25 to 22/25.
- The patient will perform tub transfers independently.

Motion sensitivity can impair functional activities. Often timed goals are useful to show improvement, such as this:

- Increase motion tolerance, as evidenced by motion tolerance of 3 minutes, to allow for ADL such as dressing the lower body.

For gait-training goals, remember to include why the distance is important to the patient. You should not simply list a goal for distance. In our example, we used 200 feet as a distance. Why is this important? Is it the distance from the house to the mailbox, or bed to bathroom? There should be a description attached to the distance we give in our goals.

Improved gait goal:

- Increase ambulation to 200 feet to allow access of the bathroom from the bedroom.

# REFERENCES

1. Erickson M, McKnight R, Utzman R. *Physical Therapy Documentation: From Examination to Outcome.* Thorofare, NJ: SLACK, Inc; 2008.
2. CareFirst. Medical records documentation standards. Available at https://provider.carefirst. com/wcmresources/Content-Provider/assets/attachments/BOK5129.pdf. Updated 2014. Accessed October 7, 2014.
3. American Physical Therapy Assocation. Defensible documentation. apta.org website. http://www.apta.org/Documentation/DefensibleDocumentation/. Updated 2012. Accessed October 7, 2014.
4. Hill E. E/M coding and the documentation guidelines: putting it all together. American Academy of Family Physicians website. http://www.aafp.org/fpm/2011/0900/p33.html. Updated 2011. Accessed October 7, 2014.
5. Jackson T. ICD-10 starts at clinical documentation. Available at http://www.healthcareitnews. com/news/icd-10-starts-clinical-documentation. Updated 2013. Accessed October 7, 2014.
6. World Heath Organization. International classification of functioning, disability and health (ICF). Available at http://www.who.int/classifications/icf/en/. Updated 2013. Accessed October 7, 2014.

# Case Study Examples

Let's review a simple case study as an example of how to think through a typical patient with problems of balance. We will use this example to demonstrate how to work through any case. We will create a patient, including a history, and walk through the process of examination findings and creation of a plan of care. There may be questions posed specific to each case example. Based on the case information, attempt to answer the questions prior to continuing.

## SAMPLE CASE STUDY

The case study patient is 70 years of age and has recently fallen while turning around in his bathroom at night. He has a history of being "dizzy." He owns a cane but does not currently use it; he lives alone in an apartment (no stairs). He takes an ACE inhibitor and diuretic medications for high blood pressure and also a medication for depression. Our examination and standardized tests reveal the following:

- Vision
  - Saccadic smooth pursuit.
  - No resting or gaze nystagmus noted.
  - Saccades are intact and within normal limits (WNL).
  - Ocular range of motion (ROM) is WNL.

Plishka CM.
*A Clinician's Guide to Balance and Dizziness:*
*Evaluation and Treatment* (pp 329-344).
© 2015 Taylor & Francis Group.

- ◦ Cover test is positive with a vertical skew during the alternate cover test.
- ◦ Vergence is WNL.
- ◦ Optokinetic nystagmus is intact, but patient complains of feeling nausea while watching the moving lines in the horizontal plane.
- Vestibular
  - ◦ Positive left Head Thrust test, negative right head thrust.
  - ◦ Positive Head Shake test with right-beating nystagmus.
  - ◦ Positive Dix-Hallpike test for the left posterior canal (canalithiasis). Nystagmus was left-rotary and upbeating, lasting 15 seconds.
- Somatosensory
  - ◦ Intact light touch.
  - ◦ Decreased proprioception, right ankle.
  - ◦ Loss of protective sensations to right metatarsal heads 1 and 3 using the 5.07 monofilament.
- Cerebellar
  - ◦ Negative cerebellar screens: diadochokinesia, finger-to-nose, point-to-point, heel-shin slide.
- Musculoskeletal
  - ◦ Strength: Bilateral hip abductors 3/5 strength, bilateral hip extensors 2/5, all other leg muscle strength grossly WNL. Bilateral UE WNL.
  - ◦ ROM: Left ankle dorsiflexion -5 degrees, right ankle dorsiflexion to neutral. Bilateral knee extension -5 degrees with tight end-feel.
  - ◦ Posture: Kyphotic trunk, slight left trunk lean.
- Standardized tests
  - ◦ Timed Up & Go: 30 seconds (fall risk).
  - ◦ Tinetti Gait & Balance test: 17/28 (high fall risk).
  - ◦ mCTSIB times: Condition 1, WNL at 30 seconds. Condition 2, loss of balance after 15 seconds. Condition 3, loss of balance after 10 seconds. Condition 4, Immediate loss of balance.
  - ◦ Barthel index: 15/20.
- Observations
  - ◦ Multiple attempts needed with use of hands to transfer sit to stand.
  - ◦ Touches furniture and walls while ambulating.
  - ◦ Has a short step length, bilaterally lacking heel strike.
  - ◦ Avoids turning head while ambulating.
  - ◦ Slow gait speed.
  - ◦ BP changes: Supine 115/80, Sitting 105/75, Standing 90/70.

Now that we have our evaluation findings, let's make our problems list (Table 13-1).

| TABLE 13-1 | | |
|---|---|---|
| **SAMPLE PROBLEM LIST** | | |
| PATIENT COMPLAINTS | PHYSICAL DEFICITS | FUNCTIONAL DEFICITS |
| • Dizziness described as light-headedness and positional vertigo<br>• Off balance while turning quickly<br>• Off balance while trying to dress<br>• Difficulty getting out of chair | • Orthostatic hypotension<br>• Left vestibular hypofunction<br>• BPPV<br>• Hip extensor and abductor weakness<br>• Limited ankle and knee joint ROM due to muscle tightness<br>• Impaired vestibular reflex<br>• Impaired somatosensory input of the lower extremities<br>• Vertical skew deviation | • Difficulty transferring<br>  ○ Sit-stand<br>  ○ Tub<br>• Balance deficits with fall risk<br>• Gait impaired<br>• Dressing lower extremity impaired<br>  ○ Sits to dress<br>  ○ Avoids bending |

**Activity Questions:** Using a note pad, answer the following questions given this patient's history and examination findings. Once you have answered all the questions, continue reading and compare your answers with the ones included here.

Answer the following questions:

1. *Do the physical findings explain the subjective complaints?*
2. *Are there any unexpected findings not explained by the previous medical history?*
3. *Is there anything in the history that may explain disequilibrium or dizziness?*
4. *Do you have any recommendations for the referring physician?*
5. *What should we do for treatments and interventions?*

Interpretation for this activity:

**Question 1. Do the physical findings explain the subjective complaints?**

Complaint:     Dizziness—light-headedness is explained by orthostatic hypotension.

Complaint:    Dizziness—positional vertigo is explained by benign paroxysmal positional vertigo (BPPV).

Complaint:    Off balance while turning quickly; may be explained by unilateral vestibular hypofunction. Contributing factors may also include the hip weaknesses, decreased joint ROM, proprioceptive loss, and decreased plantar foot sensations of pressure.

Complaint:    Off balance while dressing; contributing factors may also include the hip weaknesses, decreased joint ROM, proprioceptive loss, and decreased plantar foot sensations of pressure as well as any vertigo or light-headedness occurring during position changes while the activity of dressing.

Complaint:    Difficulty getting out of a chair; most likely due to the hip weakness and limited joint ROM but may also be hampered by the orthostatic hypotension and BPPV (depending on head position changes during the transfer).

It would appear that all of the patient's complaints are explainable by our exam findings!

*Question 2. Are there any unexpected findings not explained by the previous medical history?*

YES! There was no history of proprioceptive loss at the ankle or loss of pressure sensation to plantar surfaces. The patient may not have even been aware of the loss of sensation. There was no history of vestibular or ear, nose, and throat issues reported. What was not surprising was the orthostatic hypotension, as the patient is taking an antihypertensive medication. The balance deficits were not unexpected owing to a history of falling and also the use of an antidepressant (although the antidepressant by itself is not a big red flag if it is not new, is a low-dose prescription, and there is no history of recent dosage changes). Vertical skew finding is concerning and unexpected, as it is a central sign that will need further examination by neurology.

*Question 3. What should we do for treatments and interventions (Table 13-2)?*

Physicians may consider medications to reduce nausea/dizziness for a unilateral vestibular weakness in the short term. Keep in mind that physical and occupational therapists may address the functional and strength issues described and also perform balance and vestibular therapy, which has been shown to improve patients' symptomatology and functional status. While sedating medications may help in the short term, keep in mind that research has shown that they do slow the adaptation process. The patient may improve faster without such medications, if tolerated, while in therapy. If a patient cannot tolerate therapy without something to reduce nausea or dizziness, just expect a longer episode of care until he or she returns to previous levels of function.

*Question 4. Is there anything in the history that may explain disequilibrium or dizziness?*

- The patient is on medications, which may impair balance. Antidepressant medications have been linked to falls.

TABLE 13-2

# FINDINGS VERSUS TREATMENTS AND INTERVENTIONS

| SYSTEM | FINDING | INTERVENTION | INDICATION FOR FURTHER TESTS OR REFERRAL TO A PHYSICIAN? |
|---|---|---|---|
| Vision | Saccadic smooth pursuit | This is an age-normal finding and will probably not be greatly affected by exercise. You could choose to add smooth pursuit as an exercise with limited expectations. | No |
| | Nausea during opto-kinetics | • Optokinetic stimulation<br>• Nausea medications as needed | Yes |
| | Vertical skew | • Refer to neurology | Yes |
| Vestibular | Left unilateral vestibular loss | • Vestibulo-ocular reflex exercises (*after* confirmation using electronystagmography/audiography or physician's order)<br>• Optokinetic stimulation | Yes |
| | BPPV | Canalith repositioning | No |
| Somatosensory | Decreased ankle pro-prioception | • Calf stretches<br>• Wedge standing<br>• Proprioceptive exercises such as trunk sways and weight shifting | Yes |
| | Decreased plantar pressure sensations | • Proprioceptive exercises such as trunk sways and weight shifting<br>• Pharmacology | Yes |

*(continued)*

| | | | |
|---|---|---|---|
| **TABLE 13-2 (CONTINUED)** | | | |
| **FINDINGS VS TREATMENTS AND INTERVENTIONS** | | | |
| **SYSTEM** | **FINDING** | **INTERVENTION** | **INDICATION FOR FURTHER TESTS OR REFERRAL TO A PHYSICIAN?** |
| Musculoskeletal | Hip weakness: extensors and abductors | Strengthening exercises in functional hip positions for extensors and abductors | No |
| | Limited ROM: Ankles dorsiflexion and knee extension | • Calf stretches, wedge standing<br>• Hamstring stretches | No |
| Other | Orthostatic hypotension | • Medication adjustments<br>• Wall leaning<br>• Tilt table | Yes |
| Function | Limited transfer ability | • Therapy referral for transfer training<br>• Assess for equipment needs | Yes: for adaptive equipment |
| | Lower extremity dressing | • Therapy referral for activities of daily living training<br>• Assess for equipment needs | Possibly: for adaptive equipment |
| | Gait abnormality | • Therapy referral for gait training<br>• Assess need for assistive device for gait stability (eg, cane/walker)<br>• Vestibular therapy | Yes: for adaptive equipment |

- The patient is taking antihypertensive agents. If the patient's hypertension medications were recently changed or his kidney function recently changed, he may be having episodes of orthostatic hypotension.
- There is a central sign (vertical skew with the alternate cover test) that requires further investigation or imaging
- The vestibular hypofunction identified with the Head Thrust test may explain disequilibrium

**Question 5. *Do you have any recommendations for the referring physician?***

- The vertical skew with the alternate cover test is a significant central finding requiring further investigation (usually with neurology).
- If balance and vestibular therapy do not produce the desired improvement in balance or reduction in dizziness, a review of medications by the primary care physician may be helpful to rule out polypharmacy.

# ACUTE CARE CASE STUDY EXAMPLE

Answer the specific case questions (if any) and then answer the acute care case questions in Activity 2. Table 13-3 provides a blank form for listing problems that we will refer to as a *deficits grid*.

For each example, complete the deficits grid and answer the following questions:
1. *Do the physical findings explain the subjective complaints?*
2. *Are there any unexpected findings not explained by the previous medical history?*
3. *What should we do for treatments and interventions?*
4. *Is there anything in the history that may explain disequilibrium or dizziness?*
5. *Do you have any recommendations for the referring physician?*

## Case 1: Acute Care

Three days ago, a 15-year-old female was a restrained passenger in a motor vehicle accident. She was riding in the front passenger seat when, at a stop sign, her car was struck from behind by another car traveling at high speed. The current plan is to discharge her home with family support.

Evaluation by the emergency department reveals the following:
- Report of loss of consciousness for a few minutes postimpact
- Radiography studies reveal:
  - Fractured skull (occipital and temporal)
  - Concussion
  - No bleeding injuries of the head
  - No other fractures
  - Normal spinal alignment

| TABLE 13-3 BLANK DEFICITS GRID | | |
| --- | --- | --- |
| PATIENT COMPLAINTS | PHYSICAL DEFICITS | FUNCTIONAL DEFICITS |
| | | |

The patient is wearing a cervical collar with orders initially written in the emergency department to wear the collar until a neurologist had reviewed the case. The orders for the collar were written prior to receiving test results.

The patient's subjective complaints include headache, neck ache, dizziness, and "jumping eyes" while trying to watch TV or read.

- Prior to examination, do you need to contact any of the physicians involved in the case? If so, for what reasons?
- What tests are needed?

After answering these questions, continue reading.

Given the radiography results, did you question the need for the cervical collar? Contacting the neurologist may allow for the removal of the collar as well as reducing the complaints of neck pain. It is also possible that the patient is suffering from a whiplash, in which case a physical therapy consultation may help the complaints of neck pain.

What tests are needed? Given the history of trauma and the complaints of dizziness and jumping eyes, you should review each system that contributes to balance as well as function:

- Vision, vestibular, somatosensory, cerebellar, musculoskeletal
- Function tests (eg, fall risk, balance, ADL)

Examination revealed the following positive findings:

- Vision
  - Left gaze nystagmus > 3 beats at 45 degrees of left eccentric gaze increasing at left end range
  - Convergence insufficiency: Diplopia with vergence at 20 cm
- Vestibular
  - The Head Thrust test had to be modified since the patient still had orders to wear the cervical collar. The patient was seated in a swivel chair and the test was performed by moving her entire body left and right while she was instructed to maintain gaze on the visual target. The test result was "positive right head thrust (modified)," indicating a likely right vestibular weakness.
- Somatosensory
  - Intact light touch and proprioception
  - Negative monofilament test, indicating normal pressure sensation
- Cerebellar
  - WNL for tests of accuracy and coordination
- Musculoskeletal
  - WNL for strength and ROM for all extremities
  - Cervical ROM was not tested because of orders to wear the cervical collar. Cervical and musculature ROM needs to be further assessed once the collar is removed.
- Function
  - Functional reach results: Loss of balance at 6-inch reach indicating fall risk

- ° mCTSIB results
  - ▪ Loss of balance eyes open after 6 seconds, standing on a firm surface
  - ▪ Loss of balance eyes closed after 5 seconds, standing on a firm surface
  - ▪ Loss of balance eyes open after 3 seconds, standing on foam
  - ▪ Loss of balance eyes closed immediately, standing on foam
- Observation of gait revealed short steps bilaterally, scissoring gait, and frequent loss of balance. The patient constantly reached out to touch reference objects.

Given this case information, create problem lists for physical and functional deficits and then answer the questions listed at the beginning of the chapter in Activity 1.

## Activity 2: Questions and Answers for Case 1

- *Do the physical findings explain the subjective complaints?*

  *Partially. The patient has had a recent head injury with skull fractures and concussion. Dizziness, headache, and neck ache are not unexpected. The vestibular findings have not been previously reported, nor have the oculomotor findings, gait abnormality, or balance deficits.*

- *Are there any unexpected findings not explained by the previous medical history?*

  *Yes. There are multiple signs of vestibular loss; however, the patient has offered no history that would indicate a vestibular insult. Other than disequilibrium, she currently has no complaints of dizziness or vertigo.*

- *Is there anything in the history that may explain disequilibrium or dizziness?*

  *Yes. Recent head injury, concussion, occipital skull fracture/trauma. Vestibular loss or vestibular concussion may also contribute.*

- *Do you have any recommendations for the referring physician?*

  *Yes.*
  - ° *Report all findings.*
  - ° *A second head scan may be indicated given the central findings.*
  - ° *Referral to neuro-otology and neuro-ophthalmology may be revealing.*
  - ° *Referral to vestibular rehab is indicated.*
  - ° *Electronystagmography/audiography at a later date once the patient can better tolerate these tests.*

- *What should we do for treatments and interventions?*
  - ° *Vestibular therapy to address vestibular hypofunction and balance*
  - ° *Physical therapy for neck pain*
  - ° *Possible vergence exercises, depending on findings from neuro-ophthalmologists*
  - ° *Gait training*
  - ° *Order an assistive device (walker or cane) that best assists balance*

## Case 2: Inpatient Rehabilitation

The patient is a 68-year-old male 2 days status-post left total hip replacement (posterior approach). The exact circumstances of the fall are unknown, as the patient cannot recall what happened to cause it. He is following hip precautions for the recent surgery, and is taking an anticoagulant therapy. Previous medical history includes hypertension, hyperlipidemia, anxiety, and cardiac bypass graft. Chronic medications include alprazolam for anxiety, atorvastatin for hyperlipidemia, and atenolol for hypertension. He has been taking these medications for years. The hip replacement was necessary owing to a fall injury that fractured the femur. The patient denies a history of disequilibrium or dizziness but owns a cane that he reports he doesn't need.

The patient lives alone and has 3 stair steps without a rail at the entrance of his home. He owns no assistive devices other than the cane. There is no other information other than the operative report.

- What are possible causes for the patient's fall?
- Is the patient at risk of falling?
- Is it safe for the patient to live alone?

Examination revealed the following findings:

- Vision
  ◦ No nystagmus noted in room light or during fixation
  ◦ Right gaze nystagmus > 3 beats at end range observed with Frenzel goggles (vision removed)
- Vestibular
  ◦ Positive left head thrust
  ◦ Negative test of BPPV
- Somatosensory
  ◦ WNL for light touch and proprioception
  ◦ Negative monofilament test for protective sensations
- Cerebellum
  ◦ WNL
- Musculoskeletal
  ◦ Hip abduction strength—Left 2/5, Right 3/5
  ◦ Hip extension strength—Bilaterally estimated at 2/5 based on the patient's need for assistance to transfer sit to stand
- Function
  ◦ Timed Up & Go test score 36 seconds, indicating fall risk
- **What are possible causes for the patient's fall?**

  Unknown. The positive Head Thrust test indicates a vestibular hypofunction which may affect balance. However, there are several physical and functional deficits that may explain a fall. For example, he has already fallen, he takes medications linked to disequilibrium, and he has hip muscle weakness.

- **Is the patient at risk of falling?**

Yes. The TUG score indicates fall risk, and the patient has already fallen once, leading to the hip fracture.

- **Is it safe for the patient to live alone?**

Unknown without further tests, such as standardized tests of cognition, ADL ability, and fall risk.

## Activity 2: Questions and Answers for Case 2

- *Do the physical findings explain the subjective complaints?*

   *The patient really did not provide subjective complaints. There is, however, a history of the fall that caused a hip fracture. Findings of vestibular hypofunction and hip weakness are likely reasons to explain the fall.*

- *Are there any unexpected findings not explained by the previous medical history?*

   *Yes. There is no history offered by the patient with vestibular symptoms. This may be due to a chronic vestibular loss, and the patient does not remember a significant event with vestibular signs or symptoms.*

- *Is there anything in the history that may explain disequilibrium or dizziness?*

   *Possibly. The patient is taking medications known to cause dizziness and disequilibrium.*

- *Do you have any recommendations for the referring physician?*
   - *Medication review may be helpful to rule out medication involvement in the patient's fall risk.*
   - *Electronystagmography/videonystagmography (VNG) and audiography tests should be ordered to rule out central pathologies and confirm vestibular loss.*
   - *Standardized tests of memory and cognition may help to answer the question of whether it is safe for the patient to live alone.*

- *What should we do for treatments and interventions?*
   - *Vestibular therapy*
   - *Gait training using an assistive device*

# Case 3: Outpatient Setting

The patient is a 37-year-old male who was struck in the head while cutting branches off of a tree. He now complains of positional vertigo while getting out of bed and while tying his shoes. He has no significant previous medical history and takes no chronic medications.

- Based on this history, is there a likely etiology?
- What tests are needed?

Examination revealed the following findings:

- Vision
   - WNL

- Vestibular
  - Tests of vestibular function are WNL
  - Positive Dix-Hallpike for right posterior canal BPPV (canalithiasis)
- Somatosensory
  - WNL
- Cerebellum
  - WNL
- Musculoskeletal
  - WNL
- **Based on this history, is there a likely etiology?**
  The history and symptoms are consistent with BPPV.
- **What tests are needed?**
  - As with all patients with a complaint of dizziness, each system that contributes to balance should be assessed.
  - Screening of the transverse and alar ligaments should be included.

## Activity 2: Questions and Answers for Case 3

- *Do the physical findings explain the subjective complaints?*
  *Yes. BPPV causes positional vertigo.*
- *Are there any unexpected findings not explained by the previous medical history? No.*
- *Is there anything in the history that may explain disequilibrium or dizziness?*
  *Yes. The blow to the head with the falling branch.*
- *Do you have any recommendations for the referring physician?*
  *Only if canalith repositioning does not resolve the patient's complaints, at which time further testing would be recommended to rule out other causes of vertigo.*
- *What should we do for treatments and interventions?*
  - *Canalith repositioning.*
  - *Educate the patient on canalith repositioning maneuvers.*
  - *Reassess for BPPV after canalith repositioning and reassess again at least 24 hours after interventions.*

# Case 4: Outpatient Setting

The patient is a 70-year-old female with a history of frequent falls and a complaint of constant dizziness with no provoking factors. The previous medical history is positive for non–insulin-dependent diabetes and psychiatric issues. Medications include glyburide for diabetes, quetiapine fumarate for bipolar disorder, and alprazolam for anxiety. The patient also has a history of alcohol abuse.

- Based on this history and examination findings, is the etiology of the dizziness and disequilibrium likely to be a peripheral or central problem?

- Is the finding of "saccadic smooth pursuit" concerning?

Examination revealed the following findings:

- Vision
  - Direction-changing gaze nystagmus
  - Saccadic smooth pursuit
  - Hypometric saccades left to right
- Vestibular
  - All tests WNL
- Somatosensory
  - Decreased light touch sensations—L5 dermatomes bilaterally
  - Positive Semmes-Weinstein Monofilament test—loss of pressure sensations to the right great toe pad and first metatarsal head
- Cerebellar
  - Dysmetria with Finger-to-Nose and Point-to-Point tests
  - Negative tests of coordination
- Musculoskeletal
  - WNL
- Function
  - Dynamic Gait Index: 15/24 indicating fall risk
  - Wide-based gait pattern
- **Based on this history and examination findings, is the etiology of the dizziness and disequilibrium likely to be a peripheral or central problem?**
  - Recall, direction-changing nystagmus is a central finding, additionally, the vestibular screens were normal
- **Is the finding of "saccadic smooth pursuit" concerning?**
  - This patient is 70 years old, and saccadic smooth pursuit is not an uncommon finding for patients of this age. By itself, it is not concerning. It must, however, be considered when looking at the entirety of findings.

## Activity 2: Questions and Answers for Case 4

- *Do the physical findings explain the subjective complaints?*

  *Yes. There are several central signs that may explain disequilibrium but require further testing.*

- *Are there any unexpected findings not explained by the previous medical history?*

  *Yes. Oculomotor abnormalities may possibly be explained by the current medications for bipolar disorder and anxiety. The positive cerebellar signs may be explained by cerebellar damage secondary to alcoholism. However, testing is needed to confirm central pathology.*

- *Is there anything in the history that may explain disequilibrium or dizziness?*

  Yes. Medications known to cause disequilibrium, as well as alcoholism, may explain the disequilibrium and oculomotor abnormalities. Central findings may indicate central pathology causing the disequilibrium. Complaints of constant dizziness are often signs of central dizziness.

- *Do you have any recommendations for the referring physician?*
  - *Weaning the patient from the bipolar and anxiety medications and testing with VNG/Audiography.*
  - *Computed tomography or magnetic resonance imaging of the brain and brainstem.*

- *What should we do for treatments and interventions?*
  - *Oculomotor exercises.*
  - *Balance training.*
  - *Gait training with an assistive device.*

## Case 5: Outpatient Setting

The patient is a 21-year-old male with no previous medical history. He complains of positional vertigo that gradually worsened over the last month. He denies history of trauma, recent illness, tinnitus, or ear fullness.

Examination revealed the following findings:

- Vision
  - Direction-changing gaze nystagmus
  - Rebound nystagmus
- Vestibular
  - Positive Dix-Hallpike test bilaterally, with symptoms suggestive of posterior canal cupulolithiasis
  - Head thrust is WNL
- Somatosensory
  - WNL for light touch and proprioception
- Cerebellar
  - Negative tests of coordination, accuracy, and proprioception
- Musculoskeletal
  - WNL
- Function
  - Dynamic Gait Index: 24/24
  - mCTSIB: Stand > 30 seconds for all conditions
  - Motion Sensitivity test: Positive for 4 positions, with subjective dizziness 5/5, and nystagmus lasting > 30 seconds for each position
- What are the possible diagnoses?
- What would treatment be?

- Is bilateral cupulolithiasis likely?
- What should be the next step for treatment of this patient?

Complete the case questions and deficits grid and then continue.

- **What are the possible diagnoses?**
  - ◦ Bilateral cupulolithiasis—while possible, this is extremely unlikely. There is no trauma history, there are central signs present, and bilateral cupulolithiasis is almost unheard of. Other possible diagnoses include central pathologies such as multiple sclerosis, Parkinson's disease, stroke, and tumor.
- **What would treatment be?**
  - ◦ Initially, send for further testing. In this case, the patient was sent to neurology. A head scan revealed MS plaque.
- **Is bilateral cupulolithiasis likely?**
  - ◦ No
- **What should be the next step for treatment of this patient?**
  - ◦ Motion habituation
  - ◦ Vestibular exercises
  - ◦ Annual check for balance, or more frequently if there are complaints of disequilibrium

## Activity 2: Questions and Answers for Case 5

- *Do the physical findings explain the subjective complaints?*
  *Yes. There are vestibular signs and central signs.*
- *Are there any unexpected findings not explained by the previous medical history?*
  *Yes. Oculomotor abnormalities are unexpected for this patient, given his age and lack of medication use that could explain oculomotor abnormalities.*
- *Is there anything in the history that may explain disequilibrium or dizziness?*
  *No.*
- *Do you have any recommendations for the referring physician?*
  - ◦ *Testing with VNG/audiography*
  - ◦ *Computed tomography or magnetic resonance imaging of the brain and brainstem*
- *What should we do for treatments and interventions?*
  - ◦ *Vestibular therapy*
  - ◦ *Motion habituation*

# 14

# Quick Reference

This section provides the essentials, mostly in bullet-point fashion. More detailed information is available throughout the book.

## COMPONENTS OF THE BALANCE SYSTEM

- Inputs (information gathering): vision, vestibular, somatosensory
- Central processing: cerebellar
- Outputs: musculoskeletal

## Vision

Eye motions are used to place objects of interest on the retina (fovea). Each eye must point at the target to achieve binocular fusion.

Plishka CM.
*A Clinician's Guide to Balance and Dizziness:*
*Evaluation and Treatment* (pp 345-359).
© 2015 Taylor & Francis Group.

## Vestibular System

- Innervated by cranial nerve VIII and responsible for generating the vestibulo-ocular reflex (VOR), vestibulocollic reflex, and vestibulospinal reflex.
- Comprising 2 otolith organs and 3 endolymph-filled semicircular canals.
  - Otolith organs (actions described in the anatomical position)
    - Utricle detecting horizontal plane changes in head velocity and the pull of gravity
    - Saccule detecting vertical plane changes in head velocity and the pull of gravity
    - Pull of gravity is detected owing to otoconia (crystals) that adhere to the otolithic matrix, containing specialized hair cells (kinocilia and stereocilia)
  - Semicircular canals
    - Named for their orientation in space (anterior, posterior, and lateral or horizontal)
    - Detect angular changes in head velocity
    - Work in coplanar pairs

## Somatosensory System

Provides information regarding body movement and position, touch, pressure, pain, temperature, and vibration using cutaneous and subcutaneous receptors.

## Cerebellar System

Processes input information and is involved in motor planning. Compares intention with action.

## Musculoskeletal System

Using muscle and joint action, we carry out the motor plan. This requires adequate strength and range of motion.

# EYE MOTIONS

Table 14-1 outlines the motions of the eyes. Different eye muscles or combinations of eye muscles produce the motions shown in Table 14-2.[2]

| TABLE 14-1 EYE MOTIONS USED TO SEE OBJECTS[1] | |
|---|---|
| Directs the eyes | Saccades Smooth pursuit Vergence |
| Holds the images steady | Fixation VOR Optokinetics |

| TABLE 14-2 MUSCLES THAT PRODUCE EYE MOTION | | |
|---|---|---|
| MOTION | PRIMARY MUSCLE | CRANIAL NERVE INNERVATION |
| Adduction | Medial rectus | III Oculomotor |
| Abduction | Lateral rectus | VI Abducens |
| Elevation | Superior rectus | III Oculomotor |
| Depression | Inferior rectus | III Oculomotor |
| Intorsion | Superior oblique | IV Trochlear |
| Extorsion | Inferior oblique | III Oculomotor |

# HISTORY QUESTIONS

## Dizziness

What does *dizzy* mean to the patient?
- Vertigo (may be caused by vestibular, cerebellar, or cervicogenic pathologies)
- Light-headedness (orthostatic hypotension, arrhythmias, hypoglycemia, medication side effects, cervicogenic, and sometimes vestibular)
- Disequilibrium (multiple etiologies)
- Floating out of body (typically CNS or psychiatric)

## General Questions

- What is the current primary complaint?
- Previous medical history.
- Previous tests results.
- Previous treatments for this issue.
- Current medications and any recent medication changes.

- Under what conditions does the patient lose balance (or become dizzy)?
- When and how did the problem begin?
- How often does the problem occur?
- Any recent trauma?
- What provokes/relieves the complaint?

## Questions for Dizziness and Balance

- When did the (dizziness/disequilibrium/pain) start?
- Was onset sudden or gradual?
- Describe the (dizziness/disequilibrium/pain)
- Rate your (dizziness/disequilibrium/pain) using a scale.
- How long do sensations of (dizziness/disequilibrium/pain) last (constant/intermittent, seconds, minutes, hours, days)?
- How does your (dizziness/disequilibrium/pain) limit your function?
- It is better/worse at certain times of day?
- Is it provoked by certain positions or activities?
- Have you had any tests for this? (And results if known)
- Have you been treated for this? (If yes, how, and results of treatments)

As we mentioned, there are some additional questions that are needed in asking about dizziness. Some of these questions include the following:

- Worse with head motion?
- Worse in light or darkness? (Helps to differentiate between central and peripheral vestibular issues)
- Positional provoked? (Helps in deciding if benign paroxysmal positional vertigo [BPPV] is a possible condition)
- When did the patient last take any sedating medications?
- Provoked by visually stimulating environments (eg, TV, grocery stores, shopping malls, car traffic, and ceiling fans)?
- What does *dizzy* mean? Vertigo (sensation of movement), disequilibrium (off balance), light-headedness (presyncope), floating?
- Has the patient taken any of the following, which may mask signs and symptoms? Antihistamines, benzodiazepines, anticholinergics?
- Ears: Any recent changes to hearing? Tinnitus? Pressure/pain?
- Any contraindications to testing or treatment interventions?
- Any recent changes to vision Rx?

### Helpful Questionnaires

- Dizziness Handicap Inventory: Score interpretation
- Activities-Specific Balance Confidence
- Modified Falls Efficacy Scale
- Vestibular Disorders Activities of Daily Living Scale

Table 14-3 outlines the physical examination.

| | TABLE 14-3 |
|---|---|
| | **SEQUENCE OF PHYSICAL EXAMINATION** |
| **SYSTEM** | **TESTS** |
| Initial interview | ✓ Review previous medical history and tests results, medications, subjective complaints |
| Vision/oculomotor | ✓ Fixation, gaze, range of motion, smooth pursuit, saccades, vergence, cover tests |
| Vestibular | ✓ Transverse and Alar Ligament Screen |
| | ✓ Function tests (Head Thrust, Head Shake) |
| | ✓ Pressure tests (eg, Tragal, Valsalva) |
| | ✓ BPPV (Dix-Hallpike, Roll test) |
| Somatosensory | ✓ Light touch, proprioception, protective sensation testing (5.07 monofilament) |
| Cerebellar | ✓ Accuracy tests: finger to nose, point to point, heel to shin |
| | ✓ Coordination tests: diadochokinesia, hand clap, feet tapping |
| | ✓ VOR cancellation |
| Musculoskeletal | ✓ Strength and joint ranges of motion |
| Vitals as needed | ✓ Heart rate and rhythm, blood pressures (supine, sitting, standing) |
| Function | ✓ Standardized tests (balance, gait, fall risk, activities of daily living, memory/cognition) |

# VESTIBULAR: TESTING, FUNCTION, AND INTERVENTIONS

## *Vestibular Testing Precautions*

Make sure the patient does not have any contraindications to testing or treatment, such as the following[3]:

- Acute fractures that prevent the patient from lying down quickly or rolling
- Recent neck fracture, surgery, or instability
- History of vertebral dissection or unstable carotid disease
- Recent retinal detachment

Other patient populations that may require test/intervention care or modifications include those with cervical stenosis, severe kyphoscoliosis, limited cervical range of motion, Down's syndrome, severe rheumatoid arthritis, cervical radiculopathies, Paget's disease, ankylosing spondylitis, low back dysfunction, spinal cord injuries, and morbid obesity.

If you are ever in doubt of the patient's ability to be tested or treated, contact the appropriate medical practitioner for approval.

# TESTS FOR BENIGN PAROXYSMAL POSITIONAL VERTIGO

Common signs and symptoms of BPPV include positional vertigo/nystagmus, nausea, and sometimes vomiting.

The most common tests of BPPV for the anterior and posterior canals include
- The Dix-Hallpike test
- The Side-Lying test

The most common test of lateral canal BPPV is
- The Roll test

For positive lateral canal BPPV, the Bow-and-Lean test may help to identify which ear is involved.

Table 14-4 is a guide to the interpretation of nystagmus during testing.

# VESTIBULAR FUNCTION TESTS

Common tests of vestibular function include
- The Head Thrust test
- The Head Shake test

Specialty tests of vestibular function requiring equipment:
- Electronystagmograph/Videonystagmograph
- Rotary Chair test
- Dynamic Visual Acuity, instrumented

| TABLE 14-4 INTERPRETATION OF NYSTAGMUS DURING TESTING | | | |
|---|---|---|---|
| **SIDE** | **ANTERIOR CANAL** | **LATERAL CANAL** | **POSTERIOR CANAL** |
| Left | **Downbeating** **Left rotational** <br><br> • Canalithiasis (loose): Latency up to 45 seconds, nystagmus lasting < 1 min. <br> • Cupulolithiasis (stuck): Immediate onset, nystagmus lasting > 1 min. | **Lateral beating:** **Geotropic (loose)** <br><br> • Treat strong-symptom side <br> **Apogeotropic** (stuck or near cupula) <br> • Treat weak-symptom side | **Upbeating** **Left rotational** <br><br> • Canalithiasis (loose): Latency up to 45 seconds, nystagmus lasting < 1 min. <br> • Cupulolithiasis (stuck): Immediate onset, nystagmus lasting > 1 min. |
| Right | **Downbeating** **Right rotational** <br><br> • Canalithiasis (loose): Latency up to 45 seconds, nystagmus lasting < 1 min. <br> • Cupulolithiasis (stuck): Immediate onset, nystagmus lasting > 1 min. | **Lateral beating** **Geotropic (loose)** <br><br> • Treat strong symptom side <br> **Apogeotropic** (stuck or near cupula) <br> • Treat weak symptom side | **Upbeating** **Right rotational** <br><br> • Canalithiasis (loose): Latency up to 45 seconds, nystagmus lasting < 1 min. <br> • Cupulolithiasis (stuck): Immediate onset, nystagmus lasting > 1 min. |

# SIGNS AND SYMPTOMS OF VESTIBULAR LOSS

- Signs and symptoms of acute vestibular loss may include the following:
  - Resting or gaze nystagmus
  - Nausea
  - Vomiting
  - Disequilibrium
  - Unidirectional resting nystagmus or gaze nystagmus that begins at 45 degrees of gaze or is greater than 3 beats near end ranges

- Signs and symptoms of chronic vestibular loss may include the following:
  - Dizziness while turning
  - Disequilibrium while turning
  - Nausea in busy visual environments (eg, grocery stores, highways, action movies, near ceiling fans)
  - Unidirectional gaze nystagmus, sometimes elicited only at end ranges (> 3 beats) or in darkness
- Signs and symptoms of bilateral vestibular loss may include the following:
  - Oscillopsia
  - Disequilibrium
  - Abnormal gait pattern
  - The patient may or may not complain of dizziness
  - There is typically no resting or gaze nystagmus

## COMMON VESTIBULAR EXERCISES

- VOR x 1 view: Head remains still, target moves. Exercises typically 1 min each horizontal and vertical motions 3 to 4 times daily at a head speed of 1 to 2 Hz.
- VOR x 2 view: Head and target move in opposite directions but at the same speed (1 to 2 Hz). Typically performed 1 minute each with horizontal and vertical motions 3 to 4 times daily.
- Progress from sitting to standing on varied surfaces to moving.

## CANALITH REPOSITIONING MANEUVERS FOR POSTERIOR CANALS

- Modified Epley maneuver
- Semont liberatory maneuver
- Gans repositioning maneuver
- Brandt-Daroff exercise

## CANALITH REPOSITIONING MANEUVERS FOR ANTERIOR CANALS

- Reverse Semont maneuver
- Reverse Epley maneuver

- Rahko's maneuver
- Kim's head-hanging maneuver
- Deep head-hanging maneuver (Yakovino)

# CANALITH REPOSITIONING MANEUVERS FOR LATERAL CANALS

- Barbecue roll
- Log roll
- Lempert 360
- Gufoni maneuver (geotropic and apogeotropic variations)
- Vannucchi prolonged positioning
- Vannucchi-Asprella maneuver

# APOGEOTROPIC CONVERSION MANEUVERS

- Head-shake conversion maneuver
- Head rotation conversion maneuver

# SOMATOSENSORY TESTS

- Light touch: dermatome testing, monofilament tests
- Pressure: Semmes-Weinstein 5.07 monofilament test
- Proprioception: Discrimination Threshold test, Joint Position Matching,
- Vibration Sensation test

# CEREBELLAR TESTS

- Muscle tone: passive limb movements
- Accuracy tests: Point to Point, Finger to Nose, Heel-Shin Slide, Heel-Knee Tap
- Coordination tests: Diadochokinesia, Hand Clapping test
- VOR Cancellation test

| TABLE 14-5 |
|---|
| **COMMON CENTRAL AND PERIPHERAL PATHOLOGIES CAUSING DIZZINESS AND IMBALANCE** |

| CENTRAL | PERIPHERAL |
|---|---|
| Brainstem strokes | BPPV (vestibular) |
| Cerebellar degeneration | Cerebellopontine angle tumors |
| Head trauma | Labyrinthitis (vestibular) |
| Migraine-related | Ménière's disease |
| Multiple sclerosis | Postsurgical (labyrinthectomy) |
| Parkinson's disease | Post-trauma |
| Vestibulopathy | Schwannomas |
|  | Superior canal dehiscence (vestibular) |
|  | Vestibular neuritis |

# MUSCULOSKELETAL TESTS

- Strength: Manual Muscle tests, Isometric Dynamometer and Isokinetic Isometric Dynamometer tests
- Range of motion: goniometry
- Active cervical range of motion
- Transverse and alar ligament screens
- Posture assessment

# COMMON CAUSES OF DIZZINESS

Table 14-5 lists pathologies that can cause dizziness and disequilibrium.[4,5] There are many standardized tests. Table 14-6 lists a few of the more commonly used. Table 14-7 is a guide to the interpretation of scores from standardized tests for fall risk.

# MEDICATIONS

## Commonly Used to Treat Symptoms of Dizziness

- Antihistamines
- Benzodiazepines
- Anticholinergics

These medications may interfere with the evaluation by suppressing symptoms. They may also slow the progress of therapy aimed at vestibular compensation.

| CATEGORY | TEST |
|---|---|
| **TABLE 14-6** **STANDARDIZED TESTS** | |
| Fall risk | • Activity-Specific Balance Confidence Scale |
| | • Berg Balance Scale |
| | • Dynamic Gait Index |
| | • Falls Efficacy Scale |
| | • Four Square Step test |
| | • Functional Gait Assessment |
| | • Functional Reach test |
| | • Gait Speed |
| | • Tinetti Balance & Gait (also known as *Performance-Oriented Mobility Assessment*) |
| | • Timed Up & Go |
| Activities of daily living | • Activities of Daily Living Scale |
| | • Barthel Index of Activities of Daily Living |
| | • Physical Performance test |
| Instrumental activities of daily living | • Frenchay Index |
| | • The Lawton Instrumental Activities of Daily Living Scale |
| Cognition and memory | • The Montreal Cognitive Assessment (MoCA) |
| | • Mini-Cog |
| | • Mini-Mental State Examination (MMSE) |

## Medications That Commonly Cause Dizziness

- Anticonvulsants
- Antidepressants
- Anxiolytics
- Sedatives
- Strong analgesics
- Muscle relaxants
- Antiarrhythmic agents

| TABLE 14-7 |
|---|
| **INTERPRETATION OF SCORES FROM STANDARDIZED TESTS OF FALL RISK** |

| CATEGORY | TEST | SCORE INTERPRETATION |
|---|---|---|
| Balance and/ or fall risk | Activity-Specific Balance Confidence Scale[6] | < 50: low level of physical functioning<br>51 to 80: moderate level of physical functioning<br>81 to 100: highly functioning |
| | Berg Balance Scale[7,8] | 56: functional balance<br>< 45: risk for multiple falls<br>≤ 40: almost 100% risk of falling |
| | Dynamic Gait Index (DGI)[8] | < 19 indicative of fall risk |
| | Falls Efficacy Scale[9] | > 80 indicates increased fall risk<br>> 70 indicates a fear of falling |
| | Functional Reach test[10] | Frail elderly: < 7.28 inches indicates fall risk<br>Parkinson's disease: < 12.5 inches indicates fall risk<br>Most healthy with adequate balance: ≥ 10 inches |
| | Four Square Step test[11-13] | Older adults: > 15 seconds indicates fall risk<br>Patients with vestibular problems: > 12 seconds indicates fall risk<br>Acute stroke: failed attempt or > 15 seconds indicates increased risk for falls<br>Transtibial amputees: > 24 seconds indicates fall risk |
| | Functional Gait Assessment[14,15] | Older adults: ≤ 22 indicates fall risk<br>Parkinson's disease: ≤ 15 indicates fall risk |
| | Gait Speed[16] | < 100 cm/s are 28% more likely to fall than gait above 100 cm/s<br>< 70 cm/s are 54% more likely to fall than gait above 100 cm/s<br>Every 10 cm/s decrease in gait speed was associated with 7% increase in fall risk |

*(continued)*

| TABLE 14-7 (CONTINUED) INTERPRETATION OF SCORES FROM STANDARDIZED TESTS OF FALL RISK | | |
|---|---|---|
| CATEGORY | TEST | SCORE INTERPRETATION |
| Balance and/ or fall risk | Tinetti Performance Oriented Mobility Assessment[17] | < 19: high fall risk<br>19 to 24: moderate fall risk<br>25 to 28: less likely to fall |
| | Timed Up & Go test[18] | Community dwelling adults: > 13.5 seconds indicates fall risk |

## INTERVENTIONS FOR BALANCE IMPAIRMENT

Interventions for balance impairments should be specific to each patient's needs, based on evaluation findings. Some interventions may include
- Sensory reweighting
- Lower extremity strengthening
- Oculomotor exercise
- Weight shifting
- Stepping
- Vestibular exercises
- Performance of functional activities
- Gait training
- Adding adaptive equipment
- Varying interventions by changing the person, task, or environment

## STROKE SCREEN FOR ACUTE VESTIBULAR SYNDROME

Using these 3 test, Kattah et al created a test battery to help predict stroke and named it using an acronym, HINTS, which stands for[19]
- Head Impulse test
- Nystagmus
- Tests of Skew

They also used another acronym when using this battery, INFARCT, which stands for

- **I**mpulse **N**ormal

or

- **F**ast-phase **A**lternating (nystagmus)

or

- **R**efixation on **C**over **t**est

With these occurring with a history of 24 hours or greater of constant dizziness Kattah et al found that any 1 of these 3 danger signs (normal head thrust, direction-changing nystagmus, or vertical skew during the Alternate Cover test) for patients presenting with acute vestibular syndrome had 100% sensitivity and a 96% specificity for stroke, which was better than diffusion-weighted magnetic resonance imaging in urgently ruling out stroke.

# REFERENCES

1. Wong A. *Eye Movement Disorders.* Oxford, UK: Oxford University Press; 2008.
2. Borchert MS. Principles and techniques of the examination of ocular motility and alignment. In: *Walsh & Hoyt's Clinical Neuro-ophthalmology.* 6th ed. Philadelphia: Lippincott WIllilams & Wilkins; 2005:887-905.
3. Rabie A, Foster C, Chang A, Windle M. Canalith-repositioning maneuvers—contraindications. Available at http://emedicine.medscape.com/article/82945-overview#a05. Updated 2012. Accessed October 4, 2014.
4. Furman JWS. Central causes of dizziness. *Phys Ther.* 2000;80(2):179-187.
5. Bhattacharyya N, Baugh RF, Orvidas L, et al. Clinical practice guideline: benign paroxysmal positional vertigo. *Otolaryngol Head Neck Surg.* 2008;139(5 Suppl 4):S47-81.
6. Powell LE, Myers MA. The activities-specific balance confidence (ABC) scale. *J Gerontol A Biol Sci Med Sci.* 1995;50(1):M28-M34.
7. Berg KO, Maki BE, Williams JI, Holliday PJ, Wood-Dauphinee SL. Clinical and laboratory measures of postural balance in an elderly population. *Arch Phys Med Rehabil.* 1992;73(11):1073-1080.
8. Shumway-Cook A, Baldwin M, Polissar NL, Gruber W. Predicting the probability for falls in community-dwelling older adults. *Phys Ther.* 1997;77(8):812-819.
9. Tinetti M, Richmand D, Powell L. Falls efficacy as a measure of fear of falling. *J Gerontol.* 1990;45(6):P239-P243.
10. Duncan PW, Weiner DK., Chandler J, Studenski S. Functional reach: a new clinical measure of balance. *J Gerontol.* 1990;45(6):M192-M197.
11. Dite W, Temple VA. A clinical test of stepping and change of direction to identify multiple falling older adults. *Arch Phys Med Rehabil.* 2002;83(11):1566-1571.
12. Whitney SL, Marchetti GF, Morris LO, Sparto PJ. The reliability and validity of the four square step test for people with balance deficits secondary to a vestibular disorder. *Arch Phys Med Rehabil.* 2007;88(1):99-104.
13. Blennerhassett JM, Jayalath VM. The four square step test is a feasible and valid clinical test of dynamic standing balance for use in ambulant people poststroke. *Arch Phys Med Rehabil.* 2008;89(11):2156-2161.
14. Wrisley DM, Kumar NA. Functional gait assessment: concurrent, discriminative, and predictive validity in community-dwelling older adults. *Phys Ther.* 2010;90(5):761-773.
15. Leddy AL, Crowner BE, Earhart GM. Functional gait assessment and balance evaluation system test: reliability, validity, sensitivity, and specificity for identifying individuals with Parkinson disease who fall. *Phys Ther.* 2011;91(1):102-113.

16. Verghese J, Holtzer R, Lipton RB, Wang C. Quantitative gait markers and incident fall risk in older adults. *J Gerontol.* 2009;64A(8):896-901.
17. Tinetti ME. Performance-oriented assessment of mobility porblems in elderly patients. *JAGS.* 1986;34:119-126.
18. Shumway-Cook A, Brauer S, Woollacott M. Predicting the probability for falls in community-dwelling older adults using the timed up & go test. *Phys Ther.* 2000;80(9):896-903.
19. Kattah J, Talkad A, Wang D, et al. HINTS to diagnose stroke in the acute vestibular syndrome: three-step bedside oculomotor examination more sensitive than early MRI diffusion-weighted imaging. *Stroke.* 2009;40:3504-3510.

# Index

abduction, 193

acoustic neuroma, 94

activities of daily living, 307
  questionnaires for, 50
  tests for, 272-276, 355

Activity-Specific Balance Confidence Scale, 50, 275, 356

acute vestibular syndrome, 259-260, 357-358

adaptation exercises, for vestibular deficits, 96

adduction, 193

age
  changes with, 38-41
  smooth pursuit changes with, 200
  vestibular rehabilitation therapy efficacy and, 105

Alexander's law, 29

Alghadir, A, on vestibular interventions, 97, 106

alignment, optical, 215-221

alignment test, for eyes, 61-62

Alternating Cover test, 219-220

American Academy of Neurology, BPPV treatment and, 185-186

American Academy of Otolaryngology-Head and Neck Surgery Foundation, on vestibular testing, 120-122

American Diabetic Association, foot sensation testing recommendations of, 243

American Physical Therapy Association, Vestibular Special Interest Group of, 48-49, 227-228

ampulla, 15, 21, 113

ampullofugal endolymph flow, 28-29

Printed in the United States
by Baker & Taylor Publisher Services

Printed in the United States
by Baker & Taylor Publisher Services